Injury Epidemiology

INJURY EPIDEMIOLOGY
Research and Control Strategies

Third Edition

Leon S. Robertson

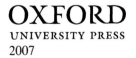
2007

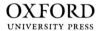

OXFORD
UNIVERSITY PRESS

Oxford University Press, Inc., publishes works that further
Oxford University's objective of excellence
in research, scholarship, and education.

Oxford New York
Auckland Cape Town Dar es Salaam Hong Kong Karachi
Kuala Lumpur Madrid Melbourne Mexico City Nairobi
New Delhi Shanghai Taipei Toronto

With offices in
Argentina Austria Brazil Chile Czech Republic France Greece
Guatemala Hungary Italy Japan Poland Portugal Singapore
South Korea Switzerland Thailand Turkey Ukraine Vietnam

Copyright © 2007 by Oxford University Press, Inc.

Published by Oxford University Press, Inc.
198 Madison Avenue, New York, New York 10016
www.oup.com

Oxford is a registered trademark of Oxford University Press

Library of Congress Cataloging-in-Publication Data

Robertson, Leon S.
   Injury epidemiology : research and control strategies / Leon S. Robertson. — 3rd ed.
      p. cm.
   Includes bibliographical references and index.
   ISBN: 978-0-19-531384-0
   1. Wounds and injuries—United States—Epidemiology. 2. Wounds and injuries—
Epidemiology—Research—Methodology. I. Title.
   DNLM: 1. Wounds and Injuries—epidemiology—United States. 2. Epidemiologic Research
Design—United States. WO 700 R651i 2007]
   RD93.8.R64 2007
   614.5'9—dc22   2006035245

Preface

This third edition of *Injury Epidemiology* includes updated data and discussion regarding the use and misuse of epidemiological methods to research injury and evaluate injury control efforts. Unfortunately, too many articles and books that rely on invalid data and logic continue to appear. Some reviewers of earlier editions considered criticism of certain studies or organizations harsh, while one accused the author of favoring the U.S. auto industry, despite numerous criticisms of some of the actions and products of U.S.-based manufacturers. In fact, the products of many corporations are unnecessarily hazardous. Various government agencies have failed to act or enforce laws and standards. Detailed illustrations and critiques of product evaluations, laws, and standards are included in appendices at the end of chapters 8, 9, 10, 12, 13, and 15.

Reluctance to criticize invites perpetuation of these practices. If injury control is to reach its full potential, we need more, not less, harsh criticism of researchers and organizations that do not do their jobs. Our profession, like many others, suffers from "pronoia," the aversion to criticism of others' work, giving them a false sense of accomplishment and self-importance (Goldner, 1982).

A major problem documented in the book is conflicting results in studies that rely on self-reports of injury and behavior. These are similar to conflicting results found in research on the health effects of certain foods, which has become a laughing stock (Shermer, 2007). It is time to stop conducting such shaky "research" before injury research meets a similar fate.

Although I have not reviewed every book, article, or Web site that may be useful to the topics discussed here, new references and links to Web sites have been added to this third edition. Some references are old but just as valid as the day they were written. Too many injury researchers apparently have no knowledge of the older literature, as indicated by their failure to reference it and, in some cases, their repetition of long-known errors.

Some references and other materials in textbooks and articles have always been a year or more out of date by the time they are edited and published. While the principles discussed here are as sound today as when they were first explicated, the data and literature on injuries change daily. To supplement the information in this text, links to data sources and other information available on the Internet will be available at http://www.nanlee.net. They will be updated as new information becomes available.

The Internet now allows access to large amounts of information and larger amounts of misinformation. My intention is to maximize the former and minimize the latter. Those who find errors or wish to suggest material to be added may do so by writing me at nanlee252000@yahoo.com. If you send me advertisements, viruses, or other useless or harmful stuff, your e-mail address will become a permanent resident of the junk file, never to be viewed again.

L.S.R.
Green Valley, Ariz.
September 2006

References

Goldner F (1982) Pronoia. *Social Problems* 30:83–91.
Shermer M (2007) Eat, drink and be merry. *Scientific American* 296:29.

Preface to the Second Edition

Injury Epidemiology, the first edition of this book, considered implications for injury control. The subtitle of the second edition, *Research and Control Strategies*, reflects this emphasis. Many new sections and references on those subjects have been added.

While the reception of the first edition by students and reviewers was mostly favorable, some readers were apparently confused or misled by the cryptic treatment given certain topics. Where this was made known to me, the sections have been rewritten or augmented in a quest for clarity. Some reviewers considered my criticism of certain studies or organizations harsh, and one accused me of favoring the U.S. auto industry despite numerous criticisms of some of the actions and products of U.S.-based manufacturers. The sad facts are that some researchers produce invalid or misleading research reports, the products of many corporations are unnecessarily hazardous, and government agencies fail to act or enforce laws and standards. Reluctance to criticize invites continuation of these practices and failures. If injury control is to reach its full potential, we need not less, but more, harsh criticism of researchers and organizations that do not do their jobs.

Epidemiologic studies of injuries have increased more rapidly in quantity than in quality in the 1990s. The collection of data with no clear research question or potentially useful results remains all too common. The revised first chapter of this book delineates specific objectives of epidemiologic studies and the data and study designs needed to attain those objectives. Each subsequent chapter has been revised and expanded with these objectives in mind to provide a more progressive step-by-step development of topics.

New analyses and updates include details on potential years of life lost from injuries, cardiovascular diseases, and cancers; effective uses of surveillance systems; clarification of the relevance of causal thinking for prevention; the misuse of behavioral inference in cases such as the C/K pickup truck fire issue; recent studies of legal intervention; the effects of motor vehicle crashworthiness relative to other factors; questions for research in prevention and rehabilitation; illustrations of cost–benefit, risk–benefit, and cost–savings analyses and evidence of confounding of estimates of effects of alcohol and seat belt use; and the effect of regulatory failure on rollovers of top-heavy vehicles and fuel economy as well as alternatives to regulation.

A number of new books that are worthwhile additions to class reading lists have appeared since the first edition was published. They are listed in the references for relevant chapters. To my knowledge, this remains the only textbook setting out general principles for research in injury epidemiology and evaluation of injury control. Good links to Internet sites are found at http://www.injurycontrol.com.

L.S.R.
Branford, Conn.
May 1997

Contents

1. Injury and the Role of Epidemiology   3
2. Energy Characteristics and Control Strategies   14
3. Research Objectives and Usable Data   23
4. Injury Severity   32
5. Injury Statistics   41
6. National Injury Surveillance   48
7. Local Injury Surveillance   59
8. The Use and Abuse of Causal Analysis   82
9. Research Designs and Data Analysis   96
10. Human Factors   119
11. Evaluation of Programs to Change Human Factors Voluntarily   137
12. Evaluation of Laws and Rules Directed at Individual Behavior   152
13. Evaluation of Agent, Vehicle, and Environmental Modifications   178
14. Evaluation of Postinjury Treatment and Rehabilitation   197
15. Injury Epidemiology and Economics   216
16. Summation of Principles   239
    Index   243

Injury Epidemiology

1

Injury and the Role of Epidemiology

For decades, injury deaths from motor vehicles, homicides, suicides, falls, poisonings, and drownings were listed in mortality statistics and largely ignored by researchers in epidemiology and public health. Near the end of the twentieth century, influential and important discussions of the future direction of epidemiological and public health research made no mention of injury (Susser and Susser, 1996; Pearce, 1996). A conference held in 2005 on the future of public health included one brief mention of injury, but more was said about Elvis impersonators than about injury prevention (University of the Sciences in Philadelphia, 2005).

Only occasionally does the issue gain some prominence. Addressing deaths among the young and a significant proportion of health care costs, the executive director of the American Public Health Association wrote "The Solution Is Injury Prevention" (Benjamin, 2004). Nevertheless, injury remains a hugely neglected public health problem.

That is not to say that injury prevention should be left exclusively to public health agencies. Epidemiology and public health bring a perspective on prevention honed from major victories in the control of infectious diseases. As was the case in those triumphs, the implementation of injury prevention requires the involvement of a wide variety of government agencies, businesses, health care providers, private voluntary organizations, and the research community. To implement an injury control agenda effectively and efficiently, the leadership and implementers in these entities must understand the epidemiological and public health perspective (Bonnie and Guyer, 2002).

Lists of numbers of deaths by type can be misleading regarding their relative importance for individual or societal well-being. Neither preventive measures nor medical treatment "saves lives," as is often claimed. If prevention or treatment is effective, it may delay death for a period of time, but everyone eventually dies. An accurate assessment of deaths and the effects of prevention or treatment on deaths would indicate potential years of life lost or preserved and years of disability avoided. Such statistics are rarely seen in medical and public health literature.

In 1985, the Committee on Trauma Research appointed by the National Research Council/Institute of Medicine published the report *Injury in America: A Continuing Public Health Problem*. The report summarized the magnitude of the problem:

> Each year, more than 140,000 Americans die from injuries, and one person in three suffers a nonfatal injury. ... Injuries kill more Americans aged 1–34 than all diseases combined, and they are the leading cause of deaths up to the age of 44. Injuries cause the loss of more working years of life than all forms of heart disease and cancer combined. One of every eight hospital beds is occupied by an injured patient. Every year, more than 80,000 people in the United States join the ranks of those with unnecessary, but permanently disabling, injury of the brain or spinal cord.

Despite reductions in the rates of fatalities and hospitalizations per population, the absolute numbers increased in the ensuing 15 years in relation to population growth. In 2000, about 149,000 U.S. residents died from injury and more that 1.8 million were hospitalized at an estimated lifetime cost of $80.2 billion in medical care costs and $326 billion in lost productivity (Finkelstein et al., 2006).

Although major new concerns about diseases such as HIV/AIDS and diabetes grab attention, injury takes about 10 times the potential years of life as each of these in the United States. The Centers for Disease Control and Prevention (CDC) separates homicide and suicide from unintentional injury, but when they are combined, injury is the leading cause of potential years of life lost through age 70. (For the latest numbers as well as state and regional data, see http://webapp.cdc. gov/sasweb/ncipc/ypll10.html, accessed August 2006.) Internationally, injury is a large proportion of the loss of life and disability in low-income countries but is seldom considered in international aid programs (Mock et al., 2004).

The 1985 Committee on Trauma Research report also pointed to the fact that injuries are highly patterned and hence subject to study and targeting of interventions, that many interventions are known to be effective but are unused, and that modest increases in funding would have large payoffs in cost savings. Eight years after the report recommended that a Center for Injury Control be established at the CDC, it was established in 1993. Although the number of professionals doing studies, teaching, and implementing injury prevention projects has grown modestly, the needs both in quantity and quality remain large. A study of 82 medical schools in 31 countries found large gaps in the injury topics addressed (Villaveces et al., 2005).

Should injuries have a higher priority? Reduction of injuries is justifiable on humane grounds, particularly since they disproportionately affect the health of the young. In a time of concern for health care costs, injury reduction is also an economic necessity. Injury control is one of the most promising ways to reduce health care costs in the immediate future. While attention to diet, increased exercise, and prevention of smoking among the young is worthwhile, the health benefits are usually not realized for decades. An injury prevented or reduced in severity has immediate benefits in reduced costs as well as grief, pain, and suffering.

Despite declines, motor vehicle injuries are the leading cause of injury deaths, while falls are the leading cause of injury hospitalizations. Firearms are the second leading cause of injury deaths in the United States but not in countries where guns are not prevalent.

This chapter lays out some of the important concepts in injury epidemiology and prevention: the distinction between accident and injury, the application of the epidemiological model for infectious diseases to injuries, and the phases of injury in relation to the factors that contribute to incidence and severity.

ACCIDENTS AND INJURIES

One aspect of injury addressed in this book is the importance of measuring severity when investigating injuries or considering injury control efforts. In the United States, motor vehicles, firearms, falls, poisonings, fire/burns, and drownings account for about 77 percent of deaths but only 36 percent of nonhospitalized injuries severe enough that their sufferers seek medical treatment (Finkelstein et al., 2006). Clearly, emphasis on prevention of all "accidents" will lead to misdirection of effort from the more serious and costly cases.

The evolution in thought about injuries is reflected in how they have been classified. Injuries often are classified as accidental or intentional. Prior to the 1960s, injury control was primarily focused on "accident prevention," and interpersonal or self-directed violence was largely left to law enforcement, psychiatry, social workers, and the clergy. That is not to say that these professions have not contributed to injury control or that all attempts to prevent "accidents" have been unsuccessful, but the extent of scientific investigation of the effectiveness of these approaches was very limited.

"Accidents" refer to a very large and fuzzy set of events, only a small proportion of which are injurious. Any unintended, incidental event that interferes in ones daily pursuits is an accident. In writing these few paragraphs, the author has had several accidents in typing, but ideally they have been corrected enough so as not to irritate the reader and thus have become irrelevant to exposure of the author to risk of injury.

The word "accident" is also intertwined with the notion that some human error or behavior is responsible for most injuries. This focus of attention on the human actors involved tends to detract from an examination of the full range of factors that contribute to injuries and, particularly, their severity.

Although the word "accident" had various meanings historically (Loimer et al., 1996), it is now primarily a euphemism for lack of intent, as though intent were a primary consideration in injury prevention. If two people have an argument that results in a brief exchange of fisticuffs, the incident usually goes unrecorded as an injury. In a similar situation, if one of the persons has a gun and kills the other with it, the case is classified as homicide as though the person intended to kill, which is often not true. While criminal law has various categories of homicide based on intent, aggregated statistics of the broad category "homicide" are included in "intentional injuries" without any data on the intent of the persons who used the weapon.

Even in the case of suicide, intent can be questioned. Some supposedly suicidal acts are attempts to get attention rather than serious attempts at self-destruction.

But if the attention-getter makes a mistake and dies, he or she will be classified as a suicide (Maris et al., 2000).

Here the term "injury" or reference to specific types of injury—amputations, burns, lacerations—indicates the phenomena of interest. Also, when referring to attempts to reduce injury, the term "injury control" is used. While "injury prevention" has been used by respectable scientists—and on occasion even by the author—and is the name of a reputable journal (http://ip.bmjjournals.com/, accessed August 2006), the term is less precise than "injury control" when severity of injury can be reduced without reducing incidence.

EPIDEMIOLOGY

The word "epidemiology" is a derivation of the classical Greek word *epidemion*, a verb meaning "to visit," used in connection with human maladies by Hippocrates circa 2400 B.C. The first known published use of the word in modern languages was in 1598, the Spanish *epidemiologia*, in a study of bubonic plague in Spain (Najera, 1988).

There are all sorts of definitions of epidemiology. The scientific study of the visitations of disease and injury on the population is as good as any. The scientific study of the distributions of diseases and injuries in populations, and their causes and "risk factors," is somewhat more descriptive of what epidemiologists do.

Historically, early epidemiologists concentrated their attention to what were later called "infectious diseases." Although the specific organisms that often infected populations were microscopic and unknown, quantification of the numbers of illnesses and deaths by location or exposure to certain environmental conditions led to actions that reduced disease and death in some instances. In nineteenth-century London, John Snow found that cholera occurred largely among people who used one water supply and not among those who used another. He did not know what was in the water that caused the disease, but he knew enough to stop the flow from that supply (Evans, 1993).

Similarly, when there are known effective means of reducing injury or severity, relatively simple studies of when, where, and how people are injured can lead to large reductions by targeting the relevant injury control measures to the circumstances to which they apply (chapter 7). This approach avoids the question of causation that is a point of both fascination and contention among epidemiologists as well as other scientists.

Some epidemiologists avoid the word "cause" and use euphemisms such as "risk factor" and "etiology." Often the incidence and severity of disease and injury are coincident with several factors, some of which may contribute to the incidence or severity and some of which may be correlates of the real causes but play no meaningful role in incidence or severity. For example, if a disease or injury is seasonal, as many are, increase in incidence may be correlated with other seasonal happenings. In northern areas of the United States, the vast majority of injuries to people while riding motorcycles occur during the season that robins are in the environment, but the correlation is known to be spurious. Few, if any, motorcyclists crash when impacting robins. The correlation occurs because both robins and motorcyclists prefer warm weather for their activities.

Since correlations thought to represent causal connections occasionally turn out to be false inferences, the embarrassment to the scientists proved wrong leads other scientists to great caution in causal inference. When dealing with maladies that kill or maim, however, one must sometimes risk embarrassment to contribute to the welfare of fellow human beings. At some point, as evidence accumulates, an attempt to change conditions coincident with the disease that would likely reduce it is appropriate. The amount, type, and quality of the evidence necessary to reach that point are matters of controversy addressed in this book, particularly in chapter 8.

A few epidemiologists believe that objective scientific investigation is incompatible with recommendations for changes in policies or practices that epidemiological research suggests would reduce harm. Some journal editors do not even allow discussions of policy implications of research results in articles reporting the results, much less recommendations for policy changes. Two important points are ignored by those stances: (1) The work of the scientist who proposes change based on research is likely to be scrutinized more carefully for bias and error. To the extent that such scrutiny weeds out invalid results, the science is improved. (2) Self-imposed or institutional bars from the policy debate of the scientists closest to the data increase the probability of misinterpretation or misuse of the data. Therefore, this book is devoted not just to the application of the theory and methods of epidemiology in injury research, but also to the uses and misuses of epidemiological data relevant to injury control.

Epidemiological methods are also applied to the study of the effectiveness of policies and practices aimed at the reduction of injury incidence and severity. Although this is called "applied" research and somehow has less prestige than "basic" research, the distinction is false. The study of human activities and other phenomena that increase the risk of injury is no more "basic" than the study of the human activities that seek to intervene in the causal process to reduce injury. Indeed, reduction of injury (or disease) by deliberately changing a factor inferred as a condition necessary for, or contributing to, specific injuries is additional evidence of causation, particularly if the change is introduced in such a way as to rule out the contribution of other factors to the reduction. Chapters 11–14 discuss the use of scientific methods to evaluate the effects of programs, laws, environmental modifications, medical care, and rehabilitation to reduce injuries or their severity.

Of course, disciplines other than epidemiology also study injury. Clinicians often describe a case or series of cases involving injury, and sciences ranging from physics to biomechanics contribute to our understanding of the mechanisms of injury. The research methods used by epidemiologists are shared by many disciplines. Statisticians, sociologists, psychologists, and physical and biological scientists use more or less the same methods. Many epidemiologists were originally trained in those disciplines as well as medicine. Nevertheless, the concepts of epidemiology provide a valuable perspective, particularly with respect to reduction of disease and injury in the population as a whole or in subsets of the population.

THE EPIDEMIOLOGICAL MODEL

Based on the experience of their predecessors in the scientific investigation of infectious diseases, many injury epidemiologists conduct their investigations mindful of a theoretical model developed by infectious disease epidemiologists. The core concepts of this model include the host (the person injured), the agent that injures, and the vector or vehicle that may convey the agent, as well as other environmental factors.

Early epidemiological investigations of what came to be known as infectious diseases showed correlations of the diseases to seasons, water sources, economic status of the populations primarily affected, and the like (Buck et al., 1988). We now know that in some cases these correlates of the diseases were carriers (vehicles or vectors) of infectious agents, and in others they were factors that increased or decreased host exposure or susceptibility to the agents—and some were spurious.

Microbiologists subsequently identified tiny biological structures (bacteria, parasites, viruses) that secreted toxins in an invaded host, or removed elements from the host, or caused other changes at the cellular or organ levels, that resulted in sickness and death. Then epidemiologists knew to look for these agents in the seasons, water, living conditions, and so on, associated with a given disease (Lilienfeld and Lilienfeld, 1980).

In some cases, the microorganism was conveyed to the host by inanimate media, such as water and milk, which came to be called vehicles. Others were carried to human hosts by insects or by animals or were directly transmitted from human being to human being. These animate carriers came to be called vectors. Living conditions, often related to economic status, increased or decreased exposure to the carriers of the agents or increased susceptibility to infection due to nutritional or other factors.

All of these discoveries had implications for control of infectious diseases. The agents could be eliminated from the media in which they reached hosts such as water and milk. In some cases, susceptibility could be reduced by modification of the immune mechanisms of the potential hosts. In others, antibiotic agents could be introduced into the infected hosts to reduce the severity of the illness. Elimination or control of certain carriers, such as rodents and insects, could be tried and, in some cases, accomplished. While diseases sometimes declined as people improved their living conditions, removing harmful agents or carriers in the process, epidemiological evidence on vehicles or vectors, as well as times, places, and populations involved, was crucial in the deliberate attempts to reduce many infectious diseases.

Although injuries can be characterized using the concepts of infectious disease epidemiology, injury epidemiology lagged in development by decades. The twentieth century was almost two-thirds past before the agents of injury were accurately identified as the various forms of energy: mechanical, thermal, chemical, electrical, ionizing radiation—or too little energy in the case of asphyxiation (Gibson, 1961). And that identification came from a psychologist, not an epidemiologist. Before and since that date, certain authors referred to motor vehicles, guns, and alcohol as agents of injury, but that is inaccurate in the epidemiological use of the concept of agent. Motor vehicles and guns are vehicles of mechanical energy in epidemiological parlance, and alcohol contributes to injury by sometimes affecting behavior that places people at greater risk of injurious energy exposure as well as perhaps increasing vulnerability of tissues to energy insults.

Prior to these insights, the research on injury was primarily focused on human characteristics and human behavior correlated with injury incidence and, more rarely, severity—with occasional studies of seasonal and geographical variations and the like. A few isolated researchers looked at human tolerance of mechanical energy as important (DeHaven, 1941; Haddon et al., 1964; Stapp, 1957).

It is not that the characteristics of the energy were unknown. The leading source of injury by far is mechanical energy, the characteristics of which have been known since Sir Isaac Newton's work on the laws of motion in the seventeenth century. Although Newton's laws of motion do not apply near the speed of light, they are applicable to moving motor vehicles, bullets, and falling human beings.

Why did it take so long to recognize energy as the agent of injury? It is more difficult to prove why something does not happen than why it does. After the great decline in death due to infectious diseases in the first half of the twentieth century, many epidemiologists turned their attention to cardiovascular diseases and cancers, at least partly due to the increases in government support of research on those diseases. Popular folklore focused on human behavior or human error as the cause of "accidents," and the small amounts of research funds available were devoted to reinforcement of that view.

Manufacturers of motor vehicles—by the 1920s the leading source of mechanical energy leading to death—deliberately supported the behavioral approach to divert attention from their vehicles (Eastman, 1984), a tradition that continues (Robertson, 1997a, 1997b; see also http://www.nanlee.net/evans, accessed August 2006). The National Rifle Association, the leading opponent of regulation of guns, coined the slogan, "Guns don't kill people. People kill people." Mosquitoes don't have lobbyists, but motor vehicles and guns do.

FACTORS AND PHASES OF INJURY

The transfer of energy to human beings at rates and in amounts above or below the tolerance of human tissue is the necessary and specific cause of injury. The amount of the energy concentration outside the bands of tolerance of tissue determines the severity of the injury.

Injury usually refers to the damage to cells and organs from energy exposures that have relatively sudden, discernible effects, although some researchers have included damage from chronic low-energy exposures, such as back strain or carpel tunnel syndrome, as injury (Waller, 1985). Chemical and radiation exposures that produce cellular changes resulting in neoplasm are usually called cancerous rather than injurious. A debate regarding the appropriateness of inclusion or exclusion of any harmful condition as injury or disease would be pointless, but at the fuzzy edges of a set of harmful consequences from energy exchanges, a given researcher should make clear the cases that are considered injuries.

Most of the concentrations of energy involved in severe and fatal injuries are the result of human inventions that alter the energy inherent in matter (Robertson, 1983). Some falls occur from heights unmodified by human construction. Lightning, tornadoes, and hurricanes kill a few hundred people annually. But motor vehicles and guns, as well as cigarettes, which cause more house fires than any other ignition source, and home swimming pools, which drown more children than other bodies of water, are examples of human inventions that are some of the major sources of serious injuries.

To alert researchers to the factors contributing to injury incidence and severity, and the timing of involvement of those factors, Haddon (1972) devised a matrix of broad categories of factors and phases of injury. This matrix, along with some examples of factors known to be important in each category, is shown in table 1-1.

Before injury, human, vehicle, and environmental factors contribute to the increase or decrease in exposure to potentially damaging energy. For example, alcohol impairs human perceptions, reactions, and judgments and may increase aggressive behavior. The weights of heavier vehicles extend stopping distances. Hedges at intersections reduce visibility of oncoming traffic.

During the energy exchange that injures, the susceptibility of the host's tissue to damage may vary. For example, a person with osteoporosis may be disabled by a fall that would hardly bruise a teenager. Sharp points and edges concentrate energy on the host. Flammable building materials increase intensity of heat and smoke in fires.

After the initial energy exchange, the condition of the host, the potential for more energy exposure, and the responses from the environment substantially affect survival and the time and extent of return to preinjury functioning of those who survive. For example, if hemorrhaging is not stopped, the host may die from loss of blood. If a gas tank is ruptured by the initial energy exchange, a spark can result in thermal energy beyond host tolerance. If emergency response is delayed, the remainder of a life that could be preserved by surgery or other intensive treatment may be lost.

Each epidemiological investigation does not have to measure all of the human, vehicle, and environmental factors at various phases to be useful, but in those cases where there is a synergistic effect of particular factors on the outcome being studied, failure to consider them can be misleading. One crucial consideration in the relevance of epidemiology for injury control is the modifiability of the factors measured.

Table 1-1. The Haddon Matrix, With Examples

| Phases | Factors | | |
	Human	Vehicle	Environment
Preinjury	1. Alcohol intoxication	4. Braking capacity of motor vehicles	7. Visibility of hazards
Injury	2. Resistance to energy insults	5. Sharp or pointed edges and surfaces	8. Flammable building materials
Postinjury	3. Hemorrhage	6. Rapidity of energy reduction response	9. Emergency medical

For example, a large number of injury investigations are limited to the distributions of rates of a particular type of injury by age and gender. It is important to know how many potential years of life are affected by injury and whether subsets of the population are disproportionately involved, but other than those considerations, age and gender distributions are uninteresting. We are not going to change the age and gender of individuals in the population.

The major modifiable factors that contribute to injury are energy and the characteristics of vehicles of energy. Human behavior that increases exposure or concentrates energy can be modified under certain conditions, but not by changing immutable factors such as age and gender (Robertson, 1983). Human tolerance to energy exposures varies among individuals by age, gender, and other factors that affect the condition of tissue, such as decalcification of bones and hemophilia. To the extent that diseases that increase susceptibility can be treated, the severity of injury can be reduced by that method, but there are substantial limits to increasing tolerance to energy.

The importance of focus on degree and type of energy exposures was most dramatically illustrated to the author while conducting a study of worker injuries. In two adjacent buildings of the same company, the injuries to the workers were remarkably different. In building A, there were virtually no injuries to the workers that were severe enough to be reported on the log required by the Occupational Safety and Health Administration (OSHA) during the eight-year period studied. In building B, about one in five workers had an OSHA-reportable injury each year. There were some age, gender, and other differences between the work forces in the two buildings, but these accounted for only a small amount of the variation in injuries among the workers in building B (Robertson and Keeve, 1983), and there was essentially no variation in injuries while at work among people in building A to investigate.

The major difference between the two buildings was the exposure to energy. In building B, some of the workers poured molten metal, heated to thousands of degrees, from large vats. Others worked adjacent to machines that rolled, shaped, and stamped the metal—forming it into wire, rods, and keys. A fall or a movement of any sort in the wrong direction would place one or another part of a worker's anatomy in contact with thermal or mechanical energy beyond the tolerance of human tissue. The people in building A also worked with machines—typewriters, photocopying machines, and computers—that contained potentially injurious electrical energy. But the manufacturers of those machines had the foresight to shield the energy from the workers so that the potential for contact with the energy was minimal.

References

Benjamin GC (2004) The solution is injury prevention. *Am J Public Health.* 94:521.
Bonnie RJ, and Guyer B (2002) Injury as a field of public health: achievements and controversies. *J Law Med Ethics.* 30:267–280.

Buck C, Llopis A, Najera E, and Terris M (eds.) (1988) *The Challenge of Epidemiology: Issues and Selected Readings.* Washington, DC: Pan American Health Organization.

Committee on Trauma Research (1985) *Injury in America: A Continuing Public Health Problem.* Washington, DC: National Academy Press. Available at: http://www.nap.edu/books/0309035457/html. Accessed August 2006.

DeHaven H (1941) Mechanical analysis of survival in falls from heights of fifty to one hundred and fifty feet. *War Med.* 2:586. Available at: http://www.mvhap.org/noteworthy_doc.php. Accessed August 2006.

Eastman JW (1984) *Styling vs. Safety: The American Automobile and the Development of Automotive Safety, 1900–1966.* New York, NY: University Press of America. Available at: http://www.mvhap.org/noteworthy_doc.php. Accessed August 2006.

Evans AS (1993) *Causation and Disease: A Chronological Journey.* New York, NY: Plenum.

Finkelstein EA, Corso PS, and Miller TR (2006) *The Incidence and Economic Burden of Injuries in the United States.* New York, NY: Oxford University Press.

Gibson JJ (1961) The contribution of experimental psychology to the formulation of the problem of safety. In *Behavioral Approaches to Accident Research.* New York, NY: Association for the Aid of Crippled Children.

Haddon W Jr (1972) A logical framework for categorizing highway safety phenomena and activity. *J Trauma.* 12:197.

Haddon W Jr, Suchman EA, and Klein D (1964) *Accident Research: Methods and Approaches.* New York, NY: Harper and Row. Available at: http://www.mvhap.org/noteworthy_doc.php. Accessed August 2006.

Lilienfeld AM, and Lilienfeld DE (1980) *Foundations of Epidemiology.* New York, NY: Oxford University Press.

Loimer H, Driur M, and Guarnieri M (1996) Accidents and acts of God: a history of the terms. *Am J Public Health.* 86:101–107.

Maris RW, Berman AL, and Silverman MM (eds.) (2000) *Comprehensive Textbook of Suicidology.* New York, NY: Guilford Press.

Mock C, Quansah R, Krishnan R, Arreola-Risa C, and Rivara F (2004) Strengthening the prevention and care of injuries worldwide. *Lancet.* 363:2172–2179.

Najera E (1988) Discussions. In Buck C, et al. (eds.), *The Challenge of Epidemiology: Issues and Selected Readings.* Washington, DC: Pan American Health Organization.

Pearce N (1996) Traditional epidemiology, modern epidemiology, and public health. *Am J Public Health.* 86:678–683.

Rice DP, and MacKenzie EJ (eds.) (1989) *Cost of Injury in the United States: A Report to Congress, 1989.* San Francisco, CA, and Baltimore, MD: Institute for Health and Aging, University of California, and Injury Prevention Center, Johns Hopkins University.

Robertson LS (1983) *Injuries: Causes, Control Strategies and Public Policy.* Cambridge, MA: DC Heath. Available at: http://www.nanlee.net. Accessed August 2006.

Robertson LS (1997a) Health policy and behavior: injury control. In Gochman DS (ed.), *Handbook of Health Behavior Research.* New York, NY: Plenum.

Robertson LS (1997b) Mistaken assertions on reducing motor vehicle injuries. *Am J Public Health.* 87:295–296.

Robertson LS, and Keeve JP (1983) Worker injuries: the effects of workers' compensation and OSHA inspections. *J Health Politics, Policy and Law.* 8:581.

Stapp JP (1957) Human tolerance to deceleration. *Am J Surgery.* 93:734.

Susser M, and Susser E (1996) Choosing a future for epidemiology: I. Eras and paradigms. *Am J Public Health.* 86:668–673.

University of the Sciences in Philadelphia (2005) *The Future of Public Health: What Will It Take to Keep Americans Healthy and Safe?* [Transcript]. Available at: http://www. usip.edu/symposium/. Accessed August 2006.

Villaveces A, Kammeyer JA, and Bencevic H (2005) Injury prevention education in medical schools: an international survey of medical students. *Inj Prev.* 11:343–347.

Waller JA (1985) *Injury Control: A Guide to the Causes and Prevention of Trauma.* Lexington, MA: DC Heath.

2

Energy Characteristics and Control Strategies

Injury epidemiologists should have at least a rudimentary understanding of the forms of energy involved in injury and the tolerance of human beings to exposure to energy. Since incidence and severity of injury are usually classified by vehicles or circumstances rather than by agent, the precise numbers attributable to a given agent are not available in many data sets. At the turn of the century in the United States, about 58 percent of fatal injuries and 62 percent of hospitalized injuries were attributed to motor vehicles, falls, and firearms (Finkelstein et al., 2006). These injuries, and a proportion of those injuries associated with factors and activities grouped into the "other" category (industrial machines, farm machines, knives, sports), indicate that mechanical energy accounts for the substantial majority of severe injury. As of 2002, each year about 1 in 110 U.S. residents was discharged from a hospital after an injury and about one in seven people in the U.S. population visited a hospital emergency room, mostly with injury from mechanical energy (see http://www.cdc.gov/nchs/about/otheract/injury/injury_hospital.htm, accessed August 2006).

Some energy releases, such as a nuclear explosion, include multiple forms of energy—mechanical, heat, chemical, and ionizing radiation. The acute effects of ionizing radiation have been rare and are not discussed in the following brief descriptions of common types of energy that cause the bulk of acute injuries.

MECHANICAL ENERGY

Any object, animate or inanimate, in motion at velocity substantially less than the speed of light has energy in relation to its mass and speed that is described by a simple formula:

$$K = mv^2/2 \qquad (2.1)$$

where

K = energy in foot-pounds
m = mass
v = velocity in feet per second

A foot-pound is the energy needed to raise a pound of material one foot from the ground at the earth's surface. Mass can be calculated at the earth's surface by dividing weight in pounds by 32. Velocity in miles per hour can be converted to feet per second by multiplying miles per hour by 1.467. Therefore, a 150-pound motor vehicle occupant traveling at 30 miles per hour has about 4,539 foot-pounds of energy, that is,

$$[(150/32) \times 44^2]/2 = 4539 \text{ foot-pounds}$$

Increase in mass or speed increases the energy, speed obviously more so than mass because it is squared in the calculation. At 60 miles per hour, the 150-pound vehicle occupant has about 18,158 foot-pounds of energy, twice the speed but about four times the energy compared with 30 miles per hour.

If the person must stop suddenly, as in a crash of the vehicle, that energy must be dissipated in the vehicle, in the environment, or in the tissues of the individual. When the vehicle stops, the occupant will continue to move at the precrash speed and collide with the interior structures or, if ejected, with materials in the exterior environment—the so-called second collision. The load on the tissue is measured in pounds per square inch. The shape and elasticity of the materials struck will determine the damage to the tissue. Inflexible, protruding or pointed objects on dashboards, for example, will penetrate the heads or other parts of the anatomy of people who move into them in crashes at common traveling speeds.

Devices such as child restraints, lap/shoulder belts, and air bags reduce the severity of injury by reducing contact with less flexible surfaces. They also increase the uniformity of deceleration of occupant and vehicle and spread the load over dozens of square inches. Energy-absorbing materials, both in the vehicle and the environment, can also dissipate energy so that the individual's deceleration is less rapid (Nahum and Melvin, 2002). Helmets used by motorcyclists, bicyclists, and in certain sports, as well as padding used in certain sports and on the hips of residents in certain nursing homes, also absorb energy if designed to do so.

The extent of damage to tissue is a function of the structure of the part of the body affected. Contact with an energy source generates forces counter to the load, called stresses. These constitute the resistance to deformation of the bonds among tissue molecules. The same tissue may have different capacity for tension stress (pulling molecules apart), compression stress (pushing molecules together), or shear stress (tearing from a tangential force).

Strain refers to the extent of deformation and may be classified as resulting from tension, compression, or shear stress. Tissues vary in elasticity—the extent to which strain is eliminated when the load is removed—and in the regenerative capability of the organism (Stephenson, 1952). Nerves do not regenerate when severed, so injuries to the brain and spinal cord are especially disabling

(Committee on Trauma Research, 1985). While a technological breakthrough in restoring nerve function may eventually occur, no reference was found that suggests it is likely to happen in the near future.

To the extent that the object striking or struck by human tissue is stressed more than the tissue, the energy will be transferred to the inanimate object and the human tissue will be damaged less. The classic study by DeHaven (1942) of people who survived falls of up to 150 feet found no major injury in some cases where the deformation in the ground, car, or other object struck was as little as a few inches.

With the exception of persons with diseases such as scurvy, osteoporosis, and hemophilia—which reduce the elasticity of important tissues—human beings are capable of experiencing substantial mechanical force with little or no injury if the load is not concentrated. Stapp (1957) conducted experiments with animals in rocket sleds and wind tunnels to test the limits of tissue tolerance and then tested healthy human volunteers, including him, within the estimated limits. Held in the sled only by three-inch-wide webbed harnesses over the shoulders and legs, and anchored to the sled, the volunteers experienced decelerations up to 35 *g* with no damage and up to 45 *g* with little damage. A *g* is the measurement of gravity at the earth's surface, 32 feet per second squared. The effective weight of a 160-pound person decelerated at 35 *g* is 5,600 pounds. Yet, because the accompanying load was distributed over the surface of the restraining belts to reduce concentration at smaller points, and was partly absorbed by the belts, the test subjects sustained no serious injury.

Biomechanical engineers study the susceptibility of animate tissues to damage from mechanical energy loads. Materials engineers study the properties of matter that increase or decrease their energy-absorbing capability. Experts in these fields should be consulted by epidemiologists who need information on the properties of tissue or other matter involved in a given set of injuries.

The velocity of the persons involved in an injury is often not known but can be estimated using another formula from elementary physics (Bueche, 1977):

$$v_t^2 = v_0^2 + 2ad \tag{2.2}$$

where

v = velocity in feet per second
t = time in seconds
a = acceleration
d = distance moved in feet

A person in a free fall accelerates at 32 feet per second every second (1 *g*). If we know the distance fallen, say, five feet from the top of a sliding board in a playground, the velocity at impact can be calculated as follows from equation 2.2:

$$v^2 = 0 + (2 \times 32 \times 5) = 320$$

Therefore, the velocity at impact is the square root of 320, which is 17.9 feet per second. If we know the maximum weight of the children who use the sliding board, then from equation 2.1 we can calculate the energy at impact in the worst-case scenario. Let's say the maximum weight of any child likely to climb onto the sliding board is 90 pounds. Then, from equation 2.1, the energy that should be managed is:

$$[(90/32) \times 17.9']/2 = 451 \text{ foot-pounds}$$

This energy, compared to that of the above-mentioned car occupant, should give more than a hint as to why motor vehicle injuries are, on average, more severe than fall injuries.

If the surface under the sliding board were designed to absorb more than 451 foot-pounds of energy over a surface of a few square inches, no damage would occur to children who fall off. If playground builders were to conduct such calculations and compare the results to the energy-absorbing properties of materials, they would find that the concrete or asphalt often placed under playground equipment does not do the job.

Faced with playground managers who do not believe the theoretical formula, an injury epidemiologist might use basic physics to do a study of injuries in falls from playground equipment. The data to be collected would include severity of injuries, weight of the injured, height of the equipment used, and surfaces under the equipment. Using an appropriate statistical model, the data would be analyzed to examine the extent to which severity of injury is a function of the type of playground surface, controlling for the energy of the falling bodies.

Unfortunately, those who study such injuries usually do not collect the data needed. For example, a report that children's falls from playground equipment result in more serious injury than their falls from standing height (Fiissel et al., 2005) will surprise no one with common sense, much less those who know basic physics. No data on the height of the equipment or the surfaces contacted were included in the study. The National Safe Kids organization claims that only 9 percent of playgrounds have energy-absorbing material under equipment but cites no reference for the claim and no assessment of the adequacy of the material (National SAFE KIDS Campaign, 2004).

The severity of the second leading cause of fatal injury, gun-related injury, is also substantially a function of the characteristics of the involved vehicles of mechanical energy—guns and bullets. In addition to high velocity applied to less than a square inch of body surface in most cases, which results in frequent deep penetration of vital organs, the extent of fragmentation after penetration increases the damage to organs affected. Muzzle velocities of bullets range widely, from 1,200 to 2,700 feet per second. They generate energy from 93 to 8,092 foot-pounds at close range (Karlson and Hargarten, 1997).

Bullets used by military forces are required by the Geneva Convention to be fully jacketed and retain their approximate original shape while moving through human tissue. Bullets sold in the United States for domestic use do not meet such a standard. Their sometimes-blunt ends and frequent fragmentation result in wounds that have an average size 27 times those caused by military bullets (DeMuth, 1966). Yet epidemiologists often study gun-related injuries as if all guns and bullets were the same.

THERMAL AND CHEMICAL ENERGY

The deaths and injuries associated with fires, heat, and smoke are the result of use of ignition sources and flammable materials, and the heat and chemical energies generated by burning or heating materials. The most common ignition source in fatal fires is a cigarette dropped in furniture or bedding, often smoldering until the occupants of a household are asleep. The extent to which a cigarette will continue to burn when dropped is a function of type of tobacco, tobacco density, paper porosity, citrate added, circumference, and second paper wrapping (Technical Study Group, 1987). Other ignition sources with variations deserving of epidemiological attention are matches, cigarette lighters, gas stoves, and electrical circuits or appliances. Heat from sources other than ignited fires most often include heated water and other liquids, heating units on stoves, and space heaters.

The physics and chemistry of combustion vary according to (1) concentration and type of heat source, (2) shape and size of a combustible, (3) oxygen concentration, (4) vaporization of gasses, and (5) presence or absence of catalysts (National Fire Protection Agency, 1981). Heat is transferred among solids, liquids, and gasses, in proximity to one another, from the medium at higher temperature to the medium at lower temperature. The effect of heat on human tissue is a function of the temperature and the time of exposure (Moritz and Henriques, 1947). Karter (2005) provides a detailed report on fires and fire-related injury.

Chemicals may be breathed, ingested, injected, or absorbed. The effect is a function of the concentration of the exogenous chemical, its interaction with body chemistry, and the rapidity of elimination relative to individual susceptibility. The dose–response curve may also vary based on genetic susceptibility, physiological development, increased or reduced tolerance resulting from previous exposure, and presence or absence of other chemicals that can have synergistic effects.

Toxicologists divide the process of harm by a chemical into three phases— exposure, toxokinetic, and toxodynamic. Epidemiologists have paid some attention to the first of these in the study of poisonings, but the second and third deserve attention regarding severity. The toxokinetic phase refers to the chemical's absorption through the organism's membranes, usually in the alimentary canal or the lungs in the case of common poisonings, as well as the distribution, metabolism, and excretion in the vascular and waste disposal systems. The interaction of the chemical with receptors in target tissues constitutes the toxodynamic phase (Ariens et al., 1976).

Researchers have given some attention to the possibility of reduction of the effects of alcohol and narcotics in the toxodynamic phase based on increased understanding of receptors, but less attention has been given to the toxokinetic phase. For example, suggestions that something could be added to alcohol to reduce absorption in the alimentary canal or make the drink taste bad after a couple have been consumed (Robertson, 1981) are often greeted with the statement that people would just drink more. Perhaps some would, but many people in the process of "partying" likely do not pay attention to the amount consumed. The issue deserves empirical research rather than offhand dismissal. (Tutorials on toxicology are available at http://sis.nlm.nih.gov/enviro/toxtutor.html, accessed August 2006.)

ELECTRICAL ENERGY

Electrical energy is inherent in matter. Atoms are made up of electrons (negatively charged), protons (positively charged), and neutrons (neutrally charged). Gain or loss of electrons in orbit about the nucleus determines whether the atom is positively or negatively charged. The flow of electrons is electrical current. The atoms of different materials, including human tissues, vary in their tendency to hold an electrical charge.

Electrical current flow over time is measured in amperes and varies as a function of the electromotive force (volts) divided by resistance to conductivity (ohms) that characterizes the materials and situation involved. The extent of damage to human tissue in contact with electrical energy increases with amperage. Muscular paralysis occurs at about 0.02 amperes, ventricular fibrillation at 0.10 amperes, and ventricular paralysis at 2.0 or more amperes. Skin resistance varies 100-fold as a function of wetness—100,000 ohms when dry but 100 ohms when soaked. The water serves as a low-resistance conductor if the water is in contact with the ground. Thus, a 120-volt electrical current in the average home socket will have low amperage (0.001) in contact with dry skin but will be high enough (0.12) to cause ventricular fibrillation if the skin is soaking wet and in contact with the ground. Deaths attributed to heart failure or other causes are sometimes found upon detailed examination to have been caused by electricity (Wright and Davis, 1980).

ASPHYXIATION

The human organism cannot function with too little energy. The absence of oxygen to sustain endogenous energy conversion, called asphyxiation, causes essential cells in the brain and heart to be damaged within minutes. Asphyxiation can occur from objects or other material blocking the nose and mouth or trachea (e.g., by a plastic bag or balloon fragment), a mechanical blow to the trachea (e.g., by a "karate chop" dash board tapered toward the occupant in a car crash), constriction of the trachea (e.g., hanging by a rope), or obstruction in the lungs. The most common fatal form of asphyxia from acute exposure to external sources, counted as injury, is water in the lungs, usually labeled as drowning or near drowning. Lung congestion from endogenous fluids, as in pneumonia and congestive heart failure, is attributed to diseases.

TECHNICAL STRATEGIES

As with cancer epidemiology and control, in injury epidemiology the varieties of energy sources involved and the differences in populations exposed to the various types of energy mitigate against a single cure for the whole problem. In contrast to cancer, however, one does not have to wait 20 years to find out if a given control strategy is having an effect on the subset of injuries toward which it is targeted.

Haddon (1970) defined 10 logically distinct technical strategies for injury control. The following is a list of the strategies, with examples relevant to some of the more commonly severe injuries:

1. Prevent the creation of the hazard in the first place: Do not allow the manufacture of particularly hazardous vehicles, such as motorcycles, minibikes, and all-terrain vehicles. These vehicles are used mainly for recreation, for which there are numerous substitutable less hazardous activities.

2. Reduce the amount of the hazard brought into being: Require that passenger vehicles have lower centers of gravity or wider track width such that track width divided by twice the height of center of gravity (*T/2H*) is not less than 1.2. Vehicles with lower *T/2H* have 3–20 times as many fatal rollover crashes as those 1.2 or greater, and the relative risk is strongly correlated to *T/2H*. Require that all motor vehicles operated on a level surface be incapable of speeds greater than 65 miles per hour. (Limitations on maximum speed would also conserve fuel and reduce emissions.) Allow sale of handguns only to police and military units. Reduce the number of pills in a prescription for drugs to a number that would not kill or disable if taken all at once. Reduce flammability of clothing. Reduce maximum temperature capability of hot water heaters, the source of heat for many scald burns.

3. Prevent the release of the hazard that already exists: Improve braking capability of motor vehicles, especially heavy trucks and sport utility vehicles that have longer braking distances than cars. Keep guns for target shooting at the shooting range rather than in homes. Provide canes and walkers for the elderly and handrails in their environments. Make matches and lighters less easy for children to ignite.

4. Modify the rate or spatial distribution of release of the hazard from its source: Use child restraints and seat belts in motor vehicles. Prohibit automatic and semiautomatic guns. Use lightly woven and smoothly finished fabrics in clothing to reduce burning rates. Install automatic sprinkler systems. Provide systems that replace air rapidly in passenger compartments of motor vehicles to prevent elevated carbon monoxide concentrations.

5. Separate, in time or space, the hazard and that which is to be protected: Remove trees and poles from near roadsides. Build pedestrian and bicycle paths separated from roads. Seat children in the back seat of motor vehicles. Prohibit large truck traffic, especially if transporting flammables or toxic chemicals, during periods of congestion. Restrict hunting and target shooting to unpopulated areas. Evacuate coastal areas at times of approaching hurricanes. Use cooking units that children cannot reach or keep children out of the kitchen while cooking.

6. Separate the hazard and that which is to be protected by interposition of a material barrier: Increase energy-absorbing capability of vehicle exteriors. Install air bags in passenger vehicles. Require motorcyclists

and bicyclists to use helmets. Use energy-absorbing barriers on the fronts and rears of large trucks that are compatible with car bumper heights. Install energy-absorbing barriers between roads and bridge abutments or other necessary rigid structures near roads. Place fences with gates that children cannot open around swimming pools and other small bodies of water in areas where children can reach them. Fit guards on boat propellers, industrial machines, and the like where moving parts can injure those in proximity. Use insulated firewalls in vehicles and buildings. Invent an additive to alcoholic beverages and other commonly ingested drugs that reduce absorption through the wall of the digestive track into the bloodstream as increasing amounts are ingested.

7. Modify basic relevant qualities of the hazard: Eliminate sharp points and edges on vehicle exteriors. Eliminate protruding knobs and "karate chop" dashboards in vehicle interiors. Use breakaway designs for utility poles and light poles along roadsides. Prohibit more than one trailer on tractor-trailer rigs. Reduce muzzle velocity of guns. Use trigger locks on guns. Apply to ammunition sold to the public the Geneva Convention regulation that prohibits flattening and fragmenting of bullets used in war. Use energy-absorbing materials of adequate depth on playground surfaces.

8. Make what is to be protected more resistant to damage from the hazard: Develop treatment of persons with hemophilia and osteoporosis to increase resistance to mechanical energy exchanges. Require physical conditioning before participation in sports that produce condition-related injuries.

9. Begin to counter the damage already done by the environmental hazard: Increase the availability of roadside emergency telephones. Place emergency response teams near areas with relatively high injury rates. Increase use of smoke detectors and carbon monoxide detectors.

10. Stabilize, repair, and rehabilitate the object of the damage: Provide prosthetic devices for amputees and wheelchairs, beds, and equipment used in work and other activities designed to optimize normal living. Provide job and self-care training.

Too often these strategies, or reference to them, are missing from published articles and books on injury control. The commonly cited Haddon Matrix (see table 1-1) is widely used to illustrate the factors and phases, but the 10 strategies are far more important in the systematic consideration of possible countermeasures.

The adoption of any one strategy is dependent on various aspects of ideology, politics, and costs. Epidemiologists can play a central role in pinpointing energy exposures, incidence, and severity among particular populations and evaluation of the effectiveness of injury control strategies. Costs of injury control can be minimized by application of the strategies to agents, vehicle or vectors, hosts, and environments in which the severity of injuries and their associated costs are most acute.

References

Ariens J, et al. (1976) *Introduction to General Toxicology.* New York, NY: Academic Press.

Bueche F (1977) *Principles of Physics.* 3rd ed. New York, NY: McGraw-Hill.

Committee on Trauma Research (1985) *Injury in America: A Continuing Public Health Problem.* Washington, DC: National Academy Press. Available at: http://www.nap. edu/books/0309035457/html. Accessed August 2006.

DeHaven H (1942) Mechanical analysis of survival in falls from heights of fifty to one hundred and fifty feet. *War Med.* 2:586. Available at: http://www.mvhap.org/ noteworthy_doc.php. Accessed August 2006.

DeMuth WE Jr (1966) Bullet velocity and design as determinants of wounding capability. *J Trauma.* 6:222.

Finkelstein EA, Corso PS, and Miller TR (2006) *The Incidence and Economic Burden of Injuries in the United States.* New York, NY: Oxford University Press.

Fiissel D, Pattison G, and Howard A (2005) Severity of playground fractures: play equipment versus standing height falls. *Inj Prev.* 6:337–339.

Haddon W Jr (1970) On the escape of tigers: an ecologic note. *Tech Rev.* 72:44.

Karlson TA, and Hargarten SW (1997) *Reducing Firearm Death and Injury: A Public Health Sourcebook on Guns.* New Brunswick, NJ: Rutgers University Press.

Karter MJ Jr (2005) *Fire Loss in the United States During 2004—Full Report.* Quincy, MA: National Fire Protection Association. Available at: http://www.nfpa.org/item-Detail.asp?categoryID=413&itemID=18238&URL=Research%20&%20Reports/ One-Stop%20Data%20Shop/Statistical%20reports/Overall%20fire%20statistics. Accessed August 2006.

Moritz AR, and Henriques CF Jr (1947) Studies in thermal injury II: the relative importance of time and surface temperature in the causation of cutaneous burns. *Am J Pathology.* 23:695.

Nahum AM, and Melvin JW (eds.) (2002) *Accidental Injury: Biomechanics and Prevention.* New York, NY: Springer.

National Fire Protection Agency (1981) *Fire Protection Handbook.* 15th ed. Quincy, MA: National Fire Protection Agency.

National SAFE KIDS Campaign (2004) *Playground Injury Fact Sheet.* Washington, DC: National SAFE KIDS Campaign. Available at: http://www.preventinjury.org/PDFs/ PLAYGROUND_INJURY.pdf. Accessed August 2006.

Robertson LS (1981) Alcohol, behavior and public health strategies. *Abstr Rev Alcohol Driving.* 2:1–4.

Stapp JP (1957) Human tolerance to deceleration. *Am J Surgery.* 93:734.

Stephenson RJ (1952) *Mechanics and Properties of Matter.* New York, NY: John Wiley and Sons.

Technical Study Group (1987) *Toward a Less Fire-Prone Cigarette: Final Report of the Technical Study Group on Cigarette and Little Cigar Fire Safety.* Washington, DC: U.S. Consumer Product Safety Commission.

Wright RK, and Davis JH (1980) The investigation of electrical deaths: a report of 220 fatalities. *J Forensic Sci.* 25:514–521.

3

Research Objectives and Usable Data

The first step in any research project is to ask a question or state a hypothesis that defines the objective of the study. The objective of the study determines the data needed. Even in very limited descriptive studies, one may have the opportunity to examine or collect data on various aspects of an injury: the severity of the injury, the energy sources involved, characteristics and behavior of the persons injured or others at the scene, the places of occurrence, the circumstances, the treatment received, and the cost of treatment.

Numerous variables describe each of these aspects, and the possible combinations of potentially measurable categories of the factors are very large. If all the possible combinations of classifications of factors were tabulated, data on an enormous number of cases would be necessary to obtain stable statistics. Obviously, a coherent and practical research project requires great care in choice of a research question, study design, and choice of variables to answer the question.

RESEARCH OBJECTIVES AND DATA NEEDS

To contribute data that are useful in the effort to reduce injury, the researcher must have a clear understanding of how the data may be used. Too many research reports describe the cross-tabulations of available data, such as the age and sex distribution of injury X, without any discernable objective. Table 3-1 presents a set of research objectives and data that would accelerate the control of injuries.

The World Health Organization's International Classification of Diseases (see http://www.who.int/classifications/icd/en/, accessed December 2006) has two types of codes for injury—so-called N-codes and E-codes. The N-codes are diagnosis codes (e.g., type and anatomical location of a fracture) and are usually coded or extractable from hospital records. E-codes are codes for broad categories of circumstances (e.g., motor vehicle, fall, gunshot, burn). E-codes are available

Table 3-1. Objectives and Data Needs of Injury Research and Control

Objective	Data Needed
1. Select the most important injuries for study or detailed surveillance	E-coded fatalities and hospitalizations
2. Efficiently apply known countermeasures	Surveillance of who, where, when, and how people are severely injured
3. Find changeable factors that will reduce injury and quantify measures of the factors and research the reduction expected	Reliable and valid designs to control for confounding factors
4. Develop causal models of homogeneous subsets of injury	Measures of all possible risk factors and specification of sequential time order
5. Evaluate the effectiveness of an intervention	Introduction of the intervention in a realistic setting, controlling for other factors, preferably with an experimental- control design
6. Evaluate the cost-effectiveness of alternative interventions	Cost of each intervention and degree of overlap in effectiveness among them

on death certificates, with greater or lesser accuracy depending on type of injury. In hospital records, however, one often cannot tell anything about how an injury occurred. For example, the record of a fracture often does not indicate whether the injury occurred in a motor vehicle crash, a fall, or an assault. Even less often is there information on where the injury occurred (geographic location, e.g., street address, highway milepost, global positioning). Without such information, one cannot adequately specify the scope of injury problems or choose those that need the most attention. Clinicians could aid injury control enormously by inclusion of when, where, and how an injury occurred in the history. E-codes and proposed changes are published online by the Centers for Disease Control and Prevention (http://www.cdc.gov/ncipc/whatsnew/matrix2.htm, accessed August 2006).

To efficiently apply known countermeasures, detailed surveillance of when, to whom, where, and how specific types of severe injuries occur is needed (table 3-1, item 2). There are two reasons for emphasizing only severe injuries, such as hospitalizations and deaths. First, large numbers of minor cuts, bruises, abrasions, and burns occur in circumstances that are substantially different from those of severe injuries (Rice and MacKenzie, 1989). Attempts to control the most frequent injuries will misdirect resources from the most severe and costly injuries. Second, including only hospitalized and fatal injuries remarkably reduces the cost of data collection.

Data on location and how the injuries occurred has led to large reductions in fall, pedestrian, and vehicle-occupant injuries in the limited instances in which such data have been collected (chapter 7). Simple pin maps of types of injury often indicate stretches of roads, intersections, or clusters of housing in which injuries occur. Obvious remedies are often revealed by visits to the sites (e.g., night lighting, sidewalks, moving or uncovering obscured stop signs, properly timed yellow lights, installation of guard rails, repair of dilapidated stairs).

In those instances where contributing factors or countermeasures are not obvious, well-designed analytic studies may specify how much a changeable factor would contribute to injury reduction if changed (table 3-1, item 3). Notice that the emphasis here is on changeable factors. Too much research focuses on unchangeable factors such as age and gender or difficult-to-change factors such as some types of behavior.

Suppose, for example, that your community has a high rate of severe injuries to children falling on stairs in households. The research question is the extent that changes in stairs would reduce the injuries. One way to answer the question is to do a case–control study comparing characteristics of stairs where children were injured and stairs in randomly selected households with similar-age children where injuries did not occur. Such a study of stairs in houses of the elderly found substantial differences in levelness, horizontal width, step width, hand rails, and lighting (Locklear, 1991). A second aspect of the research would compare the factors relevant to falls of children and the elderly to make sure that any recommended modifications of stairs would reduce injuries in both populations.

The development of elaborate causal models of the sequence of factors that lead to injury is the goal of some researchers, but it is the least productive research activity leading to injury control (table 3-1, item 4). The point of injury control research is not to specify some original cause in a sequence of factors but to specify changeable factors that reduce injuries irrespective of other factors. As noted in chapter 2, an injury cannot occur unless there is an energy exchange with the human anatomy beyond the tolerance of human tissue. Any countermeasure that reduces such energy exchanges will reduce injury severity irrespective of the factors that increased the probability of the event. The more proximate a risk factor to the energy exchanges, the greater the likelihood that changing the risk factor would have an effect on injuries (chapter 8).

The effectiveness of interventions, where unknown, can best be studied in controlled experiments (table 3-1, item 5). That includes medical care interventions, acute care, and rehabilitation (chapter 14), as well as some types of prevention (chapter 11). In the case of laws and regulations aimed at prevention, random assignment of treatments is usually not possible, so quasi-experimental designs and other approaches are necessary (chapters 12 and 13).

If there is more than one countermeasure that substantially reduces the same types of injuries, the degree in overlap of effectiveness and the relative costs of the countermeasures must be considered (table 3-1, item 6). The allocation of resources to duplicative efforts consumes the resources available to reduce injuries that are not being addressed (chapter 15).

Students choosing topics for library research papers or data for a thesis often approach an instructor with a vague statement such as "I am interested in children's injuries." A conversation usually follows, the point of which is to help the student narrow the topic to a researchable question given the time and resources available. For example, what age range is considered childhood? Since the activities of children vary by age, are there specific activities in a specific age range that you think might be related to certain types of injury? How severe are those types of injuries? Would they occur in limited number of settings? What are the energy exposures in those settings that might injure? How is the energy conveyed to the hosts? How many would receive treatment and where? Are you more interested in implications for treatment or in reduction of incidence or severity? What do you think is the most important information needed to improve treatment (or reduce incidence or severity)?

To find out what needs to be known, one must first find out what is known. The best way to choose an original research question is to survey the scientific literature on a topic and make a list of questions that come to mind in reading the literature. Literature reviews should not be confined to a search of the Internet or MEDLINE. Such a search will miss important research in the social and policy sciences on injury control. Significant research on topics such as behavioral, social, and cultural factors, violence, and the effects of laws and incentives on behavior is often found in the behavioral and social science literature not indexed in MEDLINE. If unanswered questions remain at the end of the literature survey, and they are researchable questions, the choices of potential topics for research are evident.

Before embarking on a research project in injury epidemiology, training in scientific methodology and statistics is essential. If one does not understand scientific principles of measurement and classification of phenomena, and the use of statistical methods to describe and analyze the data, the production of a publishable or useful study is very unlikely. Indeed, some of the scientific literature is unintelligible to a reader without such understanding, and some of it is easily seen as invalid, or at least highly questionable, when viewed by the informed reader (Riegelman, 1981).

One way of judging the adequacy of a published literature review is the extent to which it is critical of the research reviewed. A review that just lists studies and what they said, without indicating which are the most methodologically valid, is much less useful than a critical review. Other criteria include the dates of the studies covered in the review. If the review's bibliography lists no studies of recent vintage or no studies several decades old, the review is likely incomplete. Occasionally researchers new to injury epidemiology reinvent the wheel, sometimes in the shape of an octagon, apparently because they lack knowledge of previous studies.

Descriptive studies may be devoted to the identification of all injuries in a population, based on some minimum severity criteria, or may be focused on place of occurrence (e.g., roads), particular types of disability (e.g., spinal cord), a subset of the population (e.g., children), those associated with a given activity (e.g., swimming), or any number of other categories.

Decisions about what data are needed can be greatly facilitated by thinking at the outset how the data are to be used. Which of the objectives noted in table 3-1 is a general objective of the study? How can that objective be refined into specific aims? What specific statistical distributions of what variables are needed to reach decisions based on the conclusions? Actually constructing statistical tables that one intends to fill with data will force the identification of variables that must be measured, reveal definitional problems, and identify relevant categorizations.

FINDING USABLE DATA

Often one does not have the resources to collect original data and must find a data set that includes the variables and categories needed to answer a particular question. Many of the classification schemes used by organizations devoted to the compilation of injury statistics were developed before the application of epidemiological concepts and scientific principles. This does not mean that all of them are useless, but the uses to which the data are put are sometimes illogical and counterproductive to injury control, at least partly due to poor classification schemes.

As noted in chapter 2, injury classifications are often a mixture of vehicle, host, or circumstantial characteristics. For example, the National Safety Council for decades attempted to assemble data on "accidents" as well as injuries and reported its estimates in *Accident Facts*, an annual publication now called *Injury Facts*. The broad categories used are work, motor vehicle, public, home, farm, and school. These categories are inconsistent with one of the fundamental principles of classification: classes should be mutually exclusive; that is, a case should be classifiable in one and only one category.

Most farmers would consider their occupational activities as work, and increasing numbers of persons in nonfarm occupations work at home. Some people are injured in or by motor vehicles while engaged in their occupations. The National Safety Council is not alone in use of categories that are not mutually exclusive. In the National Health Interview Survey, conducted by the National Center for Health Statistics, similar categories were used, although in both systems the motor vehicle cases that occur while working or in the home driveway were classed systematically as motor vehicle rather than work or home (National Center for Health Statistics, 1986). The 2004 report from the survey on child health hardly mentions injury and combines injury and illness in statistics on days lost from school (National Center for Health Statistics, 2004). If one wanted to target the primary causes of school absenteeism, the data are useless.

Total numbers of deaths from injury of those who die soon after injury are probably counted in total with reasonable accuracy excepting some, such as electrocutions classified as "heart attacks" or pneumonia in the elderly bedridden because of a fall. People whose disabilities from injury shorten their lives later, such as those with spinal cord injury who die from infection, usually do not have their deaths counted as injury deaths.

Categorization problems, along with differences in data sources, can produce remarkable differences in estimates of numbers of injuries, or even deaths, the most easily countable injuries. The National Safety Council estimated 11,700 worker deaths from injury in 1984 compared to 3,740 counted by the Bureau of Labor Statistics (BLS) in its annual survey of businesses. Some of this difference is because certain small businesses and farms were excluded from the BLS survey, but that cannot possibly account for such a large difference in the estimates (Panel on Occupational Safety and Health Statistics, 1987). In India, the national railway reported 1,000 railway-related fatalities compared to more than 10,000 estimated from police reports. The railway reports only cases where a railway employee or equipment was judged at fault (Berger and Mohan, 1996). Obviously, the researcher must be aware of who is doing the counting and the definitions they use.

A second principle of classification is that the classes be exhaustive; that is, there should be a category for every case. Again looking at the National Safety

Council categories, where would one classify an injury to a child playing touch football in the field of a neighbor's farm? It would be misleading to call it a farm injury, and it did not happen anywhere in or near the child's or neighbor's home, at school, or in a public place.

Usually, the most useful injury categories are those that are relatively homogeneous as to energy source and vehicle or vector of the energy. For example, if one is interested in burns, the place of injury—home, school, restaurant, or hotel—may or may not be important. The same energy source may be the major culprit at each of these sites. Burns from heated liquids spilled from unstable cups or other containers may occur in all of these places. To control the damage, information on the extent to which the burns and other injuries (e.g., lung damage from smoke) occur from fires (specified by ignition source and material ignited), tap water, hot drinks spilled from specific types of containers, or space heaters by specific types is the most useful (McLoughlin and Crawford, 1985).

The point here is not to pick on organizations that employ scientifically inadequate or nonuseful categories. The point is to avoid using categories that are not mutually exclusive, exhaustive, and meaningful relative to the uses to which the data might be put. Injury researchers choose their projects for all sorts of reasons—personal experience with or concern about a particular type of injury, intellectual curiosity, or the need to identify a problem that will attract grant support perhaps being the most common. Whatever the motivation, consideration of the usefulness of the data to be collected would perhaps accelerate the use of categories that enhance the linkage between injury epidemiology and injury control. The definition of what constitutes a case and precision and accuracy of severity measurements are crucial.

CASE FINDING

Once one has decided the set of injuries that are to be investigated and meaningful categories to describe them, a means of finding cases must be identified and implemented. Various people and organizations, public and private, are potential sources for case identification and data on particular sets of injuries—the person injured and witnesses, private physicians and clinics, police, emergency medical responders, hospital emergency departments, hospital inpatient personnel, rehabilitation facilities, medical examiners, and coroners. Each data source has biases that must be understood and made explicit to avoid misinterpretation of the data.

Figure 3-1 presents the paths through which the vast majority of injury cases flow. Once an individual is exposed to energy sufficient to cause pain or perceptible tissue damage, that person or someone in proximity makes a decision whether to seek medical or other help. Most cases are relatively trivial cuts and bruises and are self-treated or ignored. The person who seeks help may go directly to a private physician or a hospital, or, if police or emergency medical personnel are called, the person may be examined and released or taken to a hospital emergency department or the morgue. If admitted to a hospital, the injured person may subsequently be released or sent to another hospital, a rehabilitation facility, or the morgue.

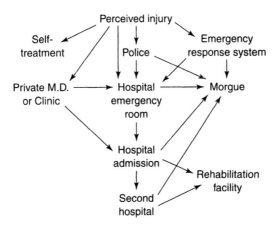

Figure 3-1. Paths of Injury Cases

Each of the arrows in figure 3-1 is a potential path that has a probability of occurrence that is related to several factors, including the circumstances of the injury and its severity. A person may not seek help because of embarrassment, threat from an assailant, knowledge of how to treat an injury, inability to pay for services, geographic remoteness from services, or attitudes regarding the services available. Private physicians and clinics, police, emergency personnel, and hospitals usually have protocols for handling or referring cases, but these are not always followed.

The flow of cases suggests various points at which data may be obtained. An epidemiologist may survey a sample of the population about injuries experienced or use the records of private physicians, emergency medical services, police, hospitals, rehabilitation facilities, and coroners or medical examiners. Each data source has potential biases that must be considered in using the data. The use of combined data sources sometimes allows an estimate of cases missing from any one and also provides data on several aspects of injury that no one source provides. Since the same injured person may have contact with more than one data source or more than one contact with the same data source, care must be taken not to count the same injury more than once.

The only way to obtain data on injuries that are not brought to medical or official attention is to contact people and question them about injury experience. There is substantial potential for bias in such surveys due to unreliable memory, embarrassment regarding certain types of injury, and differences among people in perceptions of seriousness. The National Health Interview Survey sometimes includes a few questions about injuries in its ongoing random sample survey of the population. To be included, an injury must have received medical attention or required a day of restricted activity. In one such survey, the rate of these self-reported injuries among persons 65 years and older was 19 per 100, compared to 38 per 100 among those younger than 45 years (National Center for Health Statistics, 1986). The elderly may have that many fewer injuries, or their rate could be biased by memory failure or other factors.

A general population survey is an inefficient way to identify severe injuries. The sample size would have to be huge to include significant numbers of deaths or permanently impairing spinal cord or head injuries.

The method of collecting data as well as the perception by the respondent of the persons or organizations soliciting the data may also affect the probability of the respondent's reporting an injury. For example, an annual survey of cervical spine injuries to high school football players was conducted by mailed questionnaire to high school principals and team trainers to identify cases. On the basis of identified cases, the researchers claimed that a decline in such injuries occurred from warnings to coaches about teaching players to use the head in blocking and tackling (Torg et al., 1985). These data are inadequate because only a few percent of the questionnaires were returned, and the respondents may withhold information because the researchers were previously active in issuing the warnings about head blocking and tackling. Some respondents may have been reluctant to report injuries in which they may have perceived themselves or members of their staffs as partially culpable. The researchers also used newspaper-clipping services to identify cases, but these were obtained from a limited and nonrepresentative sample of newspapers. To the author's knowledge, no comparison between cases reported in newspapers and those reported by school officials in the same communities has been reported.

One way of estimating completeness of injury reporting in interviews is to interview more than one person with probable knowledge of the injury. In a study of injuries to football players in Pop Warner leagues, coaches were asked to report injuries that required restricted participation for more than one week. At the end of the season, two players and two coaches, randomly selected from each team, were interviewed and asked to provide the names of anyone on the team who had such an injury. Of the total injuries identified, the coaches were the best source (82 percent of injuries reported), but an additional 18 percent were reported by the other respondents that would not have been found by sole reliance on coaches (Goldberg et al., 1988).

Reporting biases have also been found in official records. A substantial underreporting, despite legal requirements to do so, has been found comparing police reports of certain motor vehicle injuries and hospital records. In the United States, state governments require that motor vehicle injuries be reported to the police. Yet, in 45 percent of emergency department cases of motor vehicle injuries in five northeastern Ohio counties, no police report could be found (Barancik and Fife, 1985). The cases lost by relying on police records may be even larger in low-income countries, particularly in remote areas where police presence is minimal (Berger and Mohan, 1996).

Furthermore, in Ohio the lack of police reports was correlated with other factors. Police reports were missing for two-thirds to three-quarters of patients younger than 16 years, those who were passengers of vehicles other than passenger cars, and Medicaid recipients. Missing cases in police reports raise serious doubts about studies of seat belts, air bags, and other crash protection based on nonfatal injury data (chapter 12).

Medical records, augmented by death certificates or coroner or medical examiner records of the fatally injured, are the best sources for case identification for most studies (e.g., Kraus et al., 1975, 1984). Although many such records do not contain data on the circumstances of injury and other variables, they usually provide information on characteristics of the injury and its severity. If the injury can be disabling, the disability may not be recorded in the data from acute care hospitals. For example, some cases of spinal cord injury not identified in acute care records in one surveillance system were found in records of rehabilitation facilities (Thurman et al., 1994).

Once the case has been identified, other data can be obtained by matching to other records, if available, or by contacting the person injured or witnesses to the incident. Injuries that were not brought to medical attention will not be included, but as noted in chapter 4, the more severe injuries that are the primary targets for injury control are unlikely to be excluded.

References

Barancik JI, and Fife D (1985) Discrepancies in vehicular crash injury reporting: Northeastern Ohio Trauma Study IV. *Accid Anal Prev.* 17:147–154.

Berger LR, and Mohan D (1996) *Injury Control: A Global View.* Delhi, India: Oxford University Press.

Goldberg B, Rosenthal PP, Robertson LS and Nicholas JA (1988) Injuries in youth football. *Pediatrics* 81:255–261.

Kraus JF, Franti CE, Riggins D, and Borhani NO (1975) Incidence of traumatic spinal cord injury. *J Chronic Dis.* 28:471–492.

Kraus JF, Black MA, Hessol N, Ley P, Rokaw W, Sullivan C, Bowers S, Knowlton S, and Marshall L (1984) The incidence of acute brain injury and serious impairment in a defined population. *Am J Epidemiol.* 119:186–201.

Locklear G (1991) *A Retrospective Case-Control Study of Porch Step Falls Occurring on the Fort Apache Indian Reservation—1987 to 1989.* Phoenix, AZ: Environmental Health Services Branch, Indian Health Service.

McLoughlin E and Crawford JD Burns (1985) Ped Clinics North America. 32:61–76.

National Center for Health Statistics (1986) *Types of Injuries and Impairments Due to Injuries, United States.* Hyattsville, MD: U.S. Department of Health and Human Services.

National Center for Health Statistics (2004) 2004 National Health Interview Survey. Available at: http://www.cdc.gov/nchs/about/major/nhis/quest_data_related_1997_forward. htm#2004%20NHIS. Accessed August 2006.

Panel on Occupational Safety and Health Statistics (1987) *Counting Injuries and Illnesses in the Workplace: Proposals for a Better System.* Washington, DC: National Academy Press.

Rice DP, and MacKenzie EJ (eds.) (1989) Cost of injury in the United States: a report to Congress, 1989. San Francisco, CA, and Baltimore, MD: Institute for Health and Aging, University of California, Injury Prevention Center, Johns Hopkins University.

Riegelman RK (1981) *Studying a Study and Testing a Test.* Boston, MA: Little, Brown.

Thurman DJ, Burnett CL, Jeppson L, Beaudoin MD, and Sniezek JE (1994) Surveillance of spinal cord injuries in Utah, USA. *Paraplegia.* 32:665–669.

Torg JS, Vegso JJ, Sennett B, and Das M (1985) The national football head and neck injury registry: 14 year report on cervical quadraplegia, 1971 through 1984. *JAMA.* 254:3439–3443.

4

Injury Severity

The measurement of injury severity is an essential element of the use of injury epidemiology for injury control. In any given year, virtually everyone experiences minor injuries, such as small scratches, bruises, and burns. Most of these heal with little or no treatment and do not interfere with one's activities. The energy sources, vehicles and vectors, and other circumstances of injuries are usually not the same for those that are relatively severe and those with trivial consequences. Since trivial injuries are so common, priority in the devotion of resources to control of injuries based on total numbers in a given category can result in substantial misallocation of resources with respect to reducing the cost of injuries and the improvement of the quality of life of the severely injured and their families.

The measurement of injury severity is based on numerous clinical signs and symptoms such as respiration rate, consciousness, blood pressure, heart rate, and number and types of organ and system damage, such as area and depths of burns, ruptured spleen, and site-specified severance of the spinal cord. Researchers have developed summary scores of these factors that are meaningful in terms of decisions related to severity reduction, acute care, and rehabilitation. Several competing scoring systems have been developed, and no single one is likely to emerge that would be acceptable to everyone for the variety of potential uses.

SEVERITY SCORES

Severity scores are used in acute and follow-up medical care to triage patients (decide where and by whom patients should be treated), to plan for the different levels of care needed according to severity distributions, and to evaluate the effectiveness of treatment. Epidemiologists use severity scores to establish minimal criteria for surveillance of injury, to measure the effects of energy and other factors on injury severity for (including the effects of attempts at injury control), and to estimate injury effects on mortality, disability, and costs (Baker, 1983).

The elements of one severity scoring system, the Trauma Score, include respiration rate, systolic blood pressure, Glascow Coma score, verbal response and motor response. These signs and symptoms are widely used by emergency medical personnel for triage and by emergency care physicians for initial evaluation of patients, such that records for use in research are often available (Champion et al., 1981). The originators of the score have revised it and occasionally it is used in research by physicians (Champion et al., 1989) but not commonly by epidemiologists because the data are not routinely included in injury surveillance systems.

Examples from another severity rating system, the Abbreviated Injury Scale (AIS), are shown in table 4-1. It is based on a dictionary constructed from expert judgment of the severity of particular injuries (Committee on Injury Scaling, 1980). The AIS is seldom used for triage, but it is used in epidemiological studies as well as the evaluation of medical care outcomes and costs. The scoring procedure has been simplified into a standardized instrument that can be used in case abstraction from medical records (Barancik and Chatterjee, 1981) or to convert International Classification of Diseases diagnosis codes to AIS scores (Durbin et al., 2001). Also, comparison of AIS scores from hospital record reviews and those obtained using a computer program to compute AIS scores from computerized hospital discharge records found agreement in 48–75 percent of cases depending on the type of injury (MacKenzie et al., 1989, 1997).

A derivative of the AIS is the Injury Severity Score (ISS)—the sum of the squared AIS in each of the three most severely injured of seven defined regions of the anatomy: head, neck, thorax, abdomen and pelvic contents, spine, extremities and bony pelvis, and external skin and muscles. The ISS was developed by researchers concerned with refining the prediction of fatal injury, particularly in the case of multiple trauma (Baker et al., 1974). They noted that the probability of survival in a series of hospitalized trauma patients increased exponentially as a function of the

Table 4-1. The Abbreviated Injury Scale (AIS), With Examples

Code	Descriptor	Examples
0	No injury	
1	Minor	Superficial abrasion or laceration of skin; digit sprain; first-degree burn; head trauma with headache or dizziness but no other neurological signs
2	Moderate	Major abrasion or laceration of skin; unconscious but <15 minutes; finger or toe crush/amputation; closed pelvic fracture
3	Serious	Major nerve laceration; multiple rib fracture without flail chest; abdominal organ contusion; hand, foot, or arm crush/amputation
4	Severe	Ruptured spleen; leg crush; chest-wall perforation; unconscious <24 hours
5	Critical	Spinal cord transection; extensive/deep laceration of kidney or liver; extensive second- or third-degree burns; unconscious 24+ hours
6	Unsurvivable	Decapitation; torso transection

AIS scores in the noted regions of the body. Cross-tabulation of the three most severe injuries in different areas of the anatomy indicated that the square of these AIS scores was a strong predictor of probability of survival, particularly when corrected for age of the injured.

These scoring systems are attempts to quantify a mixture of quantitative and qualitative elements of the extent of injury. The quantitative elements of the Trauma Score, such as respiration rate and blood pressure, are strangely broken up into qualitative categories and then requantified by regression weights. Although each of these measurements could be used quantitatively without categorization in segments, mathematical modeling of them in combination to obtain a useful score would be very complex and difficult to use in emergency situations without a specially designed calculator with the logic built into it.

An index combining the Trauma Score and the ISS, as well as patient age, has been developed using logistic regression, with probability of survival as the outcome (Boyd et al., 1987). Logistic regression is a technique that assigns weights to different factors regarding their relative power to predict probability of a discrete outcome such as death versus survival (e.g., Selvin, 1991). Cases in which the patient dies despite a high probability of survival, or survives despite a low probability of survival, are suggested as worthy of peer review by the American College of Surgeons (Committee on Trauma of the American College of Surgeons, 1987). The validity of this approach has also been verified for children's injuries (Kaufmann et al., 1991). Modifications of the measurements improve prediction of death from penetrating injuries (Champion et al., 1990).

Since the ISS leaves out some injuries, a system called the Anatomic Profile (AP) was developed to summarize the AIS of all injuries. A committee of clinical experts defined sets of injuries to comprise components of a score, based on the International Classification of Diseases codes for injury in particular regions of the anatomy. The square root of the sum of the squares of the AIS of each injury in each component was related to probability of survival, and weights for each factor were obtained by logistic regression. Comparison of the AP scores and ISS scores indicated an improvement in the prediction of survival by using the AP (Copes et al., 1990). Physicians who treat trauma in children have been critical of the use of indices based on measurement of trauma and outcomes for adult patients. A Pediatric Trauma Score, the elements of which are shown in table 4-2, has been shown to have excellent correlation to the probability of survival of traumatized children (Tepas, 1989).

The AIS, ISS, and AP are indices of trauma mainly from mechanical energy. One interesting question is the feasibility and usefulness of scoring that would include heat, electrical, or chemical injuries and asphyxiations. Mortality from burns is an exponential function of surface area burned and age of the patient (Rutowski et al., 1976). Comparison of the predictability of the Trauma Score or Pediatric Trauma Score, as currently used, and statistically adjusting the weights of components in studies of mortality and disability from burns, electricity, poisonings, and asphyxiations would be useful research projects. Since survival from both mechanical and thermal energy insults to human tissue is an exponential function of the injury severity to areas of the organism, there may be common biological processes at work that could be identified and targeted in treatment. (For

Table 4-2. Pediatric Trauma Score

Component	Points		
	+2	+1	−1
Size	>20 kg	10–20 kg	<10 kg
Airway	Normal	Maintainable	Unmaintainable
Systolic blood pressure	>90 mm Hg	50–90 mm Hg	<50 mm Hg
Central nervous system	Awake	Obtunded/loss of consciousness	Coma/decerebrate
Open wound	None	Minor	Major/penetrating
Skeletal	None	Closed fracture	Open/multiple fracture

severity scoring systems and calculators, see http://www.trauma.org/scores/index.html, accessed August 2006.)

IMPAIRMENT AND DISABILITY

Study of outcomes other than death in relation to injury severity scoring has been limited. Length of hospital stays and disability from motor vehicle injuries are substantially predicted by the ISS (Bull, 1975; Schluter et al., 2005), but other scoring systems might improve predictability. It has been noted, for example, that a lesion to the eye that would be minor in another body area can cause blindness (Jorgensen, 1981), and that head and spinal cord injuries with low AIS scores can result in substantial impairment (Conboy et al., 1986; MacKenzie et al., 1986).

The severity and persistence of disabling impairments from injury have not been extensively investigated. The National Health Interview Survey periodically notes prevalence (the proportion of the population with a condition at a given point in time) of certain impairments—vision, hearing, speech, absence and deformities of extremities, and paralysis—and the percentage that occurred in the year of the survey (National Center for Health Statistics, 1986; for current information on injury from National Center for Health Statistics, see http://www.cdc.gov/nchs/fastats/acc-inj.htm, accessed August 2006). However, the severity and prognosis of these impairments would require more detailed data.

Special studies of certain types of long-term disability have indicated the substantial excess of particular circumstances for certain types of injury. For example, the Utah Health Department's surveillance of spinal cord injury found that, during 1989–1991, 65 percent of nonfatal spinal injuries to motor vehicle occupants occurred in rollovers (Thurman et al., 1995), about twice what would be expected from the proportion of occupant deaths that occur in rollovers.

The proposed impairment and disability measurement in table 4-3 is an attempt to develop scales analogous to the AIS (States and Viano, 1990). The developers adopted a 7-point scale, like the AIS, despite the fact that they could not identify seven points on some dimensions. As was the case in the development of the Trauma Score and the AIS, the categories were formed based on clinical experience

Table 4-3. Proposed Impairment and Disability Scales

Mobility/Dexterity Impairment

1. *Minor:* Detectable impairment of mobility or dexterity but with intact functional ability, e.g., minor limp due to knee with degenerative arthritis, mild tremor, limitation of motion in some but not all digits, thumb normal, detectable weakness in hands.

2. *Moderate:* Walking distance limited to less than 1/4 mile. Uses cane occasionally. Can use stairs; difficulty in balance. Hands weak or usefulness impaired by tremor or spasticity. Typing and driving difficult.

3. *Serious:* Cane, crutches, prosthesis, and/or walker are necessary for walking except in dwelling. Stairs are difficult; railing is essential. Motor deficit of hands or extremities. Cannot type or use hand tools. Unilateral hand amputee.

4. *Severe:* Wheelchair is used by choice, but patient can stand and walk with apparatus, i.e., crutches or walker. Severe motor weakness, incoordination, or spasticity; self-feeding slow or uncertain.

5. *Very Severe:* Wheelchair is required for ambulation although patient can stand and walk short distances with assistance. Virtually complete motor paralysis. Virtually no hand function. Bilateral hand amputee.

6. *Totally Immobile and Dependent:* Requires hoist for transfer; cannot stand; requires aide for activities of daily living. Has no useful function in upper extremities.

Cognitive/Psychological Impairment

1. *Minor:* Mild inappropriate behavior; occasional errors in language and arithmetic.

2. *Moderate:* Noticeable memory loss; difficulties with simple arithmetic; difficulty in self-expression; infrequent disorientation and dizziness. Mild mental retardation.

3. *Serious:* Occasional disorientation, significant memory loss or language impairment, and occasional signs of psychosis. Moderate mental retardation.

4. *Severe:* No memory for recent events; disoriented, psychotic, requires sheltered home, and speech unintelligible. Severe mental retardation.

5. *Very Severe:* No memory, total loss of speech; psychotic; usually requires institutional care. Profound mental retardation.

6. *Coma:* Vegetative; no purposeful response to stimuli; brain dead.

Cosmetic/Disfigurement Impairment

1. *Minor:* Normally covered, amenable to cosmetic makeup. Readily covered orthosis.

2. *Moderate:* Can be covered by cosmetics and/or forces change in dress; may require orthesis but not prosthesis.

3. *Serious:* Prothesis or cover-up required.

4. *Severe:* Readily observable, not amenable to cosmetic, prosthetic, or clothing cover-up.

Sensory Impairment

	Vision	Hearing	Sensation	Taste and Smell
1. *Minor:*	Minor loss but does not interfere with usual activities; correctable with readily available aids such as glasses, hearing aids.			
2. *Moderate:*	Correctable to 20/100 in best eye.	Hearing loss not fully correctable.	26–50% loss to special senses or limbs.	Complete loss of taste or smell.

Table 4-3. Proposed Impairment and Disability Scales

	Vision	Hearing	Sensation	Taste and Smell
3. *Serious:*	Complete loss of vision in one eye, partial in other eye.	Total hearing loss.	Greater than 50% loss.	Complete loss of both taste and smell.
4. *Severe:*	No vision.			

Pain Impairment

1. *Minor:* Occasional pain; analgesics not required or used; no interference with sleep.

2. *Moderate:* Occasional pain; more frequent or occasional use of nonnarcotic analgesics.

3. *Serious:* Constant or occasional severe pain; nonnarcotic analgesics required for sleep, work. Narcotic analgesics occasionally required.

4. *Severe:* Constant or severe occasional pain requiring narcotics or invasive therapy. Sleep poor; unable to work. Recreation and socialization severely limited.

5. *Very Severe:* Constant or severe pain requiring narcotics or invasive therapy. Sleep poor; unable to work. No recreation or socialization.

6. *Uniformly Causes Total Impairment:* Constant and/or occasional pain uncontrolled except with large doses of narcotics that affect the central nervous system. Incomplete control with invasive therapy.

Sexual/Reproduction Impairment

1. *Minor:* Decreases frequency of intercourse because of occasional pain or decreased libido.

2. *Moderate:* Inability to have satisfactory erection; loss of libido. Pain with intercourse. Reduced fecundity.

3. *Serious:* Complete loss of capability for an erection; loss of libido. Pain precluding intercourse. Complete absence of fecundity.

Disability Scale

0. *No Disability:* Self-support (full-time work and full recreational activity compatible with patient's age).

1. *Minor:* Self-support with reduced recreational activity.

2. *Moderate:* Self-support with no recreational activity.

3. *Serious:* Independent living (limited or no assistance with activities of daily living); may be capable of part-time work.

4. *Severe:* Living at home but with assistance of aide less than four hours per day and/or assistance with shopping, meal preparation, and medications.

5. *Very severe:* Full care at home with aid more than four hours per day or institutional care but with ability to perform some activities of daily living.

6. *Extreme:* Institutional care with external life support systems such as mechanical respiratory assistance or tube feeding.

Source: States and Viano (1990).

Reprinted from *Accident Analysis and Prevention*, Vol. 22, States JD and Viano DC. Injury impairment and disability scales to assess the permanent consequences of trauma. Pp. 151–160, Copyright (1990) with permission from Elsevier.

but must be studied in terms of reliability and validity and revised accordingly before widespread use.

Reliability (sometimes called precision) refers to the repeatability of a measurement. For example, do different people who interview the same patient or review the same medical record produce the same score? Validity (sometimes called accuracy) refers to whether the dimension that one is attempting to measure is actually being measured. Reliability of data is often easily assessed by comparing independent recording of the data, but the determination of validity is much more difficult.

If a scale is to measure injury severity relevant to survival, and it is strongly predictive of survival, it satisfies a major criterion for validity. A major validity test of an impairment scale is the extent to which it predicts degree and permanence of disability.

One problem evident in the proposed impairment and disability scales (table 4-5) is the presence of the same or similar criteria in both scales. Notice that ability to perform tasks such as typing, hand tool use, and work are included in the mobility/dexterity and pain impairment scales; and self-support, which may require these activities, is in the disability scale. Similarly, "usually requires institutional care" is in the cognitive/psychological impairment scale and "institutional care" is included in the disability scale. Thus, the scales are not independently determined and will, by definition, be correlated. Also, the disability scale does not have exhaustive categories; in the "extreme" group, persons may be institutionalized that do not require life support systems or tube feeding.

These scales need revision before being studied empirically, as recognized by the proponents who suggested that they be examined by expert consensus panels (States and Viano, 1990). Field tests to assess potential problems and establish weights for the effects of impairment on disability are also recommended before use in a full-scale research project. One obviously should not just add up scales that may not be additive in effect and double counting of particular elements should be eliminated.

The Functional Capacity Index is a somewhat simpler attempt to measure limitations of normal function and has been subjected to field testing. Also designed to mirror the AIS, it has three to seven levels of indication of ability to perform 10 activities: eating, excreting, sex, ambulation, use of hands and arms, bending/lifting, seeing, hearing, talking, and thinking. To assess interrater reliability, weights were assigned by raters from convenience samples of experts and white- and blue-collar workers. Although raters assigned similar weights within dimensions, clinical experts tended to underestimate the importance of various activities relative to the other raters. There was also large variation in intrarater reliability among some scales when the ratings were repeated after a two-week period (MacKenzie et al., 1996).

Studies of disability in activities of daily living among the elderly indicate a hierarchy of factors (Dunlop et al., 1997). One type of scale worth investigating is one in which a number indicates a cumulative effect (Guttman, 1946). For example, if the data so indicated, a 1 would indicate "cannot walk," a 2 would indicate "cannot walk" and "cannot transfer from chair to bed," and so forth. Such are among numerous disability scales that have been developed. (For a list and references, see http://www.gwu.edu/~cicd/toolkit/function.htm, accessed August 2006.)

The researcher should not adopt any injury or disability scoring system without careful consideration of what is being measured relative to the hypotheses and possible uses of the research (MacKenzie, 2001). The injury severity scales mainly indicate probability of death and are not very useful as measures of probability of impairments and disabilities among those who survive (MacKenzie et al., 1996). Some disability measures may be distorted because they are related to eligibility for insurance or governmental benefits (Aarts and DeJong, 1992; Bloch, 1982).

The extent to which a particular limitation is disabling depends on an individual's desires for specific activities and the environment in which they are pursued. There are three stages prior to disability that offer the opportunity for prevention: (1) pathology (e.g., traumatic denervation of an arm); (2) impairment (e.g., atrophy of muscle); and (3) functional limitation (e.g., no pulling strength). The effect on the person's life depends on the extent that pulling strength is necessary for work, recreation, and other activities (Pope and Tarlov, 1991).

References

Aarts LJM, and DeJong PR (1992) *Economic Aspects of Disability Behavior.* Amsterdam: North Holland.

Baker SP (1983) Panel: current status of trauma severity indices. *J Trauma.* 23:193–196.

Baker SP, O'Neill B, Haddon W Jr, and Long WB (1974) The Injury Severity Score: a method for describing patients with multiple injuries and evaluating emergency care. *J Trauma.* 14:187–196.

Barancik JI, and Chatterjee BF (1981) Methodological considerations in the use of the Abbreviated Injury Scale in trauma epidemiology. *J Trauma.* 21:627.

Bloch FS (1982) *Disability Determination: The Administrative Process and the Role of Medical Personnel.* Westport, CT; Greenwood Press.

Boyd CR, Tolson MA, and Copes WS (1987) Evaluating trauma care: the TRISS method. *J Trauma.* 27:370–378.

Bull JP (1975) The Injury Severity Score of road traffic casualties in relation to mortality, time of death, hospital treatment time and disability. *Accid Anal Prev.* 7:249–255.

Champion HR, Sacco WJ, Carnazzo AJ, Copes WS, and Fouty WJ (1981) Trauma score. *Crit Care Med.* 9:672–676.

Champion HR, Sacco WJ, Copes WS, Gann DS, Gennarelli TA, and Flanagan ME (1989) A revision of the trauma score. *J Trauma.* 29:623–629.

Champion HR, Copes WS, Sacco WJ, Lawnick MM, Bain LW, Gann DS, Gennarelli T, MacKenzie E, and Schwaitzberg S (1990) A new characterization of injury severity. *J Trauma.* 30:539–544.

Committee on Injury Scaling (1980) *The Abbreviated Injury Scale, 1980 Revision.* Park Ridge, IL: American Association for Automotive Medicine.

Committee on Trauma of the American College of Surgeons (1987) Appendix G. Quality assurance in trauma care. In *Hospital and Prehospital Resources for Optimal Care of the Injured Patient.* Chicago, IL: American College of Surgeons.

Conboy T, Barth J, and Boll T (1986) Treatment and rehabilitation of mild and moderate head trauma. *Rehabil Psychol.* 31:202–215.

Copes WS, Champion HR, Sacco WJ, Lawnick MM, Gann DS, Gennarelli T, MacKenzie E, and Schwaitzberg S (1990) Progress in characterizing anatomic injury. *J Trauma.* 30:1200–1207.

Dunlop DD, Hughes SL, and Manheim LM (1997) Disabilty in activities of daily living: patterns of change and a hierarchy of disability. *Am J Public Health.* 87:378–383.

Durbin DR, Localio AR, and MacKenzie EJ (2001) Validation of the ICD/AIS MAP for pediatric use. *Inj Prev.* 7:96–99.

Guttman L (1946) An approach for quantifying paired comparisons and rank order. *Ann Math Stat.* 17:144–163.

Jorgensen K (1981) Use of the Abbreviated Injury Scale in a hospital emergency room. *Acta Orthop Scand.* 52:273–277.

Kaufmann CR, Maier RV, Kaufmann EJ, Rivara FP, and Carrico CJ (1991) Validity of applying adult TRISS analysis to injured children. *J Trauma.* 31:691–697.

MacKenzie EJ (1997) *ICDMAP-90 Computer Software.* Bel Air, MD: Tri-Analytics.

MacKenzie EJ (2001) Measuring disability and quality of life postinjury. In Rivara FP, et al. (eds.), *Injury Control: A Guide to Research and Program Evaluation.* Cambridge, UK: Cambridge University Press.

MacKenzie EJ, Damiano A, Miller T, and Luchter S (1996) The development of the Functional Capacity Index. *J Trauma.* 41:799–806.

MacKenzie EJ, Shapiro S, Moody M, Siegel JH, and Smith RT (1986) Predicting post trauma functional disability for individuals without severe brain injury. *Med Care.* 24:377–387.

MacKenzie EJ, Steinwachs DM, and Shankar B (1989) Classifying trauma severity based on hospital discharge diagnoses: validation of an ICD-9CM to AIS-85 conversion table. *Med Care.* 27:412–422.

National Center for Health Statistics (1986) Types of Injuries and Impairments Due to Injuries, United States. Hyattsville, MD: U.S. Department of Health and Human Services.

Pope AM, and Tarlov AR (1991) *Disability in America: Toward a National Agenda for Prevention.* Washington, DC: National Academy Press.

Rutowski W, Nasilowski W, Zietkiewicz W, and Zienkiewicz K (1976) *Burn Therapy and Research.* Baltimore, MD: Johns Hopkins Press.

Schluter PJ, Cameron CM, Purdie DM, Kliewer EV, and McClure RJ (2005) How well do anatomical-based injury severity scores predict health service use in the 12 months after injury? *Int J Inj Contr Saf Promot.* 12:241–246.

Selvin S (1991) *Statistical Analysis of Epidemiologic Data.* New York, NY: Oxford University Press.

States JD, and Viano DC (1990) Injury impairment and disability scales to assess the permanent consequences of trauma. *Accid Anal Prev.* 22:151–160.

Tepas JJ III (1989) Update on pediatric trauma-severity scores. In Haller JA Jr (ed.), *Emergency Medical Services for Children.* Columbus, OH: Ross Laboratories.

Thurman DJ, Burnett CL, Beaudoin DE, Jeppson L and Sniezek JE (1995) Risk factors and mechanisms of occurrence in motor vehicle-related spinal injuries: Utah. Acc Anal Prevent 27:411-415.

5

Injury Statistics

The simplest statistical description of injuries is the distribution by severity, obtained by counting the numbers in specific categories, such as fatal, hospitalized, and ambulatory, or on the severity scale of interest. For example, injury severity is sometimes described as distributed in the shape of a pyramid, with deaths at the top, hospitalizations in the middle, and others at the base. More refined categories of injuries by type and severity scales, however, are not pyramid shaped by severity. For example, there are substantially more deaths from motor vehicles than there are nonfatal, critical injuries (Abbreviated Injury Scale code 5; see table 4-2). Drowning and near drowning tends to result in death or a much lower number of severely brain-damaged and impairment cases from oxygen deficits, or persons survive without injury.

Among the most commonly reported distributions of injury are by age and sex. While such distributions of injuries of a given type may be of use in targeting age groups for prevention, another important way of looking at age of the fatally injured is by years of potential life lost. This is calculated by multiplying the number of deaths at a given age times the years persons of that age would be expected to live (from a life table) and summing the total number of years lost. (For a life table based on deaths in the United States, see http://www.ssa.gov/OACT/STATS/table4c6.html, accessed August 2006.)

Although more people die from heart diseases and cancers, injuries are the leading cause of years of life lost through age 70 (chapter 1). That is because those who die from injury are, on average, decades younger than those who die from the "leading" causes of death. Some researchers subtract age of death from 65 to obtain "productive years of life lost," but that practice implies that the only value of life is economic. The years lost from injury prior to age 85 (6.0 million in 2003) were nearly as many as those lost each from cardiovascular diseases (6.5 million) or cancers (8.4 million).

Such comparison of potential years of life lost has resulted in more attention given to injuries but is seldom used in detailed research. Potential years of life lost by type of injury would also be suggestive of the importance of concentrating on certain types of injury that take more years than the total numbers of fatal injuries in a given category would indicate.

INJURY RATES

Injuries are often reported as rates per population, or some other denominator, such as per miles driven for motor vehicle injuries or per hours flown for injuries in aircraft. The population rate is calculated by dividing the number of people injured by the number of people in the population:

$$\text{Rate} = \frac{\text{Number of injuries in a year in the population}}{\text{Number of people in the population}}$$

This rate is usually multiplied by 100,000 to get rate per 100,000 population, or by 10,000 or 1,000 if the injuries of interest occur in larger numbers.

To be accurate, the people injured in the numerator must have come from the population in the denominator, and both must be counted accurately. Most such calculations are approximations based on estimates of the population from the census or some other source. Some of the injured during the year, or whatever time period chosen, may be visitors from outside the population, and some of the population may have been outside the area all or part of the year.

These potential biases may not be important in total population estimates when the visitors' injuries or the numbers of the population that are outside the area are small relative to the total numbers involved. Estimates of injury rates per population for smaller areas such as cities, counties, or even states may be substantially affected by seasonal influxes of tourists or students, roads carrying large amounts of nonlocal traffic, and the like.

The basic principle in calculating population rates is that cases in the numerator should come only from the population in the denominator. This is a major problem in hospital trauma registries, where the population from which the injuries come is often difficult or impossible to define (Waller, 1988). To calculate rates for segments of the population, or using some other denominator such as miles driven in the case of motor vehicle injuries, one must be able to place cases in the numerator and denominator into the same mutually exclusive and exhaustive categories. For example, if the injury cases are classified by age in years, such as 0–4, 5–9, 10–14, and so on, and the population data are classified by age as 0–3, 3–6, 7–10, and so forth, the rates for each age group cannot be calculated without reclassifying one or the other.

Use of denominators other than population is an attempt to obtain a more refined estimate of rate per exposure. For example, the Federal Aviation Administration reports injuries in aircraft crashes per hours flown. Obviously a person who does not travel in airplanes will not crash in one, although crashing aircraft occasionally injure people on the ground. Aircraft usually crash during attempts to take off or land. In the same make and model of airplane, a person who flies the same number of hours over shorter distances is at greater risk per hour flown than when flying the same number of hours over longer distances. Therefore, rate per hours flown can be a misleading indicator of risk. (For data on exposure to various forms of transportation, see http://www.bts.gov/, accessed August 2006.)

Measuring hours of exposure becomes even more problematic when considering numerous activities. For example, drowning of young children often occurs in home swimming pools. How do we estimate hours of exposure of young children to home swimming pools? Hours in or by the pool are inadequate because many wander into the pool from the house or yard at times when use of the pool is unintended by their adult supervisors. Some wander into a neighbor's pool. Do we count the number of hours the children are awake? Do we multiply the number of hours awake times the number of pools in the neighborhood? What constitutes the neighborhood in defining the likelihood of home pool exposure?

Trends in rates of motor vehicle fatalities are sometimes based on total deaths per million total miles driven, the latter based on self-reports, periodic odometer monitoring, road use surveys, or sales of fuel. The deaths per mile are often decreasing even in periods when the population rate is not changing or increasing. This occurs, for example, when use of vehicles in urban areas is increasing faster then use in rural areas. In urban areas, the speed limits are lower and congestion of traffic during the misnamed "rush hours" also reduces speeds, thus lowering the energy exchange in crashes. Crashes in urban areas are more frequent per mile but are less severe, and vehicle occupant death rates are lower than in rural areas.

An auto industry analysis of occupant fatalities in cars and light trucks by hour of day and day of week noted that 32 percent of such fatalities occurred between 11:00 P.M. and 5:00 A.M., while diaries of personal vehicle use indicate that only 4.5 percent of total mileage was accumulated during those hours (Schwing and Kamerud, 1988). Unfortunately, the authors went on to speculate about "risk-taking behavior," which they did not measure, as the explanation. It is difficult to believe that behavior during those hours is so radically different than during the remainder of the day. As further noted in chapter 7, lighting roads at sites where severe crashes clustered at night virtually eliminated the problem, which suggests that visibility at night may explain a substantial proportion of the diurnal variation in fatalities per mile. Nevertheless, mileage as exposure does not necessarily indicate that quality of exposure is a valid point.

When considering separately other road users struck by motor vehicles, such as pedestrians and bicyclists, rates per mile of motor vehicle use in urban areas are higher than in rural areas. This is probably because more people walk or use bicycles in urban areas, but miles walked or bicycled are difficult to estimate accurately and are rarely used.

The point here is that there is no absolutely right or wrong measure of exposure. The issue under consideration should determine the choice of denominators to be researched and what can be learned about injury reduction from the results.

The use of one or another measure of exposure has various implications for interpretation that may not be obvious.

RELEVANCE AND IRRELEVANCE OF RATES

One focus in the collection of data on incidence, severity, and other aspects of injury is to specify the risk of the injury in question. Risk is the probability that the injury, or a specific level of severity, will occur in use of a given product or participation in a given activity. Risk is an estimate of what will happen in the future, while a rate is an indication of relative frequency in the past. Risk is usually derivable from rates based on the assumption that the previous relative frequency will continue, adjusted for the deaths that eliminate future participation (Kelsey et al., 1986), but interpretation is sometimes difficult depending on how accurately the denominator reflects quality of exposure. For very rare events, such as nuclear power plant meltdowns, estimates of risk are based on probability of various combinations of failures in the technology rather than the previous frequency (Gould et al., 1988).

The scientist who calculates injury rates using whatever denominators should be aware of poor methodology and tricky interpretations that have been applied to the data. Particularly in regulatory and product liability forums, the word "risk" is often preceded by adjectives such as "reasonable" or "acceptable." From a technical standpoint, an injury rate is the occurrence per specified unit of exposure and merely reflects the occurrence per exposure during the specified period of time. Standing alone, the rate does not indicate anything about whether it could be reduced by the manufacturer of an involved product, except by not manufacturing the product, or by the user of the product.

The risk of a product is the expected number of injuries per product during its use. If a given make and model of motor vehicle has an occupant death rate of 20 per 100,000 vehicles per year, and if it will be in use an average of 10 years per vehicle, its occupant fatality risk is $(10 \times 20)/100,000$ or 0.002, or stated in the inverse, 1 occupant death per 500 vehicles. Too many "risk analyses" fail to account for the lifetime risks of products or practices. Failure to understand the difference between annual risk and cumulative risk over the life of products has resulted in grotesque errors in estimating the effects of potential preventive measures (see appendix 15-1).

Manufacturers and others opposed to regulation, or "experts" and attorneys involved in product liability lawsuits, often cite the injury rate from the product in question relative to injury rates from other products as indicative of reasonableness or acceptability. Given the variety of denominators available to calculate rates and the difficulty in measuring exposure, the placement of a given rate in an array of rates of injury by products or users can be very different, depending on the denominator used and the comparability of the research methods in case finding and exposure measurement.

An interesting case of such arguments about rates and risk occurred regarding the consideration of regulation of all-terrain vehicles (ATVs) by the U.S. Consumer Products Safety Commission (CPSC). These vehicles are propelled by modified motorcycle-type engines at speeds up to 60 miles per hour. They have three or four balloon tires and are steered by handlebars similar to those on a motorcycle. The steering is not as easy as it looks, however, requiring weight shifts by the rider different from those on a bicycle or motorcycle. The vehicles are unstable when in motion and will roll over at low speeds, sometimes onto the rider, if the rider does not apply the weight shift at the moment needed (Deppa, 1986).

These vehicles are marketed in the United States as a recreational vehicle for families, including children, and sales increased rapidly in the early 1980s to the point that about 2.5 million were in the hands of consumers by 1986. The CPSC estimates of deaths on the vehicles increased from 26 in 1982 to 268 in 1986, and estimates of injuries from a survey of those treated in hospital emergency departments increased from about 8,600 in 1982 to 86,400 in 1986. Congress and consumer groups pressured the CPSC to ban the vehicles or issue safety standards for them.

Arguments ensued among the staff and commissioners of the CPSC as to whether the rate of injuries to occupants of ATVs should be compared to those of occupants of other motorized, off-road vehicles such as snowmobiles and mini/trail bikes. Initial comparisons indicated that the rate of injury for ATVs was twice that for mini/trail bikes and four to five times that for snowmobiles. Based on a few anecdotal reports of hours of use per vehicle in public hearings, however, the rates per hours of use for ATVs were said to be less than those for the other vehicles (Verhalen, 1986). A majority of the commissioners voted that the comparison was irrelevant to the issue of whether ATVs should be regulated (General Accounting Office, 1986), but the industry commissioned research on injuries per hours of participation in other recreational activities in an attempt to justify the risk of ATVs.

An economist formerly employed at the CPSC was hired by the industry to conduct a survey of hours of use of mini/trail bikes and snowmobiles. Based on these data and CPSC counts of injuries, he argued that the injury rate per hours of use were no different among the three types of vehicles (Heiden, 1986). In subsequent congressional hearings (Heiden, 1990) and in lawsuits against manufacturers, comparisons were also made to injuries per hour for people engaged in other activities such as organized football, use of motorcycles and other on-road vehicles, general aviation, snow skiing, swimming, and other activities. With the exception of organized football games and general aviation, the estimates of hours of participation were extrapolated from surveys that used categories for time of participation such as "daily or almost daily," "about once or twice a week," "about once or twice a month," and "less than once per month." These are useless for estimation of hours of participation, and given the problems of remembering hours of participation, questions regarding more specific hours of participation in most activities are likely to be unreliable or invalid (Robertson, 2006).

Aside from methodological issues, this case illustrates some of the uses or misuses of epidemiological data of which the researcher should be aware. While it may be useful to present the public with information about risks of engaging in activities that are substitutable one for the other per hour, per person, per vehicle, per product, or whatever, the comparison of descriptive injury rates per whatever exposure unit among various activities or products does not tell us whether the risks are "reasonable" or "acceptable" or whether products involved are defective.

Two products may have the same injury rate, one of which could have been reduced by product modifications at less cost, no cost, or little cost, while the cost of modification of the other may be very large. The calculation of cost savings, cost-effectiveness, risk–benefit, or cost–benefit of injury reduction modifications to products, or injury control programs generally, is not based on risk per hour or risk per product or activity. These calculations should be based on total costs of the injuries relative to the total costs of product modifications or programs to reduce them (chapter 15).

If a product or activity were to be considered "reasonable" or "acceptable" as long as its injury rate were less than the most risky products and activities, manufacturers and promoters of products and activities would be free to add one new risk after another with impunity. The fact that more risky products are for sale does not indicate user acceptability of a less risky product when the vast majority of purchasers do not have any way to assemble the data on relative rates.

One methodology that has been used to assess public acceptability of risk is to compare perception of current restrictions or regulations to desired restrictions or standards for motor vehicles, guns, commercial aviation, industrial chemicals, nuclear power generation, and nuclear weapons. In random sample surveys of the population in Connecticut and the Phoenix metropolitan area, the respondents rated desired restrictions and standards far above restrictions and standards prevalent in 1982–1983, a period of severe economic recession and strong anti-regulation political sentiment (Gould et al., 1988).

Epidemiological data on injury rates is relevant to the issue of modifiability of products and activities when and if the specific characteristics of the products and activities that increase or decrease the rates are delineated using sound epidemiological research. The methods for such analytical epidemiological studies are discussed in chapter 8. Chapters 6 and 7 deal with a special case of descriptive epidemiology that is useful for problem identification and targeting control strategies—injury surveillance.

References

Deppa RW (1986) *Report on the Engineering Evaluation of All Terrain Vehicles.* Washington, DC: U.S. Consumer Product Safety Commission.

General Accounting Office (1986) *Consumer Product Safety Commission: Concerns About Staff Memorandum Relating to All-Terrain Vehicles.* Washington, DC: U.S. Congress.

Gould LC, Gardner GT, DeLuca DR, Tiemann AR, Doob LW, and Stolwijk JAJ (1988) *Perceptions of Technological Risks and Benefits.* New York, NY: Russell Sage Foundation.

Heiden EJ (1986) *Some Additional Evidence on Comparative Safety for ATVs and Related Vehicles.* Washington, DC: Heiden Associates.

Heiden EJ (1990) *Statement. Washington, DC: Commerce, Consumer, and Monetary Affairs Subcommittee of the House Government Operations Committee.* Washington, DC: U.S. House of Representatives.

Kelsey JL, Thompson WD, and Evans AS (1986) *Methods in Observational Epidemiology.* New York, NY: Oxford University Press.

Robertson LS (2006) *The Expert Witness Scam.* Available at: http://www.lulu.com/content/296817. Accessed December 2006.

Schwing RC, and Kamerud DB (1988) The distribution of risks: vehicle occupant fatalities and time of week. *Risk Anal.* 8:127–133.

Verhalen RD (1986) *ATV Project: Comparative Injury Tables.* Washington, DC: U.S. Consumer Product Safety Commission.

Waller J (1988) Methodologic issues in hospital-based injury research. *J Trauma.* 28: 1632–1636.

6

National Injury Surveillance

The word "surveillance," with its connotation of police watching the residences of suspects, or someone's phone being tapped, may not be the best word to describe an epidemiological activity. The epidemiological use of the term refers to collection of data on who, when, where and, sometimes, how people become diseased or injured. The data are purged of individual identifiers so that the individuals involved are anonymous.

Collection of detailed data on who, when, where, and how people are injured can be used to target injury control measures to relevant circumstances and populations and increase cost-effectiveness of resource allocation. Identification of relatively homogeneous subsets of injuries in defined locations and populations coupled with a systematic review of Haddon's technical options for injury control (see chapter 2) can lead to substantial reductions if implemented. Some examples of the power of surveillance data in injury control are given at the end of chapter 7. This chapter provides a description of some important surveillance systems.

Several governmental and private agencies in the United States maintain surveillance systems that continually or periodically collect data on injuries. Some of these systems include data useful for more detailed study than simply following trends. The purpose of this chapter is to identify major national injury surveillance systems, note some of their strengths and weaknesses, and suggest improvements for usefulness in injury control.

The criteria for judging the adequacy of a surveillance system depend on its intended use and other possible uses (Klaucke, 1992). The measurement of trends in injuries of a given type requires that the definition of the type remain constant during the time period studied and, where all injuries of the type are not counted, the sampling method remains constant so as not to alter the comparability of the count during segments of the time period. For example, the International

Classification of Diseases (ICD) includes two types of codes for injury, diagnosis codes—sometimes called N-codes—and codes for "external causes," called E-codes. Addition to the E-codes in 1968 of a category for "injuries undetermined whether accidental or purposely afflicted" resulted in discontinuity in the trend in infant homicides. Apparently, a number of cases that would have been called homicide before the new category was added were placed in the undetermined category thereafter (Jason et al., 1983). The process for updating the codes has been described elsewhere and should be read by anyone using these codes (Fingerhut and McLoughlin, 2001).

As noted in chapter 5, using surveillance or any data to correlate injuries to other factors requires attention to issues of classification and relevance to injury control. If rates are calculated, changes in the population exposed or changes in measurement of exposure during the period examined must be considered. For example, trends in injury per population are sometimes adjusted for changes in the age distribution of the population but not for other factors that may also have changed. Even population age adjustments can be misleading. In the case of motor vehicle injuries, for instance, the proportion of the population that is licensed in an age group may change such that population age adjustment is inadequate to account for changes in exposure by age. (Data on licensure by age are available at http://www.fhwa.dot.gov/policy/ohpi/qfdrivers.htm, accessed August 2006.)

Finding clusters by geographic areas is of major importance in targeting certain injury control efforts. Distributions of injuries in certain regions may suggest very different priorities from those indicated by national or other larger areas. The reader may be surprised to learn, for example, that during 1988–1992 drowning was the second leading cause of injury mortality in Alaska (Lincoln et al., 1996). In one hospital in rural Ghana, burns were the second leading cause of admissions (Moch et al., 1995). Complete counts of severe injuries during a period of time, rather than samples, are required to reveal clusters, particularly if the areas are small. Usually, the smaller the area, the longer the time period required for stable numbers. (For a discussion of methodological issues, see http://ehp.niehs.nih.gov/members/2004/6735/6735.html, accessed August 2006.)

A number of sources of injury surveillance data have been evaluated on a variety of criteria, including public health importance, usefulness/cost, acceptability to the persons who must record the data, timeliness of reporting, prevalence of injuries in a defined population, sensitivity (identification of all cases), specificity (misclassification of noncases as cases), simplicity of data collection and management, and flexibility in inclusion of injuries not originally included (Graitcer, 1987). That evaluation is not repeated here, but each of those attributes of a surveillance system affects its use or usefulness.

GENERAL SURVEILLANCE

The National Center for Health Statistics assembles mortality records that provide information on trends and clusters of fatal injuries by age, gender, state, city, and county (Baker et al., 1992). The data are based on death certificates that are usually filled out by physicians at the time of pronouncement of death or soon thereafter. Nosologists code the clinical nature of injury and area of the body injured (N-codes) and "external cause" (E-codes). (For the latest data available, see http://www.cdc.gov/nchs/products/elec_prods/subject/mcompres. htm, accessed August 2006.)

Researchers who investigate cases in detail question the accuracy of reporting of certain types of injury on death certificates. In one state, about one in four cases of child deaths coded as intentional homicides were of questionable validity. It is unlikely that the death was intended in a variety of circumstances, for example, that homicide was the appropriate category in the cases of pedestrians killed by hit-and-run drivers and children killed while playing with guns (Lapidus et al., 1990). Fatal motorcycle injuries were underestimated by 38 percent on death certificates when checked against police reports (Lapidus et al., 1994). In another state, a study of asphyxiation by food found that data on the death certificates were substantially incomplete, apparently due to the rush to complete the certificate so that the body could be released to the family (Salmi et al., 1990).

The advantage of death certificate data is that they are available nationally on computers, and counts can be generated for local areas, but detailed examination of medical examiner and coroner records is often more useful in areas where a thorough investigation is routine. In some cities or counties, an autopsy by a qualified forensic pathologist is required in cases of violent death, intentional or unintentional, but the results are usually in narrative form with no computerized coding (Raasch, 1985). The data, if coded and computerized, would be very useful for increased understanding of injury circumstances. In many jurisdictions, however, a coroner, sometimes with no medical or other qualifications, is in charge of the investigation, which may be no more thorough than acceptance of the information on the death certificate. The wise researcher will examine the records in detail and conduct an independent investigation of their reliability and validity before assuming that they are coded accurately.

Hospital records are an important source of identification of severe, nonfatal injuries. The extent of use of ICD codes on hospital discharge records varies widely among hospitals. The National Hospital Discharge Survey provides computerized data on a national probability sample of 200,000 hospital discharges annually, including all discharges, not just those associated with injury. Data on hospitalized injuries at the local level are available in hospitals that maintain a trauma registry, but in communities with more than one hospital, one or more may not have a registry, and the patients in those that do may not be representative of all injured patients from the area of interest (see http://www.cdc.gov/nchs/about/major/hdasd/nhds.htm, accessed August 2006).

Even in hospitals where the injury coding is done systematically, the E-codes are often missing, particularly in cases with so many N-codes that there is no room for E-codes on computer files as the data are structured (Marganitt et al., 1990). In many cases, the medical history and notes by physicians and nurses in hospital records do not contain enough detail about the circumstances of an injury to classify it by E-code or specific geographic location.

The Council of State and Territorial Epidemiologists advocates universal E-coding of hospital discharge records, and several states now require them.

The Indian Health Service routinely requires such coding in its hospitals, and E-codes for injuries were found on 99.3 percent of its injury case records, although 25 percent lacked sufficient information for validity of detailed three-digit codes. Comparison of the codes and detailed examination of a sample of hospital records indicated excellent reliability in general categories (motor vehicle, fall), but discrepancies increased in the more refined subcategories (Smith et al., 1990).

Although universal E-coding would provide much better information on trends and clusters of injuries by type, severity, and a few demographic characteristics, it would mainly serve as a source to identify cases of particular types of injury for more detailed investigation. Cases without E-codes are identifiable as injuries by N-codes, which are much more complete.

Since the codes are revised periodically, the researcher must be careful in examining trends in data that bridge a revision. The codes are relatively specific for some causes of injury, but in other cases, the aggregation of causes is frustrating to the researcher when more refined categories are needed. Also, new products and activities that are introduced after the latest revision will not have specific E-codes.

The available general surveillance systems of injuries that do not require hospitalization are valuable only for indication of frequency and overall cost estimates. Given the priority to reduce death and severe injury, and the often-differing circumstances that contribute to severe and nonsevere injuries, devotion of resources to collection of more detailed data on less severe injuries is difficult to justify. Exceptions may occur in work or other settings where very severe injuries are rare but musculoskeletal injuries result in inability to work or drawn-out pain and suffering.

SPECIAL SURVEILLANCE SYSTEMS

Governmental agencies with statutory responsibility for monitoring certain types of injuries, or regulating products and activities that are associated with injuries, maintain special surveillance systems. Some of these provide sufficient detail for analytic as well as descriptive epidemiological studies.

Motor Vehicles

Among the best surveillance systems in terms of detailed data on vehicles and vectors as well as environmental circumstances is the Fatality Analysis Reporting System (FARS) of the National Highway Traffic Safety Administration (NHTSA). Begun in 1975 as the Fatal Accident Reporting System, this system collects data on virtually all fatalities related to motor vehicles that occur on public roads in the United States for cases in which the fatally injured person died within 30 days. Most of the data are from police reports, but additional information is included from motor vehicle licensing agencies, hospitals, and coroners or medical examiners. (The raw data and Statistical Analysis System (SAS) data sets can be downloaded at ftp://ftp.nhtsa.dot.gov/fars/, accessed August 2006.) The categories for some variables have changed from time to time, so the user is warned to check them carefully before doing year-to-year comparisons or pooling data among years.

The completeness and accuracy of FARS data are specific to each variable and vary among states and over time for some variables. For example, measurement of blood alcohol concentration of fatally injured drivers increased in the 1980s and has been completed for more than 80 percent of such drivers in more than half of the states since 1984 (National Highway Traffic Safety Administration, 1988). In years and states where blood alcohol is not tested as systematically, the possibility of bias in selection of those tested is of concern. NHTSA uses imputation methods to infer alcohol, or lack thereof, in missing cases. Such methods may be useful to gain a more accurate description of alcohol involvement but should not be used in causal analysis. To the extent that causal factors are used in the imputation, the reasoning is circular.

Speeds of vehicles in crashes are missing in more than half of FARS cases, and where it is found, the reliability is questionable. Fault-finding by police is also questionable since such judgments are made after the fact of the crash and may be based on reports by biased or unreliable eyewitnesses or lack of knowledge of vehicle factors and conditions. For example, the driver may be blamed for a rollover that would not have happened if the vehicle were more stable, or a mechanical failure may be obscured by the destruction of evidence by crash forces.

An unusual attribute of the NHTSA files, FARS and others, is the specificity of vehicle information. Codes for vehicle makes and models, as well as vehicle identification numbers that can be decoded as to make and model for verification, are included in the data. When matched with data on vehicles in use by make and model, this allows characteristics of specific vehicles, coded in the vehicle identification number or obtained from other sources, to be examined in relation to fatal injuries.

A system with data similar to that in FARS, but based on a sample of motor vehicle crashes on public roads reported to police, is the National Automotive Sampling System (NASS)—formerly the National Accident Sampling System—which is made up of the Crashworthiness Data System (CDS) and the General Estimates System (GES). The CDS contains detailed data on injury severity and mechanisms of injury. It was pilot tested in 1978 and has collected data supposedly representative of the defined crashes in the United States since that year. Since many motor vehicle injuries are not reported to police (see chapter 3), the numbers of injuries estimated from the NASS are underestimates and are undoubtedly biased.

Also, selection of cases included in the CDS is partly based on police codes of injury severity that are often invalid (see http://www-nrd.nhtsa.dot.gov/departments/nrd-30/ncsa/NASS.html, accessed August 2006). The police in most states use A, B, and C as codes for more to less serious injury in addition to K for persons killed. Figure 6-1 shows the K (fatal) and A (incapacitated) injuries of passenger car and light truck drivers in the NASS distributed by the clinically based Maximum Abbreviated Injury Score (MAIS). The deaths increase with injury severity, but the police judgments of "incapacitating" injury are not reflective of injury severity. Obviously, NASS sampling, based on selection of cases by police codes of injury is unwise. Any claim to national representation of the distribution of injury severity is false.

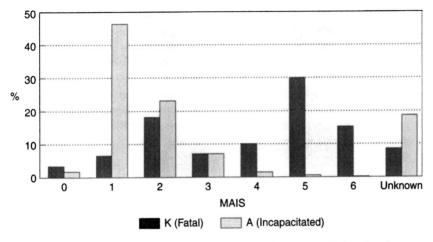

Figure 6-1. Maximum Abbreviated Injury Score (MAIS) of Police-Reported K (Fatal) and A (Incapacitated) Injury Codes

The data in the NASS CDS files include more detail on injuries than does FARS, including injuries by area of the anatomy, abbreviated injury scores, and Injury Severity Scores, but their use for analytic studies is dubious given the potential biases in sampling as well as substantial missing data on key variables, which is noted in subsequent chapters. The same problems in many variables in FARS are also present in NASS, such as unusable police codes of injury severity, missing alcohol and speed data, and falsely classified seat belt use. Ignorance of the latter resulted in publication of implausible estimates of seat belt use and effectiveness in prestigious journals (see appendix 12-1).

Since the CDS is based on a sample of a limited number of counties or clusters of counties around the country (about 8,400 crashes per year are in the sample), it is obviously not useful for local injury surveillance unless the area of interest is in one of the sampling areas. Most states and many smaller jurisdictions have computerized files of motor vehicle cases investigated by police. Injury codes in these state and local files are not considered refined enough for adequate indication of injury severity other than death. There are too many cases in which a bloody but superficial cut is coded as severe, while in other cases a person with an severe internal injury is coded at the scene as suffering a nonsevere injury. In a comparison of police rating of injury and hospital records of children struck as pedestrians or bicyclists, for example, the Injury Severity Score ranged from 0 to 30 in the least severe police code and 1 to 40 in the most severe nonfatal code (Agran et al., 1990).

Police files are used in some areas for identification of clusters of crashes on sections of roads, but the clusters of all reported crashes do not necessarily reflect the sites of the more severe injuries. A system still used in several states weights a fatal crash as only 9.1 times as important as a crash that involved only property damage (Federal Highway Administration, 1981). Site modifications based on such systems are too often directed to sites where crashes without injury are frequent, at the neglect of sites where severe injuries are clustered.

Beginning in 1988, the NHTSA initiated the GES, a program to sample a larger number of police-reported crashes among the states. The GES is an area probability sample of crashes reported to police throughout the country (National Highway Traffic Safety Administration, 1990). The data are exclusively those recorded by police. The advantage of the sample is the larger number of cases (about 48,000 per year) compared to the CDS. The disadvantage is that the data on injury have not been augmented from other sources, as was the case in the CDS, and suffer from the poor indicators of injury severity in all police data. Also, the vehicle identification number is missing in a third of the cases.

Assaults and Homicides

The Federal Bureau of Investigation (FBI) collects data from local police on several crimes, including assaults reported to police and homicides that are deemed criminal, in its uniform crime reporting system (http://www.fbi.gov/ucr/ucr.htm, accessed August 2006). Comparison of death certificates and deaths attributed to homicide in the FBI system indicate about 9 percent fewer homicides in the FBI files, at least partly because presumed noncriminal homicides, such as a felon killed by a law enforcement officer, are not included, and 4 percent of local jurisdictions do not report to the FBI (Rokaw et al., undated).

The FBI data include valuable information on trends in weapons used, demographic characteristics of victims, and relationship to assailants where known, but no data on nature of the injuries. Medical examiner or coroner files can be used to identify homicide cases at the local level and are usually adequate for indicating trends, or clusters in certain neighborhoods, bars, or other places.

Since nonfatal assaults are often not reported to police, ongoing interview surveys of the population—the National Crime Surveys—are sometimes used as sources of data on trends and some of the correlates. The trends in assault rates per population from the FBI reports and the National Crime Surveys moved in opposite directions during 1974–1988, apparently because of increased reporting of assaults to police (Jencks, 1991). Similar differences have been reported in other countries (Shepherd and Sivarajasingam, 2005). Data on nature and severity of injury are inadequate in the National Crime Surveys, and children younger than age 12 are not interviewed. These files are available from the National Criminal Justice Reference Service. The sampling system is complex, with households interviewed seven times and then replaced in the sample. Before using the data, consultation with experts familiar with the files is recommended. (Reports based on the data can be searched by keyword online at http://www.ncjrs.gov/App/search/AdvancedSearch.aspx, accessed August 2006.)

Hospital records are the best source of serious nonfatal assault cases at the local level, although assaults are probably underestimated from these sources, and the inaccuracy spills over into other categories. Assaults are sometimes reported to hospital personnel as falls or gun "accidents."

Suicides as well as homicides are reported in the National Violent Death Reporting System that was initiated by the Centers for Disease Control and Prevention (CDC) in seven states in 2003. As of 2006, the CDC funds 17 states to contribute data (http://www.cdc.gov/ncipc/profiles/nvdrs/facts.htm, accessed September 2006). Some preliminary data from states participating in the first two years have been reported (Patel et al., 2006), hardly the "United States" as billed, but it remains to be seen whether this system improves on those with a longer history.

Suicides and Attempts

Surveillance of suicides is based on death certificates (Centers for Disease Control and Prevention, 1986). Since there may be doubt as to intent in some cases and pressure to protect families in others, the numbers recorded as suicides are thought to be undercounts. Nonfatal suicide attempts in hospital records are subject to substantial misidentification as "accidents" for the same reasons. Because suicides can also cluster, apparently from imitative behavior, the CDC urges local communities to establish means of monitoring suicides and attempts, but the extent to which this is done is unknown. (An interagency suicide prevention effort, including reports and data sources, can be accessed at http://www.mentalhealth.samhsa.gov/suicideprevention/surveillance.asp, accessed August 2006.)

Occupational Injuries

The Bureau of Labor Statistics (BLS) conducts an annual survey of employer summaries of injuries that meet reporting regulations according to standards of the Occupational Safety and Health Administration (OSHA). The evidence of underreporting in some cases and overreporting in others, as well as the lack of detail on machines, work practices, or worker characteristics, severely limits the usefulness of the data (Panel on Occupational Safety and Health Statistics, 1987).

Users of these data should be aware that some of the categories do not make any sense clinically. For example, repetitive motion injuries are classified as illness, unless they result in back strain, which is always called injury. (OSHA data are available at http://www.osha.gov/oshstats/work.html, accessed August 2006.) BLS collects more detailed data on worker injuries from worker compensation records in industries subject to worker compensation laws (data are available at http://www.bls.gov/iif/home.htm, accessed August 2006). Important variables such as nature of injury, body part affected, occupation, and aspects of circumstances are included routinely, but others such as age, time of injury relative to time work began, and extent of disability are optional. Lost work time is a misleading indication of severity because it is strongly related to maximum compensation in a given state for certain injuries (Robertson and Keeve, 1983). Also, industries and even plants within the same company vary in the practice of assigning workers to other duties that can be performed after certain injuries, as opposed to having the worker take time off until he or she can return to regular duties.

The National Institute for Occupational Safety and Health (NIOSH) attempts to estimate fatal occupational injuries in its National Traumatic Occupational

Fatality database (Centers for Disease Control and Prevention, 1987), but the case identification is dependent on accurate coding of occurrence at work. Whether or not a death is work related is supposed to be recorded on the death certificate, but the data are often missing. Fatal injuries in agriculture, for example, were undercounted by 20 percent when compared to independent sources (Murphy et al., 1990). One study that identified cases of fatal farm injuries from both death certificates and newspaper clippings found 14 percent in newspaper clippings that were not identified in death certificates (Hayden et al., 1995), and newspaper clippings are undoubtedly incomplete. Data at the NIOSH Web site are mostly out-of-date as of August 2006 (see http://www.cdc.gov/niosh/injury/traumadata.html).

Investigation of adequacy of death certificates at the local level is recommended before they are used. Similarly, hospital records often do not contain data on the place of injury. Also, nonhospitalized emergency department records are inadequate for finding cases of worker injuries because larger industries have their own clinics to treat less serious injuries.

Consumer Products

The U.S. Consumer Product Safety Commission uses a sample of hospital emergency departments and also uses death certificates to identify trends in product-related injuries and emerging problems. Major products were excluded at the outset—alcohol, motor vehicles and firearms—but assaults and motor vehicle injuries, as well as injuries such as falls with no mention of a product, were added in 2000 (http://www.cpsc.gov/cpscpub/pubs/3002.html, accessed August 2006). Occasional special studies are conducted, such as the study of all-terrain vehicles discussed in chapter 5. In the general survey and specific studies, brand names and models of the products are not identified, precluding the comparison of injury incidence and severity by product characteristics. The sample of hospitals is small relative to the number in the country and cannot be used for identification of local injury clusters. (For data on consumer products, see http://www.cpsc.gov/cpscpub/pubs/3002.html., accessed August 2006.)

Fire-Related Injuries

The National Fire Data Center collects data based on reports from local fire marshals. Several important aspects of these data are computerized, including location, date, response time of the fire department, type of construction, and type of injury. A detailed comparison of these records and death certificates, coroner or medical examiner records, and hospital records is needed to determine the completeness and reliability of reporting (for data and links, see http://www.usfa.fema.gov/statistics/, accessed August 2006).

Boat-Related Injuries

The Coast Guard maintains records of deaths and some injuries related to use of boats. Probably no more than 10 percent of nonfatal injuries related to boat use are reported to the Coast Guard. The data include boat type, "cause of accident," and alleged alcohol use as well as demographic variables. The data on "causes" may not be reliable, and alcohol use is usually not confirmed by toxicology testing. A study of completeness of reporting of deaths, and reliability of other codes, should be undertaken before using these data. (For Coast Guard reports on injury, see http://www.uscgboating.org/statistics/stats.htm, accessed August 2006.)

References

Agran PF, Castillo DN, and Winn DG (1990) Limitations of data compiled from police reports on pediatric pedestrian and bicycle motor vehicle events. *Accid Anal Prev.* 22:361–370.

Baker SP, O'Neill B, Ginsburg M, and Li G (1992) *The Injury Fact Book.* 2nd ed. New York, NY: Oxford University Press.

Centers for Disease Control and Prevention (1986) *Youth Suicide Surveillance.* Atlanta, GA: U.S. Department of Health and Human Services.

Centers for Disease Control and Prevention (1987) Traumatic occupational fatalities— United States, 1980–1984. *Morbid Mortal Wkly Rep.* 36:461–470.

Federal Highway Administration (1981) *Highway Safety Engineering Studies: Participant Notebook.* Washington, DC: U.S. Department of Transportation.

Fingerhut LA, and McLoughlin E (2001) Classifying and coding injury. In Rivara FP, et al. (eds.), *Injury Control: A Guide to Research And Program Evaluation.* Cambridge, UK: Cambridge University Press.

Graitcer PL (1987) The development of state and local injury surveillance systems. J Safety Res 18:191–198.

Hayden GJ, Gerberich SG, and Maldanado G (1995) Fatal farm injuries: a five-year study utilizing a unique surveillance approach to investigate the concordance of reporting between two data sources. *J Occup Environ Med.* 37:571–577.

Jason J, Carpenter MM, and Tyler CW (1983) Underrecording of infant homicide in the United States. *Am J Public Health.* 73:195–197.

Jencks C (1991) Is violent crime increasing? *Am Prospect.* 1(Winter):98–109.

Klaucke DN (1992) *Evaluating public health surveillance systems.* In Halperin W, and Baker EL Jr (eds.), *Public Health Surveillance.* New York, NY: Van Nostrand Reinhold.

Lapidus GD, Braddock M, Schwartz R, Banco L and Jacobs, L (1994) Accuracy of fatal motorcycle-injury reporting on death certificates. Acc Anal Prevent 26:535-542.

Lapidus GD, Gregorio DI, and Hansen H (1990) Misclassification of childhood homicide on death certificates. *Am J Public Health.* 80:213–214.

Lincoln JM, Perkins R, Melton F and Conway GA (1996) Drowning in Alaska waters. Pub Health Rep 111:531–535.

Marganitt B, MacKenzie EJ, Smith GS, and Damiano AM (1990) Coding external causes of injury (E-codes) in Maryland hospital discharges 1979-88: a statewide study to explore the uncoded population. *Am J Public Health.* 80:1463–1466.

Murphy DJ, Seltzer BL, and Yesalis CE (1990) Comparison of two methodologies to measure agricultural occupational fatalities. *Am J Public Health.* 80:198–200.

National Highway Traffic Safety Administration (1988) *Fatal Accident Reporting System 1987.* Washington, DC: U.S. Department of Transportation.

National Highway Traffic Safety Administration (1990) *General Estimates System 1988.* Washington, DC: U.S. Department of Transportation.

Panel on Occupational Safety and Health Statistics (1987) *Counting Injuries and Illnesses in the Workplace: Proposals for a Better System.* Washington, DC: National Academy Press.

Patel N, Webb K, White D, Barker L, Crosby A, DeBerry M, Frazier L, Korch N, Lipskiy N, Shaw K, Steenkamp M, and Thomas S (2006) Homicides and suicides—National Violent Death Reporting System, United States—2003–2004. *Mortal Morbid Wkly Rep.* 55:722–724.

Raasch FO Jr (1985) Forensic analysis of trauma. In Nahum AM, and Melvin J (eds.), *The Biomechanics of Trauma.* Norwalk, CT: Appleton-Century-Crofts.

Robertson LS, and Keeve JP (1983) Worker injuries: the effects of workers' compensation and OSHA inspections. *J Health Politics Policy Law.* 8:581–597.

Rokaw WM, Mercy JA, and Smith JC (undated) *Comparability and Utility of National Homicide Data From Death Certificates and Police Records.* Washington, DC: Centers for Disease Control and Prevention.

Salmi LR, Dabis F, Rogier C, and McKinley T (1990) Quality of death certificates: studying or burying? *Am J Public Health.* 80:751.

Shepherd J, and Sivarajasingam V (2005) Injury research explains conflicting violence trends. *Inj Prev.* 11:324–325.

Smith SM, Colwell LS, and Sniezek JE (1990) An evaluation of external cause-of-injury codes using hospital records from the Indian Health Service. Am J Public Health 80:279–281.

7

Local Injury Surveillance

Some states and other entities have established systems of surveillance for particular types of injury outcome, such as spinal cord or brain injuries. For example, in response to congressional mandate, the Centers for Disease Control and Prevention (CDC) funds traumatic brain injury surveillance in 12 U.S. states (Langlois et al., 2005). Focus on such injuries may be useful because of the effects on mortality (e.g., Salassie et al., 2005) and the lives of the injured and those who must care for them, as well as the costs. Surveillance of injury from activities such as skiing is obviously not applicable to areas where the activity is not done but provides useful insights into prevention in areas where it is relevant (Xiang et al., 2004).

When a complete census of such conditions is problematic, as in low-income jurisdictions because of costs or where hospitals are not cooperative, sampling methods originally used for estimating animal, bird, and insect populations are being employed. Called "capture–recapture," analysis of the number of cases found repeatedly in different samples gives an indication of the incidence (or prevalence, depending on the sampling methods) of the outcome conditions (Chiu et al., 1993).

HOSPITAL-BASED SURVEILLANCE

Certain hospitals have increased the recording of data on injuries in trauma registries, partly for use in monitoring quality of care and partly as a database for research (Scheib et al., 1989). The use of hospital data for surveillance is limited by the differential case mix among hospitals and the lack of specification of the source population (Payne and Waller, 1989). If the population served uses more than one hospital, and the preference for a given hospital or the criteria of the emergency response system for using a given hospital change over time, the trends in injuries in the registry can be misleading. Epidemiologists call this selection bias.

Hospitals in the same community or region sometimes refuse to share data because they do not want the competition to have information about their "market."

In at least one state, an attempt to adopt uniform data recording among hospitals designated as trauma centers in Pennsylvania resulted in substantial compliance— 81.5 percent (Gillott et al., 1989). While this system allows for a larger sample size for studies to increase quality assurance, the exclusion of hospitals that are not trauma centers limits the usefulness of the data for surveillance and other epidemiological studies.

Several states have contracted with the National Highway Traffic Safety Administration (NHTSA) to match hospital and police records of motor vehicle injury in a system called the Crash Outcome Data Evaluation System (CODES). Data from his system have been used to mislead the U.S. Congress regarding the effectiveness of seat belts because of invalid reporting of belt use to police. One report claimed 85 percent belt effectiveness in reducing injuries to motor vehicle occupants, which is absurd (see appendix 12-1). NHTSA has refused requests under the Freedom of Information Act by outside researchers to gain access to the data, despite the fact that it was collected using taxpayer money. Apparently, state authorities must clear each such request (see http://www-nrd.nhtsa.dot.gov/departments/nrd-30/ncsa/codes.html, accessed August 2006). Matched hospital, police, and other data are potentially useful for targeting countermeasures and analytic studies, but if the data are not available to the research community, the uses are limited and the results are not subject to independent study.

There is a fundamental issue that people collecting surveillance data must address: How is the data being used? Taxpayers, the medically insured, and other patients are paying for what is often a formidable effort in data collection. Are they getting anything for their money? What changes in emergency response or treatment have been made based on the data? How many miles of road have been modified or lights installed based on concentrations of cases at specific road sites at specific times? What changes in police deployment and arrest policies occurred based on data regarding concentrations of assaults in space, time, public places, or recidivism of spouse and child abuse? What changes in laws regarding alcohol, guns, or use of personal protection have been considered or enacted based on the data? Indeed, have the data been given to anyone in a position to do something to reduce injury incidence and severity? If so, was it given to them in a form that gave them some notion of what to do?

RISK FACTOR SURVEILLANCE

The CDC coordinates a telephone survey in numerous states that attempts to measure behavioral risk factors, including several related to injury, such as smoking, alcohol use, and seat belt use (Anda et al., 1990). Despite research indicating that self-reports of these behaviors are invalid, articles based on them are prevalent in the literature with no caveats regarding validity (e.g., Escobedo et al., 1995; Wechsler et al., 1995). A comparison of self-reported belt use from that survey and observed seat belt use from the annual observational survey of the NHTSA illustrates the importance of not relying on self-reports of behavior.

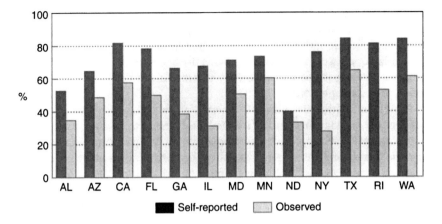

Figure 7-1. Self-Reported and Observed Belt Use

As displayed in figure 7-1, self-reported belt use was substantially more than that observed in the vicinity of large cities from each state from which data were available—an average difference of 21.5 percentage points in 1988. Belt use is lower in rural areas than in and around cities, so the actual difference could be larger (Robertson, 1992).

Self-reported driving while intoxicated and other claims of heavy alcohol use in the behavioral risk factor survey also was not predictive of alcohol in fatally injured drivers. As shown in figure 7-2, there was a sixfold variation among states regarding claimed driving after drinking, but less than a twofold variation in actual percent alcohol measured by toxicologists in fatally injured drivers. Alcohol in

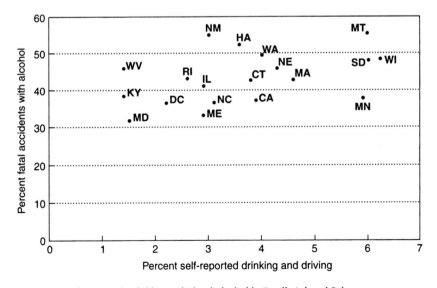

Figure 7-2. Self-Reported Drinking and Blood Alcohol in Fatally Injured Drivers.

fatally injured drivers was used for this comparison because it is objectively measured in more than 80 percent of fatally injured drivers in the states indicated. It does not include those who survived while killing other road users because alcohol is not measured objectively in such drivers often enough to avoid selection bias, but there is no reason to believe that the ratio of dead to surviving drunk drivers varies among states.

A high correlation between self-reported alcohol use in the behavioral risk factor survey and alcohol sales in 21 states has been reported, but the correlation of alcohol sales and self-reported drinking and driving was poor (Smith et al., 1990). The funds used for collecting data on self-reported behavior would be better used to improve surveillance of objectively measured risk factors. For example, belt use, child restraint use, and motorcycle and bicycle helmet use are easily observable, and an estimate of use in a given area can be obtained by observations at randomly selected sites and times.

PREVENTION-ORIENTED SURVEILLANCE

Previous successful efforts in injury control based on surveillance have included the following steps:

1. Surveillance of injury incidence and severity to identify clusters of similar injuries and the hazards that increase incidence and severity
2. Identification of one or more technical strategies to eliminate or reduce the hazard
3. Implementation of the technical strategy among the populations at high risk
4. Continued surveillance to monitor the trend in the injuries

An outstanding example of the application of this approach occurred in the study and subsequent reduction of fatal falls to children in New York City. Epidemiologists from the health department devised a surveillance system of the circumstances of the falls and found that 66 percent of injuries in fatal falls to children up to 5 years of age occurred when the children crawled out of windows in high-rise buildings. The research also identified the areas of the city where these deaths most frequently occurred (Bergner et al., 1971).

A barrier that could be placed over windows, preventing children from crawling out, was the technical approach identified as most feasible under the circumstances. A campaign was launched in high-risk neighborhoods to persuade the parents or landlords to install the barriers (Spiegel and Lindaman, 1977). Eventually, the health department required landlords to install such barriers when requested by tenants. In association with these efforts, the deaths from children's falls from high-rise windows declined from about 30–50 per year in the 1960s to 4 in 1980. Total reported falls declined proportionately during the same period (Bergner, 1982; Barlow et al., 1983). Subsequently, as attention to the issue declined, the falls and fatalities increased somewhat. In July 1986, the city changed the regulation to require barriers in buildings where there were children younger than 11 years (Bijur and Spiegel, 1996).

In addition to illustration of the steps necessary for efficient injury control, the New York experience with children's falls from heights suggests the local nature of certain hazards. In cities and towns with few or no high-rise buildings (indeed, in the boroughs of Queens and Staten Island, as the researchers found in New York), a campaign to install barriers in windows would be inappropriate because the problem is rare relative to other types of injury. Therefore, local injury surveillance is necessary to identify major injury problems that vary widely among local areas, and their circumstances and specific locations within the areas. The local health department is an appropriate agency for such an activity, but other agencies, such as hospitals or emergency medical service crews, could also do the work (e.g., Short, 2002).

Numerous technical strategies are available for injury control, but efficient use requires data on the extent to which they are needed where the problem is most acute (chapter 2). For example, certain road modifications, signaling systems, and lighting reduce relevant injuries by more than 50 percent (Federal Highway Administration, 1982). Yet modifying every mile of road with every possible modification would be very expensive.

By conducting detailed surveillance of the circumstances, frequency, and locations of serious injuries, the health department or other organization can recommend action to agencies or organizations in a position to implement, require, or distribute technology or other approaches. For example, if particular road intersections were found to have high rates of severe injury crashes, the data and suggestions for changes, such as extension of the yellow phase of traffic control lights at the specified intersections, would be forwarded to the road or police department that has jurisdiction. If skid strips on stairs, hand rails, or other approaches were identified as likely ameliorative strategies for specific types of falls found among the elderly, the recommendations for specific modifications could be made to vulnerable community residents by visiting nurses or other persons who provide services to the elderly.

Investigation of the circumstances of drowning of young children in one state revealed that all of the drowning in bathtubs occurred with young siblings but no adults present. All drowning in pools and larger bodies of water were from falls into the water, not swimming or wading. These results indicate the need for adult supervision of young children's baths and the need for barriers to prevent children from falling into larger bodies of water (Jensen et al., 1992). In areas with year-round warm climates, such as Maricopa County, Arizona, drowning rivaled motor vehicles as a cause of death among toddlers at the turn of the century. Most drowning in this environment occurred in in-ground swimming pools (http://www.azdhs.gov/phs/phstats/meddir/pdf/cpsc03.pdf#search='drowning%20 surveillance, accessed August 2006).

Geographic distributions of injuries have been used to designate the placement and staffing of emergency medical services and trauma treatment centers. For example, one emergency medical service that covered a metropolitan area of 600 square miles found that 25 percent of the calls occurred in two 13.5 square mile sections, less than 5 percent of the metropolitan area. The severe injuries were distributed similarly (Pepe et al., 1990). Geographic clusters of child pedestrian injuries combined with information about the children and the neighborhoods suggest modifications to reduce the problem (Braddock et al., 1994).

As indicated in the discussion of extant surveillance systems, few include data in sufficient detail to identify specific types of injury by specific locations, and none directly identify environmental modifications that could have reduced incidence and severity. To provide such information, a supplementary data collection system was developed for the Indian Health Service (IHS) (Robertson, 1985). The data to be gathered are indicated on the forms in appendices 7-1 through 7-7, one form each for injury from motor vehicles, burn or smoke, drowning or near drowning, a fall, assault, suicide attempt, and others. The forms include not only the circumstances of the injury but also a list of possible actions that might have prevented the injury or reduced severity. The surveillance is not simply for the collection of data but is also prevention oriented.

Confining the initial effort to the more severe cases was deemed appropriate to avoid excessive effort expended on relatively trivial injuries that may occur in large numbers but are relatively unimportant in terms of long-term consequences for the persons injured and use of community resources. The definition of "serious" is somewhat arbitrary and can be changed as progress is made in prevention of the more severe cases. Fatalities and hospitalized injuries should receive first priority in most instances.

Since the IHS provides outpatient as well as inpatient and preventive services in many Native American communities, access to cases by injury prevention specialists is no doubt easier than it would be in communities with more fragmented services. Nevertheless, the potential cost savings to be obtained by targeted injury control efforts informed by data should be appealing to hospitals. Reimbursement systems based on average costs for diagnosis-related groups have resulted in insufficient payments to hospitals for certain severe injuries because of the skewed distributions of costs (e.g., Jacobs, 1985).

Initial experience with the use of the IHS system indicated that lack of expertise in identifying potentially effective environmental modifications was a problem. A fellowship program to train injury control specialists and a series of seminars for other users of the system were instituted (Smith, 1988), and the graduates and others implemented many successful injury control projects.

Technical assistance to state and local communities not served by the IHS is available from the injury control centers funded by the CDC, or from CDC. (A current list of injury control centers is available at http://www.naicrc.org/, accessed August 2006.)

The IHS developed computer software that allows easy entry of the data from the surveillance system. The program can be edited for use in any community. As sufficient numbers accumulate, a summary of the circumstances tabulated by the suggested actions that might have had a preventive effect provides a priority list for action.

Development of detailed computerized codes for injury locations to identify geographic clusters may be cumbersome, but good database management systems, such as Epi Info used by the IHS, allow listing of case identifiers by other variables. (Epi Info can be downloaded free at http://www.cdc.gov/epiinfo/, accessed August

2006.) Once high-priority actions have been identified, cases that would have been reduced by a given action can be listed and the locations marked on detailed maps of local areas by referring to the location information on the original forms.

Location can be a powerful factor in concentrating resources. In Stockholm, Sweden, 47 percent of assaults on public streets occurred on 3 percent of all streets in a single year, and street homicides in a 40-year period were highly concentrated on the same streets as those identified in the assault study. The assaults were near places of "entertainment" such as bars and theaters (Wikstrom, 1995). In one U.S. city, 45 percent of child pedestrian injuries were located in 16 percent of the census tracts (Lapidus et al., 1991).

The IHS undertook numerous projects based on local surveillance data (Smith and Robertson, 2000). Injury control specialists on the White River Apache Reservation in Arizona found a cluster of severe pedestrian injuries that occurred at night on a 1.2-mile section of road in a two-year period. The tribal government and IHS collaborated in the installation of lights that illuminated the road section at night (D. Aiken and G. Rothfus, personal communication, 1989). Comparison of the installation site and adjacent sites during the five years before and five years after the installation, controlling for average daily traffic and the removal of a liquor store in the area, indicated that about six fewer pedestrian injuries than expected occurred after the installation (A. Dellapena and J. Peabody, personal communication, 1997).

In Browning, Montana, 59 severe motor vehicle injuries, including 13 fatalities, occurred in a two-mile stretch of road during a seven-year period. Overhead lighting and curbs that channeled parking lot traffic to controlled entry points were installed. In the two-year period year after lighting and curbs were installed, only two severe injuries occurred in that stretch of road (J. Lee and L. Beck, personal communication, 1991).

After being shown data on a cluster of 22 fatal pedestrian injuries at night on a two-mile section of the road between Gallup, New Mexico, and the Navajo Nation, state authorities agreed to put night lighting of the road section in their five-year plan for road modifications. No fatalities occurred in the lighted section in the two years after installation (N. Bill, personal communication, 1995).

The Hoopa Health Association Emergency Medical Services gathered data on motor vehicle fatalities that occurred on the 100 miles of road through and adjacent to the Hoopa, Yurock, and Karok reservations in northern California. The primary cause of death was vehicles plunging over steep embankments. Comparison of the sites where the state installed guardrails to noninstallation sites, 10 years before and 10 years after the installation, corrected for average daily traffic, indicated some 21 fewer deaths than expected in the period after installation (Short and Robertson, 1998).

A visit to the site of each severe injury to consider environmental modifications that might have reduced the injuries is strongly recommended. For example, visits to the sites of child pedestrian injuries on the Pine Ridge Reservation in South Dakota indicated that the surfaces and equipment on nearby playgrounds were in such poor condition that the children apparently preferred to play in the streets or driveways of homes (Price, 1990).

The choice of recommended ameliorative actions should not necessarily be confined to the more obvious ones that can be fitted on a one-page form. The narratives and comments may suggest others. Those included on the forms are oriented to actions that can be initiated at the local level and do not include actions delegated to federal regulatory agencies. A review of the literature on the technical strategies for specific injuries provides expertise in the identification of additional options (e.g., Federal Highway Administration, 1982; Haddon, 1970; Robertson, 1983).

Ideally, every community would have an injury surveillance system analogous to that of the IHS. If the numbers in a given community were too limited for generalization, small communities in similar areas could pool the data to assess patterns for their environment. A system for accumulating data from the local systems at the state (or provincial) and national levels would give each level of government, or private entity, information on injury patterns relevant to agencies or organizations under its purview. Since national systems may be long in coming, local communities that are concerned about their injury problems can take the initiative.

Use of the IHS or similar forms could be required of medical examiners, coroners, and hospitals. The mechanism of enforcement of quality of data from medical examiners and coroners is not evident, but hospitals could be required to obtain the data to qualify for reimbursement by Medicare, Medicaid, or private insurance. A former emergency medical service coordinator has written a useful guide for surveillance and injury control activities by first responders (Short, 2002).

If and when a national system is developed, the information gathered in local surveillance systems must be made uniform on certain variables. For use by national regulatory agencies and independent researchers, the specific identification of product brand names and other identifiers such as serial numbers should be included. Where structures or other facilities that are, or could be, subject to local codes and ordinances are involved, the builders or maintainers should be identified. The mere fact that the data are being collected could serve as motivation for some organizations to undertake injury control actions. The data would give them better information on actions to take.

References

Anda RF, Waller MN, Wooten KG, Mast EE, Escobedo LG, and Sanderson LM (1990) Behavioral risk factor surveillance, 1988. *Morbid Mortal Wkly Rep.* 39(June):1–21.

Barlow B, Niemirska M, Gandhi RP, and Leblanc W (1983) Ten years experience with falls from a height in children. *J Pediatr Surg.* 18:509–511.

Bergner L (1982) Environmental factors in injury control: preventing falls from heights. In Bergman AB (ed.), *Preventing Childhood Injuries.* Columbus, OH: Ross Laboratories.

Bergner L, Mayer S, and Harris D (1971) Falls from heights: a childhood epidemic in an urban area. *Am J Public Health.* 61:90.

Bijur PE, and Spiegel C (1996) Window fall prevention and fire safety: 20 years of experience in New York City. *Pediatr Res.* 39:102A.

Braddock M, Lapidus G, Cromley E, Cromley R, Burke G, and Banco L (1994) Using a geographic information system to understand child pedestrian injury. *Am J Public Health.* 84:1158–1161.

Chiu W, Dearwater SR, McCarty DJ, Songer TJ, and LaPorte RE (1993) Establishment of accurate incidence rates for head and spinal cord injuries in developing and developed countries: a capture-recapture approach. *J Trauma.* 35:206–211.

Escobedo LG, Chorba TL, and Waxweiler R (1995) Patterns of alcohol use and the risk of drinking and driving among U.S. high school students. *Am J Public Health.* 85:976–978.

Federal Highway Administration (1982) *Synthesis of Safety Research Related to Traffic Control and Roadway Elements.* 2 Vols. Washington, DC: U.S. Department of Transportation.

Gillott AR, Thomas JM, and Forrester C (1989) Development of a statewide trauma registry. *J Trauma.* 29:1667–1672.

Haddon W Jr (1970) On the escape of tigers: an ecologic note. *Tech Rev.* 72:44.

Jacobs LM (1985) The effect of prospective reimbursement on Trauma patients. *Bull Am Coll Surg.* 70:17–22.

Jensen LR, Williams SD, Thurman DJ, and Keller PA (1992) Submersion injuries in children younger than 5 years in urban Utah. *West J Med.* 157:641–644.

Langlois JA, Marr A, Mitchko J, and Johnson RL (2005) Tracking the silent epidemic and educating the public: CDC's traumatic brain injury-associated activities under the TBI Act of 1996 and the Children's Health Act of 2000. *Head Trauma Rehabil.* 20:196–204.

Lapidus GD, Braddock M, Banco L, Montenegro L, Hight D, and Eanniello V (1991) Child pedestrian injury: a population-based collision and injury severity profile. *J Trauma.* 31:1110–1115.

Payne SR, and Waller JA (1989) Trauma registry and trauma Center biases in injury research. *J Trauma.* 29:424–429.

Pepe PE, Mattox KL, Fischer RP, and Matsumoto CM (1990) Geographic patterns of urban trauma according to mechanism and severity of injury. *J Trauma.* 30:1125–1132.

Price D (1990) *Motor-Vehicle Related Pedestrian Injuries on the Pine Ridge Indian Reservation.* Unpublished MPH thesis. New Haven, CT: Yale University.

Robertson LS (1983) *Injuries: Causes, Control Strategies and Public Policy.* Lexington, MA: DC Heath.

Robertson LS (1985) *Epidemiological Assessment of the Contributing Factors of Injury Mortality and Morbidity Among Native Americans.* Springfield, VA: National Technical Information Service.

Robertson LS (1992) On the validity of self-reported behavioral risk factors. *J Trauma.* 32:58–59.

Scheib BT, Thompson ME and Kerns TJ (1989) Federal influences on the development of trauma registries. J Trauma 29:83–841.

Selassie AW, McCarthy ML, Ferguson PL, Tian J, and Langlois JA (2005) Risk of post-hospitalization mortality among persons with traumatic brain injury. South Carolina 1999–2001. *Head Trauma Rehabil.* 20:248–260.

Short D (2002) *Quick Guide to Effective Injury Prevention: Saving Lives With Proactive Emergency Services.* Washington, DC: U.S. Department of Health and Human Services Maternal and Child Health Bureau. Available at: http://www.nanlee.net/ems/quickguide.htm. Accessed August 2006.

Short D, and Robertson LS (1998) Motor vehicle death reductions from guardrail installations. *J Transport Eng.* 124:501–502.

Smith PF, Remington PL, Williamson DF, and Anda RF (1990) A comparison of alcohol sales data with survey data on self-reported alcohol use in 21 states. *Am J Public Health.* 80:309–312.

Smith RJ (1988) IHS fellows program aimed at lowering injuries, death of Indians, Alaska natives. *Public Health Rep.* 103:204.

Smith RJ, and Robertson LS (2000) Unintentional injuries and trauma. In Rhoades ER (ed.), *American Indian Health.* Baltimore, MD: Johns Hopkins University Press.

Spiegel CN, and Lindaman FC (1977) Children can't fly: a program to prevent childhood morbidity and mortality from window falls. *Am J Public Health.* 67:1143.

Wechsler H, Dowdall GW, Davenport A, and Castillo S (1995) Correlates of college student binge drinking. *Am J Public Health.* 85:921–926.

Wikstrom PH (1995) Preventing city-center street crimes. In Tonry M, and Farrington DP (eds.), *Building a Safer Society: Strategic Approaches to Crime Prevention.* Chicago, IL: University of Chicago Press.

Xiang H, Stallones L, and Smith GA (2004) Downhill skiing injuries among children. *Inj Prev.* 10:99–102.

Appendix 7-1
Motor Vehicle Injury Form

Community _____ Census tract _____

Location of the incident (specify road, street, or intersection and distance to an identifiable reference point such as an intersection, business, or milepost number):

_____

_____

_____

Severity: _____ Fatal _____ Hospitalized _____ Ambulatory (fracture, loss consciousness only—exclude others)

Age: _____   Gender: _____ M   _____ F

Single-vehicle occupant

If fixed object: _____ Tree _____ Utility pole _____ Bridge abutment

_____ Light pole _____ Sign pole _____ Other

_____ Rollover

_____ Animal on the road _____ Other (What? _____)

Multiple vehicle occupant: _____ Frontal _____ Side _____ Rear

Motorcyclist: _____ Single vehicle   _____ Multiple vehicle

Pedestrian: _____ Crossing intersection   _____ Crossing elsewhere

               _____ Walking along road   _____ Vehicle came off road

               _____ Laying in road   _____ Other (What? _____)

Bicyclist: _____ Crossing intersection   _____ Crossing elsewhere

               _____ On road parallel to traffic _____ On road against traffic

               _____ Motor vehicle came off road

               _____ Other (What? _____)

Lighting: _____ Daylight   _____ Dark   _____ Dark but lighted

_____ Dawn or dusk

Signals: _____ None   _____ Flashing warnings   _____ Red-yellow-green

_____ Stop sign   _____ Yield sign   _____ Other (What? _____)

Crash protection: _____ Seat belt   _____ Child restraint   _____ Crash helmet

Roadway jurisdiction: _____ City or town   _____ County   _____ State

_____ Federal

Modification that might have prevented the injury or reduced severity (check all that apply):

_____ No pass stripe   _____ Roadside hazard removal

_____ Rumble strips   _____ Signal or sign at intersection

_____ Lengthen yellow phase at signalized intersection

_____ Install or lengthen pedestrian walk signal

_____ Median barrier   _____ Reflectors on curve

_____ Snow removal   _____ Improve road skid resistance

_____ Separate pedestrian walkway from road

_____ Reflectors on vehicles or clothing

_____ Lighted roadway   _____ Curb to limit road access

_____ Other (What? _____)

_____ Additional observations

Appendix 7-2
Burn or Smoke Injury

Community _____ Census tract _____

Address _____

Severity: _____ Fatal _____ Hospitalized ___ Ambulatory (loss of consciousness and/or immobilization only—exclude others)

Age: _____   Gender: _____ M   _____ F

Victim sleeping when fire began? _____ Yes _____ No

Place of fire: ____ Home ____ Car ____ Other (Where? _____)

If home, number of door exits to the home _____

Location of the victim: _____ Bedroom _____ Living room

_____ Bathroom _____ Kitchen

_____ Other (Where? _____)

Ignition or heat origin: ____ Cigarette ____ Cooking unit

____ Wood-burning space heater _____ Kerosene space heater

_____ Other space heater _____ Chimney _____ Electrical wiring

_____ Arson _____ Household water _____ Food or drink

_____ Other (What? _____)

Material first ignited: _____ Chair or sofa _____ Bed _____ Loose papers

_____ Clothing on person _____ Other clothing _____ House framing

_____ Cooking grease _____ Other (What? _____)

If in a building, smoke detector installed? _____ Yes _____ No

　　　　If yes, did detector give alarm? _____ Yes _____ No

Was a fire extinguisher available? _____ Yes _____ No

　　　　If yes, was it used? _____ Yes _____ No

Modifications that might have reduced injury or severity (check as many as apply):

_____ Additional exit　　　_____ Fire ladder

_____ Smoke detector   _____ Batteries in detector

_____ Fire extinguisher   _____ Sleeping nearer exits

_____ Fire-resistant clothing   _____ Fire-resistant furniture

_____ Fire-resistant mattress or sheets

_____ Automatic sprinkler system

_____ Properly installed cooking unit

_____ Properly installed wood stove

_____ Properly installed kerosene heater

_____ Cleaned chimney _____ Reduced hot water temperature

_____ Less tip-prone food or drink container

_____ Other (What? _____)

_____ Additional observations

Appendix 7-3
Drowning or Near Drowning

Community _____ Census tract _____

Directions to location _____

_____

_____

Severity: _____ Fatal _____ Hospitalized _____ Ambulatory (loss of consciousness only—exclude others)

Age: _____   Gender: _____ M   _____ F

Victim know how to swim? _____ Yes _____ No

Water temperature at time of the incident: _____

Body of water involved: _____ Bathtub _____ Supervised beach

_____ Unsupervised beach _____ River nonbeach _____ Lake nonbeach

_____ Ocean nonbeach _____ Irrigation ditch _____ Drainage ditch

_____ Swimming pool

_____ Flood _____ Other (What? _____)

Watercraft involved: _____ None _____ Motorboat _____ Sailboat _____ Surfsail

_____ Rowboat _____ Canoe _____ Motorized raft _____ Nonmotorized raft

_____ Other (What?_____)

Preventive gear available: _____ Lifeline _____ Life jacket

_____ Floating cushion _____ Nonsinkable boat _____ Fenced area

_____ Flares _____ Boat-to-shore communication

_____ Other (What? _____)

Modifications that might have prevented the incident or reduced severity:

_____ Fenced swimming pool _____ Other fencing

_____ Lifeline _____ Life jacket _____ Floating cushion

_____ Nonsinkable boat _____ Supervised swimming area

_____ Flood warning and evacuation _____ Flare

_____ Boat to shore communication

_____ Other (What? _____)

_____ Additional observations

Appendix 7-4
Injury from a Fall

Community _____ Census tract _____

Directions to the site _____

_____

_____

Severity: _____ Fatal _____ Hospitalized _____ ambulatory (include only if loss of consciousness or fracture)

Age: _____   Gender: _____ M   _____ F

Type of fall: _____ Same level _____ Different level (approximate number of feet _____)

Same level location: _____ Bathtub _____ Other bathroom

_____ Bedroom _____ Kitchen _____ Living room _____ Basement

_____ Attic _____ Home yard _____ Sidewalk _____ Street

_____ Public building _____ Private building _____ Sports field

_____ Other (Where? _____)

_____ Not applicable

Different level location: _____ Exterior stairs to house entrance

_____ Stairs to upper floors _____ Stairs to attic

_____ Stairs to basement _____ Stairs in public building

_____ Stairs in nonresidential private building _____ Home porch or landing

_____ Window _____ Roof _____ Tree _____ Cliff or other dropoff

_____ Ladder _____ Horse

_____ Other (Explain _____)

Modification that might have prevented injury or reduced severity:

_____ Skid strips in tub _____ Skid strips on stairs

_____ Nonskid rug _____ Nonskid shoes _____ Handrail

_____ Snow or ice clearance _____ Soft carpet

_____ Stair repairs _____ Fence or other barrier

_____ Sports equipment (What? _____)

_____ Other (What? _____)

_____ Additional observations

Appendix 7-5
Assault Injury

Community _____ Census tract _____

Directions to the site _____

_____

_____

Severity: _____ Fatal _____ Hospitalized _____ ambulatory (include only if loss of consciousness or fracture)

Age: _____   Gender: _____ M   _____ F

Where did the assault occur? _____ Home _____ Other house

_____ Bar _____ Other business _____ Elsewhere

Assailant relation to the injured: _____ Spouse _____ Father

_____ Mother _____ Child _____ Sibling _____ Other relative

_____ Other family _____ Acquaintance _____ Stranger _____ Unknown

Weapon used in the assault: _____ Body (fists, feet, etc.)

_____ Gun _____ Knife _____ Other sharp object

_____ Blunt object _____ Fire or heat _____ Poison

_____ Other (What?_____)

Apparent reason for the assault: _____ Rage _____ Robbery

_____ Mental illness _____ Other (What? _____)

Modification that might have prevented injury or reduced severity:

_____ Limit number of drinks purchasable in bars

_____ Metal detector at door of bar and refuse service to those armed with gun or knife

_____ Do not allow bottles that shatter as containers for alcoholic beverages

_____ Provide lighting in high-risk area

_____ Arrest of the assailant involved in previous incident

_____ Remove assailant from the home

_____ Remove person assaulted from the home

_____ Other (What? _____)

_____ Additional observations

Appendix 7-6
Self-Inflicted Injury

Community _____ Census tract _____

Directions to site _____

_____

_____

Severity: _____ Fatal _____ Hospitalized _____ Ambulatory (include only if loss of consciousness or fracture)

Age: _____   Gender: _____ M   _____ F

Where did the attempt occur? _____ Home _____ Relative's home

_____ Other home _____ Jail _____ Other public building or business

_____ Out of doors

_____ Other (Explain _____)

Weapon used: _____ Gun _____ Knife _____ Other sharp instrument

_____ Carbon monoxide _____ Prescription drug

_____ Other drug _____ Other poison _____ Rope

_____ Jump _____ Other (What? _____)

Circumstances: _____ Physical illness _____ Mental illness

_____ Copying recent real event _____ Copying television event

_____ Copying other fictional event _____ Financial loss

_____ Reaction to rejection by spouse or lover

_____ Reaction to difficulty with other family member

_____ Other (What? _____)

Modification that might have prevented injury or reduced severity:

_____ Encourage seeking of treatment for depression

_____ Increase awareness of depression symptoms in families and sources of help especially if friend or popular figure recently attempted suicide

_____ Encourage families with depressed members to limit access to guns, drugs, etc.

_____ Encourage families not to leave depressed members alone in circumstances or areas where previous suicide attempts occurred

_____ Reduce incarceration for nonserious offenses that result in jailhouse suicide
attempts

_____ Increase surveillance of incarcerated persons

_____ Other (What? _____)

_____ Additional observations

Appendix 7-7
Other Severe Injury

(Use specified forms for motor vehicles, drowning, fire, falls, assaults, and suicide attempts; this form is for other injuries that were hospitalizations, fatalities, and ambulatory cases that involved loss of consciousness, fractures, or worse conditions.)

Community _____ Census tract _____

Directions to the site _____

_____

_____

Severity: _____ Fatal _____ Hospitalized _____ Ambulatory (fracture or lost consciousness)

Age: _____   Gender: _____ M   _____ F

Type of energy that caused the damage to the person:

_____ Mechanical _____ Heat or lack _____ Chemical

_____ Electrical

What conveyed the energy to the person (be specific; e.g., if farm tractor, machine, or other product, give make, model, moving part that caused injury):

_____

_____

_____

_____

List as many strategies you can think of that could be employed to reduce the incidence or severity of this type of injury in the future:

_____

_____ Additional observations

8

The Use and Abuse of Causal Analysis

On an exam in a course on the use of epidemiology for injury control, the author asked the students, "What is wrong with this statement: 'Alcohol is consistently associated with unintentional injury deaths; therefore, alcohol abuse must be reduced to lower rates of death and disability due to injury'?" Only 1 in 20 came close to writing a correct answer. Yet in the course, numerous instances to the contrary were noted. Motor vehicle injuries have been reduced, for example, by improved vehicle crashworthiness, lighting dark sections of road, and channeling traffic, without reducing alcohol or otherwise changing drivers.

In explaining the answer to the students, the statement was rewritten: "Gender is consistently related to injury; therefore, gender must be changed to reduce injury." The nervous laughter, particularly from the gender often at higher risk (males), suggested that some might have got the point.

The statement about alcohol on the exam was not original. Prominent leaders in public health published the statement (Brown et al., 1990). There is an assumption inherent in much public health literature that specification of complex interaction of factors—sometimes called causal webs—is key to injury and disease reduction (Krieger, 1994). To the contrary, while the notion of the causal web may be useful to call attention to the complexities of multiple causes of diseases and injuries, it may disable our minds in thinking about prevention (Renwick, 1973).

The "public health model" is usually presented as follows: (1) identify the problem (surveillance), (2) identify risk factors, (3) develop and test interventions, (4) implement interventions and measure effectiveness (e.g., Powell et al., 1996). In fact, many interventions and therapies have been successful without the second step. One does not need to know the "risk factors" for a headache to use an analgesic. Focusing on multiple risk factors in causal webs may lead one astray rather than toward injury control.

Consider the New York Health Department's study of children's fatal falls that resulted in barriers over windows and a huge reduction in child deaths (chapter 7). What would have happened if the researchers had attempted an analysis of numerous "risk factors" that could contribute to children falling from windows, such as no adult present, intoxicated adults, numerous factors that distracted adults, and inquisitiveness, hyperactivity, or numerous other characteristics of children? Would there have been attempts to change those factors rather than install window barriers? If so, it is unlikely that the falls would have declined nearly to the extent produced by the window barriers.

Multiple causation of disease and injury, for which the causal web is the most common metaphor, is repeatedly demonstrated. It does not logically follow, however, that multifactorial theory or analysis leads to rational prevention policy. This was recognized in the original conceptualization of the "causal web" (McMahon et al., 1960), but it is commonly forgotten. Those of us who study injuries in the United States are not fond of metaphors involving gun imagery, but there were instances in which "magic bullets" were found despite multiple causation of infectious diseases (Evans, 1993).

If we have to deal with causal webs, perhaps we need a metaphor for something more effective than bullets against webs and spiders—perhaps brooms. To Krieger's (1994) provocative question regarding causal webs, "Has anyone seen the spider?" should be added, "Has anyone seen the housekeepers with the preventive brooms?"

Proponents of the search for complex causes before consideration of preventive action argue that, without understanding of causes, prevention may fail because of confounding factors or may have unintended consequences. Confounding refers to the attribution of risk to a factor that has little or no effect but is mistakenly thought to have an effect because it is correlated to a factor that is important.

In rare instances, confounding has misled preventive efforts, and adverse "side effects" have also occurred, but the nature of certain types of causes is such that the potential for unintended consequences is minimized. Complete understanding is an elusive goal that is yet to be accomplished for most phenomena. How much, then, do we need to know for injury control?

To eliminate an injury (or anything else that is undesirable), one need only find a controllable necessary condition for the outcome and then control that condition. Even the least resilient of human anatomies can tolerate some mechanical energy load (commonly measured in pounds per square inch or kilograms per square centimeter). In the road environment, any combination of energy management by vehicle components or the surrounding environment that keeps loads below that tolerance will eliminate injury. While energy management to that extent has not been accomplished, and may not be feasible in the extreme for economic or other reasons, substantial reduction in motor vehicle death rates occurred due to increased vehicle crashworthiness. There are claims of unintended consequences in increased risky driving by those protected, but these claims are not supported by the better research (chapters 12 and 13).

Causal analysis of injury can inform preventive approaches when it specifies factors that are substantially changeable and that account for a proportion of a given type of injury, and rules out factors that are spuriously correlated to injury. Attention to the nature of types of causes gives guidance to the extent that a given injury might be reduced if a given factor were changed.

In examining data on potential causes of injuries, it is useful to bear in mind the types of statistical distributions of injuries that are found when conditions are necessary, sufficient, or contributing factors. Examples are shown in tables 8-1 through 8-3, where the designations "none," "some," and "more" cases refer to a proportion of all cases in the table.

If A is a necessary condition for B, then B will not occur in the absence of A, and the joint distribution of A and B will look like that in table 8-1 when the measurement of both is accurate. For example, keeping the height of playground equipment below the level that can produce enough energy in a fall to injure the heaviest users will eliminate such injury (chapter 2). On the other hand, if A is sufficient for B, then B will always occur in the presence of A, but the absence of A does not imply the absence of B unless A is also necessary for B (table 8-2). A competently used guillotine will behead anyone placed under it, but all beheadings are not by guillotine. Occupants of cars that run under trailers of tractor-trailer rigs are sometimes beheaded.

In table 8-3, if the lower left and upper right cells both contained zero, factor A would be both necessary and sufficient for B, but such effects are very rare. In table 8-3 as shown, A increases the probability of B, and more cases of B are found in the presence of A, but A is neither necessary nor sufficient for B. Some people who drink and drive are not in crashes, and many drivers in crashes

Table 8-1. Distribution of Observations When A Is a Necessary Condition for B

	B	Not B
A	Some	Some
Not A	None	Some

Table 8-2. Distribution of Observations When A Is a Sufficient Condition for B

	B	Not B
A	Some	None
Not A	Some	Some

Table 8-3. Distribution of Observations When A Increases the Probability of B

	B	Not B
A	More	Some
Not A	Some	More

have not consumed alcohol, so alcohol is a contributing factor, neither necessary nor sufficient to cause a crash.

Since prevention of a necessary condition for harm completely reduces the harm, the more closely the distribution of injuries of a given type and severity (B) in relation to the presence of some factor (A) resembles the distribution in table 8-1, the greater the number of such injuries that will be prevented if A is eliminated.

CRITERIA FOR CAUSATION

The old Henle-Koch criteria for attributing causes to infectious diseases required that a microorganism or other factor be found both necessary and sufficient to produce a given infectious disease, but clearly those criteria were too stringent. Many microorganisms were found necessary but not sufficient for the infection to occur (Kelsey et al., 1986). Nevertheless, by controlling the microorganism, its access to the host, or host resistance, the disease could be controlled.

Similarly, as noted in chapter 2, an energy exchange with the human organism is a necessary and specific condition for injury, but the degree of the energy exchange necessary in individual cases may vary by the nature of the tissues affected, which makes them more or less tolerant of energy insults. Nevertheless, if the energy exchange can be kept below the tolerance of the most vulnerable tissue, injury will not occur. Where it is not possible to reduce energy exchanges to that degree, it is nevertheless possible to greatly reduce severity by reducing energy exchanges.

Several criteria must be met to make a strong inference of causation. First, the cause must precede the effect in time. For example, a study of alcohol measured in the breath of emergency room patients found that some claimed to have consumed alcohol after the injury (Wechsler et al., 1969). In those cases, if true, alcohol could have not contributed to the incidence, although it might affect recovery.

Second, the hypothesized cause must be correlated with the effect; that is, they must have joint distributions similar to one of those in tables 8-1 through 8-3, or in the case of noncategorical variables such as blood alcohol concentration, there should be a dose–response covariation. The cliché among some scientists that "correlation doesn't mean causation" is not precise. Correlation is a necessary but not sufficient condition for inference of causation.

The absence of correlation does not totally rule out causation if measurement is unreliable, biased, or invalid or if other factors intervene in such a way as to mask the correlation. Occasionally, claims of lack of correlation are disproved when better research designs controlling for other factors are used (e.g., Zador et al., 1984). In other cases, the effect may be under- or overestimated for lack of control of relevant factors. For example, the National Highway Traffic Safety Administration (NHTSA) estimated that placement of fuel tanks in front of rear axles of passenger cars reduced fatal rear impact fires by 29 percent (Tessmer, 1994). The analysis did not account for the fact that cars were being reduced in size during the period that gas tanks were being relocated. When vehicle size and tank location were considered simultaneously in a multivariate analysis, forward-located tanks were found to reduce rear fire fatalities by more than half (Robertson, 1993).

Third, the correlation must be demonstrated to be large enough, given the numbers of observations in the sample, that it is unlikely to have occurred from random fluctuations in drawing samples of that size. If the sample size is too small, however, a causal connection may be falsely rejected. Statistical power is a function of sample size. Studies often lack a large enough sample to detect magnitudes of covariation that would have practical use if detected. One study of prominent medical journals, such as the *Journal of the American Medical Association*, found that 70 percent of articles with statistically insignificant results did not discuss the issue of statistical power; that is, the number of cases studied was often not large enough to detect important differences beyond chance variation (Hebert et al., 2002). Textbooks in statistics contain criteria for sampling and tests for random fluctuation in samples (e.g., Armitage, 1971; Selvin, 1991). Computer programs such as Epi Info (chapter 7), used for data entry and statistical calculations, include features for estimating statistical power before a study is undertaken (e.g., Dean et al., 1994).

Fourth, the research design must be adequate to rule out covariation between the hypothesized cause and other factors that could explain the same variation, or specify how such covariation represents a causal sequence. This is the previously mentioned problem of "confounding." Research projects that demonstrate a non-random correlation between A and B are often criticized by statements such as, "You didn't control for X." The criticism may be legitimate if X could reasonably be expected to affect both A and B strongly enough to account for their correlation, but some such criticisms have no basis in terms of plausible causal mechanisms or potential magnitude of the effect.

Fifth, the mechanism of the causation should be plausible in terms of what is known about the phenomena in the relevant discipline. Occasionally, the theories of physics, chemistry, biology, or behavior are revolutionized by some seemingly implausible research finding, but often such a finding is subsequently shown to be the result of faulty research methodology. See appendix 8-1 for an analysis of an implausible claim of the cause of a divergence in trends of motor vehicle fatality rates among countries.

CAUSAL MODELS

The more plausible hypotheses are those that are deduced from what is known. Some important discoveries occur as a result of hypotheses based on hunches, observations of a few cases in a clinic or morgue, and the like, but the odds of finding something useful are greater when the hypothesis to be tested provides a plausible link in a causal model.

In the case of injury, a hypothesis is more plausible if the proposed cause has a likely connection to the concentration of energy, an energy exchange with tissue, or the vulnerability of tissue. If the hypothesized cause could not directly affect one or more of these factors, it is likely to be a relatively weak and indirect contributor to the incidence or severity of injury. To aid thinking about the research that is needed to fill gaps in knowledge, a diagram of the hypothesized causal paths of a given set of injuries is often useful.

For example, it is well known that age is correlated to severe motor vehicle injuries, but age is merely a measure of how often one has circled the sun. While age indicates differential risk that can be used to target injury control efforts, it is not a cause of injury. Age is an inexact proxy measure of human limitations and behaviors, including exposure to more or less risky energy sources (knowingly or unknowingly), which result in concentration of energy or energy exchanges, and physical conditions that affect tissue vulnerability.

Correlating such factors as age and gender to injury rates has been called "black box" epidemiology (Susser and Susser, 1996). Without precise knowledge of the exposures to energy and behaviors in the presence of those exposures, by age and gender, the causal mechanisms involved are lumped in a box, the contents of which are unknown. Figure 8-1 illustrates some possible paths of causation whereby correlates of age may contribute to the necessary and specific causes of injury and severity of injury to motor vehicle occupants. The direction of the arrows represents the known or hypothesized direction of effect of a given factor on another.

Energy generated by speed and mass interacts with vulnerable tissue in a crash, exacerbated by insufficient room for vehicle occupants to decelerate as indicated by vehicle size. The power of an engine, measured as horsepower in given increments, is necessary for given increments in speed. Vehicle size and horsepower accounted for about 55 percent of the variation in occupant fatalities per 100,000 passenger cars of particular makes and models in the 1980s (Robertson, 1991). Observations of age, gender, and speed of drivers at sites where vehicles rolled over indicated that younger drivers were driving faster than the average speed at the sites, but there was no correlation of speed and gender. Age, however, was not correlated with rollover, and speed was not correlated with vehicle stability. Therefore, speeding or young drivers did not confound the effect of vehicle stability on rollover (Robertson and Maloney, 1997).

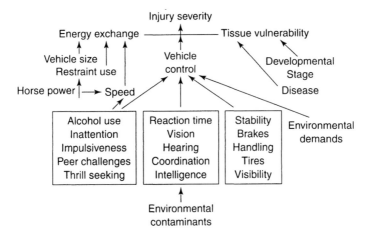

Figure 8-1. Causal Model of Motor Vehicle Injury

Loss of control of one or more vehicles usually precedes a crash. Loss of control is affected by vehicle stability, steering characteristics, braking capacity, and tire characteristics in interaction with inputs from the driver—speed, steering, braking. Vehicle stability accounts for about 62 percent of the variation in fatal rollover crashes per 100,000 utility vehicles, independent of other major known risk factors. These vehicles have stability less than the vast majority of cars (Robertson, 1989).

Inputs to the vehicle by the driver are known to include impairment or other effects of alcohol and other drugs and variations in human limitations such as reaction times (time from signal of need to change inputs to actual behavior), vision, hearing, intelligence, and coordination of senses and motor function. The effect of each is not known precisely and is more or less contingent on the demands of the driving environment. Therefore, the extent of reductions in injuries that could be achieved by changing the factors that are changeable is in more or less doubt for each one. The other listed behavioral factors may affect speed, reaction time, steering or braking, and degree of vehicle use, but how often is largely unknown. Factors related to age may also affect tissue vulnerability, including developmental stages, alcohol or other drugs, and certain diseases.

As depicted in figure 8-1, the effects of given variables are straightforward in causal chains, but some of the links among factors may be more complicated. While the effect of alcohol is usually referred to as impairment, there are several aspects of the correlation of alcohol and injuries that suggest a more complex causal pattern. Alcohol in drivers in motor vehicle crashes is more correlated with injury severity than with incidence (Haddon et al., 1968). Alcohol is found more often in the victims of assault and homicide than in drivers killed in motor vehicle crashes (Wechsler et al., 1969; Baker et al., 1971). Therefore, it is unlikely that the effect of alcohol is just to impair performance or make tissue more vulnerable. Based on these and other findings, a more elaborate model of alcohol use and its effects has been suggested (Robertson, 1983), as displayed in figure 8-2.

In biological and other systems, the system goes out of control when there is positive feedback; that is, factor A increases factor B, which in turn increases factor A, directly or through its effect on other factors. In the model, alcohol use

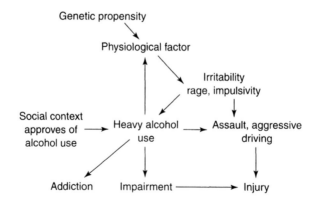

Figure 8-2. A General Theory of Alcohol Use and Effects

is hypothesized as partly a consequence of inherited biological factors that affect emotions, which may then contribute to increased drinking in an uncontrolled feedback. If such feedback occurs, the individual effects in the loop do not have to be large to have an enormous effect in a few iterations. For example, if $b = 1.02a$, $c = 1.03b$, and $a = 1.02c$, the three factors will about double in 10 cycles and about quadruple in 20 cycles.

If the alcohol model is supported by research evidence, then elimination of alcohol might not eliminate all of the injuries with which it is associated. The emotions that contributed to drinking may also contribute to the behaviors leading to injuries and would be present in the absence of alcohol, albeit to a lesser degree (McClelland, 1984). Chapter 15 includes an analysis that indicates that removal of all alcohol from drivers would reduce fatal crashes about half the amount presumed from data on alcohol "involvement." Too often, the human mind converts "involved in" to "caused."

This dynamic model of the causes and consequences of alcohol use is more comprehensive regarding the possible reasons for the involvement of alcohol in assaults as well as other injuries, and for eventual alcohol addiction. It suggests that if the physiological factor possibly intervening between the genes and increased use can be identified and controlled, a variety of problems would be alleviated.

These are relatively simple examples of causal models. Numerous variations have been suggested just for driver factors in motor vehicle injury (Michon, 1985). The value of a model is not necessarily its complexity or completeness, but whether or not it suggests testable hypotheses regarding variables that have a major influence, particularly variables that are controllable for injury prevention or severity reduction.

APPENDIX 8-1

False Inference of Causation

A retired General Motors employee, Leonard Evans, published a book in which trends in motor vehicle death rates in the United States were compared to those in other countries (Evans, 2004). The decline in U.S. rates slowed in the 1990s compared to those of several other industrialized countries. As a result, the United States no longer holds its historically leading position—the lowest motor vehicle death rate. Evans said the trends indicated a "Dramatic Failure of U.S. Safety Policy." His "analysis" was confined to eyeballing the trends and assertion regarding the cause. The changed slope in U.S. rates he attributed to personal injury lawyers who, he said, have an interest in focusing on vehicles to the neglect of programs to change driver behavior. He said that the emphasis on vehicle factors that resulted in the Motor Vehicle Safety Act of 1966 was the beginning of the problem and singled out the airbag controversy of the 1970s and 1980s as the recent major culprit.

Actually, the National Traffic and Motor Vehicle Safety Act of 1966 was inspired by a book co-edited by a physician and two social scientists, who had no interest in injury lawsuits (Haddon et al., 1964). That book emphasized that the energy in car crashes (and other injurious events) could be managed by product and environmental modifications to reduce injury severity. Based on that analysis,

Senator Abraham Ribicoff began hearings on vehicle manufacturer responsibility to improve vehicle safety. When private detectives hired by General Motors were caught trying to entrap Ralph Nader in a scandal, and GM's chairman apologized in a Senate hearing, the issue gained wider public attention. Although Nader, a consultant to the Senate committee, was a lawyer, his career had nothing to do with product liability lawsuits. He had served in government and was the author of a book highly critical of a General Motors product. (Nader, 1966; McCarry, 1972). Whether the National Traffic and Motor Vehicle Safety Act would have been enacted without that incident is uncertain, but it was a positive step to reduce vehicle fatalities. The initial regulations substantially improved the crashworthiness of passenger cars. The manufacturers subsequently improved crashworthiness, possibly in response to publicized crash tests (Robertson, 1996).

Evans says Joan Claybrook (lawyer) in the Carter administration, egged on by Ralph Nader (lawyer), imposed the "air bag mandate" in the United States. In fact, the only air bag mandate was introduced by nonlawyers Douglas Toms, head of the NHTSA and a former state motor vehicle administrator, and John Volpe, Secretary of Transportation and a former owner of a construction company, in the Nixon administration. Because their mandate was not a performance standard as required by U.S. law, the standard was later revised to require minimum forces on crash dummies in frontal impacts at 30 miles per hour, which is not an "air bag mandate." The Reagan administration tried to overturn the standard but was overruled by the courts as a result of a lawsuit by insurance companies and others, not personal injury lawyers. Automakers chose to use air bags to meet the standard but were not compelled to do so if they had chosen to design the vehicles differently.

Even more bizarre than the false assertions were the favorable reviews of Evans's book in leading medical and other journals. The reviewer in the *Journal of the American Medical Association* called the chapter on U.S. policy failure a "showstopper" and devoted most of the review to an uncritical repetition of Evans's allegations regarding the history of vehicle regulation (Eisenberg, 2005).

So what are the available data that Evans failed to analyze? One prominent trend in U.S. vehicle sales in the 1990s was the increase in large sport utility vehicles (SUVs) built on pickup truck frames. (Readers outside the United States unfamiliar with SUVs may see pictures by typing SUV in any Internet search engine.) Evans mentioned a possible effect of SUVs but said they could not make a difference of more than "a few thousand" deaths per year, "up or down." He did not mention the fact that pickup trucks also increased in sales. It has long been known that higher weight vehicles contribute disproportionately to the deaths of occupants of other vehicles, as well as pedestrians and bicyclists, the latter probably because of longer braking distances of heavier vehicles (Robertson and Baker, 1976).

Vehicles with centers of gravity too high relative to their width also have excessive rollover death rates (Robertson and Kelley, 1989). Stiff frames in certain SUVs, pickup trucks, and vans are also a factor in increased risk (Gabler and Hollowell, 1996).

Using data from the countries that Evan claims are superior in safety policy to the United States, trends in the sales of trucks were examined to see if those countries had a similar increase in truck use compared to the United States (Binder, 1990–2003). The major separation in the rates of the United States and other countries occurred in the 1990s. Figure 8-3 illustrates the change in truck and SUV sales, which are classified as trucks, during that period. In the United States, trucks and SUVs were 25 percent of sales in 1991 and steadily increased to more than 40 percent of sales in 2002. None of the other countries experienced a parallel increase. In Japan, the percentage of trucks sales declined substantially, but the trend was relatively flat in most countries. Trends among other European countries mentioned by Evans (Denmark, Finland, Luxembourg, and the Netherlands) were similar to those of their nearby neighbors shown here. The Canadian percentage started lower, rose similar to that of the United States until 1998, and then declined. These trends led to substantial differences in vehicle mix among the countries.

Of course, we cannot say with certainty that trends in truck sales explain the differences in fatality trends among countries without additional data, but the facts that trucks have a higher death rate than other vehicles and that truck sales increased in the United States disproportionately favor this explanation over the lawsuit explanation, which has no plausible causal nexus.

More convincing data are available based on Canadian vehicle sales. Evans gives special emphasis to the decline in Canadian death rates because, he claims, Canada has the same mix of vehicles and drivers as the United States. The Canadian motor vehicle death rate per vehicles in use declined 63 percent from 1979 to 2002, similar to other industrialized countries, compared to a reduction of 46 percent in the U.S. rate.

Canada does not keep records of the makes and models of vehicles in fatal crashes, but the data from death rates for each make and model in the United

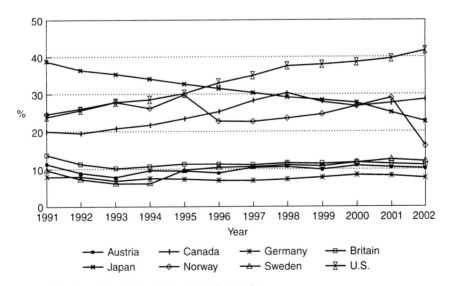

Figure 8-3. Truck Sales 1991–2002—Selected Countries

States can be applied to the same make-models in use in Canada to calculate an expected death rate, adjusted for average miles traveled per vehicle. The following steps were undertaken to obtain an expected death rate for Canada:

1. Count the number of deaths of each make and model in use in the United States and divide by the number in use during 2001–2002.
2. Multiply the death rate for each make and model in the United States times the number of each make and model in use in Canada during the same period to obtain expected deaths for each make and model in Canada.
3. Sum the number of expected deaths across makes and models and divide the total by the total number of vehicles in use in Canada. Multiply the expected rate per 100,000 vehicles by the ratio of annual miles in Canada to annual miles in the United States.

The fatalities in the United States by make and model of vehicle in the years 2001–2002 were obtained from the NHTSA's Fatality Analysis Reporting System. Only 1991 and later models were included. All deaths in a fatal crash in which a given vehicle was involved were counted. In collisions of two or more vehicles, only the occupants who died in each vehicle were counted for that vehicle to avoid double counting. Vehicles in use in the United States and Canada were estimated by tabulating the annual sales by make and model in each country during 1991–2002 and subtracting the number scrapped before 2002, using published data on vehicles remaining after a given number of years of use for cars and trucks separately in each country (Binder, 1990–2003).

Differences in types of vehicles in use in 2001–2002 between the United States and Canada are shown in table 8-4, based on examination of specific make-model sales from 1991–2002, discounted for scrapped vehicles. Drivers in the United States used proportionately heavier cars that had somewhat lower death rates than lighter cars, while Canadian drivers disproportionately used vans—the vehicles with the lowest aggregate death rates. (See appendix 9-1 for an analysis of the effects of weight controlling for size). Drivers in the

Table 8-4. Percent Vehicles in Use in the United States and Canada and U.S. Fatality Rates: 2001–2002

	Percent Use		Total Deaths/100,000 Vehicles	Occupant Deaths/100,000 Vehicles
	U.S.	Canada		
Cars <3,000 lbs	30.4	38.8	18.2	16.5
Cars ≥3,000 lbs	25.9	17.5	16.9	14.0
Vans	9.6	16.5	13.4	9.7
SUVs	12.8	8.4	19.9	14.4
Pickup trucks	18.0	16.3	22.7	15.0
Motorcycles (single vehicle)	3.1	2.4	33.4	33.4

United States used proportionately more SUVs and pickup trucks that have higher total death rates mainly because of their higher involvement in deaths to road users other than their occupants. The higher weights of trucks and SUVs result in longer stopping distances, contributing to increased deaths of pedestrians, bicyclists, and motorcyclists. Motorcycles are also used more in the United States. Even with deaths to motorcycle riders counted in the total rate of other vehicles that collided with motorcycles, the single-vehicle death rate of motorcycles is higher than the total death rate of the other classes of vehicles.

Drivers in the United States drove an average 12,655 miles in 2002 compared to 10,733 miles driven by Canadian drivers. Applying the U.S. rates for each make-model to the numbers of vehicles of the same make model in use in Canada, and correcting for mileage differences, results in an expected death rate in Canada of 15.9 per 100,000 vehicles compared to 18.9 per 100,000 in the United States. That difference is exactly the difference in the total death rates between the countries in 2002.

Contrary to Evans's assertion, the United States and Canada did not have the same mix of vehicles. The difference in death rates between Canada and the United States is predicted by the difference in vehicle mix and miles driven between the two countries. The results suggest that if Canadian drivers had driven the same mix of vehicles the same miles per vehicle as U.S. drivers, they would have the same total death involvement rate as U.S. drivers.

One of the possible reasons that Canadians drive less is a higher gasoline tax. Gasoline taxes in the United States are the lowest among the industrialized countries (Parry, 2002). The attenuation in the decline in U.S. fatality rates in the 1990s was at least partly attributable to increased miles driven due to the decline in gasoline prices, adjusted for inflation. Controlling for various state laws and economic factors, "a 10 percent decrease in the real gasoline price is associated with a 1.6 percent increase in fatal crashes per capita" (Grabowski and Morrisey, 2004).

There is no evidence for Evans's claim that the differences between the United States and Canada resulted from too little emphasis on behavioral factors in the United States. Indeed, the U.S. federal government spends large amounts on such programs. According to officials at Transport Canada, the national government's transportation agency, there is no Canadian federal government expenditure on behavior programs. In addition to the National Traffic and Motor Vehicle Safety Act, in 1966 the U.S. Congress enacted the Highway Safety Act that provides grants to the states for safety programs. Study of the early effects of such grants found an adverse effect on state motor vehicle fatality rates of high school driver education expenditures but a favorable effect of other programs (Robertson, 1984). Driver education is no longer federally funded. The grants more than doubled in the 1990s. From 1998 to 2002, the grants were incremented from $236.1 million to $556.8 million—targeted substantially toward alcohol abuse, seat belt use, and child restraint use. States and provinces in the United States and Canada may have spent additional funds, but there was certainly no paucity of attention to behavioral factors in the United States.

NOTE

The appendix is adapted from Robertson LS (2006) Motor vehicle deaths: failed policy analysis and neglected policy. *J Public Health Policy.* 27:182–189.

References

Armitage P (1971) *Statistical Methods in Medical Research.* New York, NY: John Wiley and Sons.

Baker SP, Robertson LS, and Spitz WU (1971) Tattoos, alcohol, and violent death. *J Forensic Sci.* 16:219–225.

Binder AK (ed.) (1990–2003) *Automotive Yearbook.* Southfield, MI: Ward's Communications.

Brown ST, Foege WH, Bender TR, and Axnick N (1990) Injury prevention and control: prospects for the 1990s. *Annu Rev Public Health.* 11:251–266.

Dean AD, Dean JA, Coulombier D, Burton JH, et al. (1994) *Epi Info Version. 6: A Word Processing, Database, and Statistics Program for Epidemiology on Micro-computers.* Atlanta, GA: Centers for Disease Control and Prevention.

Eisenberg D (2005) Review of "Traffic Safety." *JAMA.* 294:746–747.

Evans AS (1993) *Causation and Disease: A Chronological Journey.* New York, NY: Plenum.

Evans L (2004) *Traffic Safety.* Bloomfield Hills, MI: Science Serving Society.

Gabler HC, and Hollowell WT (1996) *Aggressivity of Light Trucks and Vans in Traffic Crashes.* Paper No. 980908. Warrendale, PA: Society of Automotive Engineers.

Grabowski DC, and Morrisey MA (2004) Gasoline prices and motor vehicle fatalities. *J Policy Anal Manag.* 23:575–593.

Haddon W Jr, Kelley AB, and Waller JA (anonymously) (1968) *1968 Alcohol and Highway Safety Report.* Washington, DC: U.S. Government Printing Office.

Haddon W Jr, Suchman EA, and Klein D (1964) *Accident Research.* New York, NY: Harper and Row.

Hebert RS, Wright SM, Dittus RS, and Elasy TA (2002) Prominent medical journals often provide insufficient information to assess the validity of studies with negative results. *J Negat Results Biomed.* 1:1.

Kelsey JL, Thompson WD, and Evans AS (1986) *Methods in Observational Epidemiology.* New York, NY: Oxford University Press.

Krieger N (1994) Epidemiology and the web of causation: has anyone seen the spider? *Soc Sci Med.* 39:887–903.

McCarry C (1972) *Citizen Nader.* New York, NY: Saturday Press Review.

McClelland DC (1984) Drinking as a response to power needs in men. In McClelland DC, *Motives, Personality, and Society.* New York, NY: Praeger.

McMahon B, Pugh TF, and Ipsen J (1960) *Epidemiologic methods.* New York, NY: Little, Brown.

Michon JA (1985) A critical view of driver behavior models: what do we know: what should we do? In Evans L, and Schwing RC (eds.), *Human Behavior and Traffic Safety.* New York, NY: Plenum.

Nader R (1966) Unsafe at Any Speed. New York, NY: Pocket Books.

Parry IWH (2002) Is gasoline undertaxed in the United States? *Resources.* 148:29–33.

Powell EC, Sheehan KM, and Christoffel KK (1996) Firearm violence among youth: public health strategies for prevention. *Ann Emergency Med.* 28:204–212.

Renwick JH (1973) Analysis of cause—long cut to prevention. *Nature.* 246:114–115.

Robertson LS (1983) *Injuries: Causes, Control Strategies and Public Policy.* Lexington, MA: DC Heath.

Robertson LS (1984) Federal funds and state motor vehicle deaths. *J Public Health Policy.* 5:376–386.

Robertson LS (1989) Risk of fatal rollover in utility vehicles relative to static stability. *Am J Public Health.* 79:300–303.

Robertson LS (1991) How to save fuel and reduce injuries in automobiles. *J Trauma.* 31:107–109.

Robertson LS (1993) Fatal fires from rear-end crashes: the effects of fuel tank placement before and after regulation. *Am J Public Health.* 83:1168–1170.

Robertson LS (1996) Reducing death on the road: the effects of minimum safety standards, publicized crash tests, seat belts and alcohol. *Am J Public Health.* 86:31–34.

Robertson LS (2006) Motor vehicle deaths: failed policy analysis and neglected policy. *J Public Health Policy.* 27:182–189.

Robertson LS, and Baker SP (1976) Motor vehicle sizes in 1440 fatal crashes. *Accid Anal Prev.* 8:167–175.

Robertson LS, and Kelley AB (1989) Static stability as a predictor of overturn in fatal vehicle crashes. *J Trauma.* 29:313–319.

Robertson LS, and Maloney A (1997) Motor vehicle rollover and static stability: an exposure study. *Am J Public Health.* 87:839–841.

Selvin S (1991) *Statistical Analysis of Epidemiologic Data.* New York, NY: Oxford University Press.

Susser M, and Susser E (1996) Choosing a future for epidemiology: I. Eras and paradigms. *Am J Public Health.* 86:668–673.

Tessmer J (1994) *An Analysis of Fires in Passenger Cars, Light Trucks and Vans.* Washington, DC: National Highway Traffic Safety Administration.

Wechsler H, Kasey EH, Thum D, and Demone HW Jr (1969) Alcohol level and home accidents. *Public Health Rep.* 84:1043–1050.

Zador PL, Jones IS, and Ginsburg M (1984) Fatal front-to-front car collisions and the results of 35 mph frontal barrier impacts. In *28th Annual Proceedings of the Association for the Advancement of Automotive Medicine*, Barrington, IL: Association for the Advancement of Automotive Medicine.

9

Research Designs and Data Analysis

The choice of study designs to investigate a given set of factors is affected by numerous considerations. What is the unit of analysis (people, vehicles, environments)? In what population should the study be conducted? To what population of people, vehicles, or environments will the results be generalized? What measurements of the factors are available or could be obtained? How reliable and valid are the measurements? Can the data be collected without violating ethical guidelines? How can the study isolate the effects of given factors independent of, or in combination with, other relevant factors? How much time will be needed to complete the study? How much will the study cost?

No single study will specify degree of effect of all the factors in a causal model. The goal of a prevention-oriented research project is to specify the extent to which injury or injury severity would be reduced by changing a given factor hypothesized to contribute to the injury or severity, other things being equal. A study design should be chosen that eliminates or minimizes the probability that factors other than the changeable factor of interest somehow bias that estimate. See appendix 9-1 for an example of elimination of alternative explanations.

Students of epidemiology are familiar with the general descriptive terms that are used to describe study designs, but they are noted here for readers unfamiliar with them. A cohort is a sample or population of units of analysis on which the researcher collects data continuously or periodically over a period of time. In a retrospective study, the researcher attempts to obtain data on a cohort accumulated in the past. In a prospective study, the data are gathered for a period of time after the generation of hypotheses and identification of the cohort to be studied.

CONTROLLED EXPERIMENTS

The most definitive results of research are produced by data gathered prospectively in controlled experiments where a modification is introduced in one or more groups of whatever units of analysis (the experimental groups) but not in one or more others (the control groups). Any change in outcomes, such as injuries, is attributable to the introduced modification if the experimental and control groups were otherwise equal at the outset. That design requires the researcher to have control of one or more hypothesized causal factors, at least to the extent of being able to assign units of analysis (people, vehicles, environments) to experimental and control groups. The assignment is usually randomized such that effects of other factors on injury or other relevant outcomes are random.

The controlled experiment is appealing not only because it maximizes the confidence that other factors are equalized by random assignment but also because it illustrates that the causal factor in question is controllable, although control in an experiment does not necessarily imply that control is possible to the same degree in the natural occurrence of the factor of interest.

If the experimental manipulation of a given variable has more than an extremely remote possibility of increasing injury, ethics dictate that the experiment should not be conducted (McGough and Wolf, 2001). For example, most researchers would not consider an experiment in which drivers in the experimental group would be given alcohol and then sent out to drive in traffic, although a few such studies have been conducted on environmentally benign driving ranges or roads without other traffic. Of course, vehicle crash tests can be done experimentally with instrumented crash dummies rather than with human subjects.

The effects of alcohol on various behaviors, including driving in environments simulated by motion pictures and other devices, have been studied by controlled experimental designs. These studies have specified the effects of alcohol on impairment of various behaviors—reaction time, steering, and so forth—and on certain emotions (e.g., Loomis and West, 1958). Apparently, no experiment has yet been undertaken to disaggregate the effects of alcohol and emotions, separately and in combination, on behaviors highly predictive of injury.

Whether laboratory experiments can be generalized to the "real world" can always be questioned. Use of experimental and control groups stratified on other factors such as age, gender, and impulsiveness not only allows the researcher to test for effects of combinations of factors but also addresses the issue of generalization to segments of the population. Such more complicated experimental designs increase the numbers of persons (or other units of analysis) needed for statistical power, and associated costs of the research. A textbook on experimental designs should be consulted regarding varieties of designs for efficiency and statistical power (e.g., Lundquist, 1953).

CASE–CONTROL STUDIES

A study design that can approximate the conditions of a controlled experiment is the case–control design. A case may be an injured person, a vehicle that rolled over, or a section of road where a vehicle hit a tree. The analogous controls would be persons not injured, vehicles that did not roll over, or sections of road that the vehicle traversed without hitting trees. The research question is how relevant individual, vehicle, or environmental factors differ between cases and controls. The controls may be matched on certain factors (age, gender, time, place) or unmatched.

For example, the important role of alcohol in motor vehicle injuries was demonstrated by case–control studies (e.g., Haddon et al., 1961). Alcohol was measured in fatally injured pedestrians and in randomly selected persons at the same places, walking at the same time of day and same day of week, and moving in the same direction as the fatally injured. Therefore, these environmental factors were the same for the cases and controls and could not account for the large differences in alcohol found in the cases and controls. The same design was also used with drivers as the unit of analysis (McCarroll and Haddon, 1962).

One way of studying the alcohol issues mentioned in chapter 8 would be to replicate these case–control studies and measure hypothesized biological factors that might contribute to alcohol use, other behaviors, or both jointly. Two major problems would be encountered in such a study. First, while measurement of alcohol in breath samples of controls may be allowed by sufficient numbers of persons selected as controls, requests for blood or other biological specimens might not be acceptable. Second, good evidence that trauma does not change the hypothesized biological factor is necessary before assuming that a difference between cases and controls is indicative of causation.

Selection of people engaged in the same activity at the same site, time of day, and day of week may not be possible for activities that occur at the case sites infrequently, such as use of all terrain vehicles or snowmobiles. A child injured in a home may have no siblings close enough in age to serve as controls within the household, although children in reasonable proximity in the same neighborhoods may serve as controls, depending on the factors of interest. For example, children who were killed in a cluster of unsolved child homicides were compared to children from the same neighborhood regarding potential risk factors. Several factors indicative of greater exposure (time and specific hours away from home alone, running errands for money) were identified as placing the killed children at greater risk (Goodman et al., 1988).

Within-household controls are inappropriate if the hypothesized hazard is common to all members of the household. A study of risk of having a gun in a household, for example, used as controls households in the neighborhood surrounding those households with a fatal shooting and statistically controlled for such factors as illicit drug use and a history of physical fights. The study documented that gun ownership increased the risk of homicide, given the same history of drug use and fighting (Kellerman et al., 1993).

The selection of controls in case–control studies requires careful thought, and measurement of certain factors retrospectively can be quite problematic. In clinical situations, it is tempting to select controls from patients who have arrived at the same clinic or hospital for reasons other than injury. If the hypothesized causal factor contributes in some way to problems other than injury that lead people to seek medical care, however, the comparison of cases and controls will underestimate the contribution of that factor to injury. If the hypothesized causal factor were reduced by factors that also lead to the seeking of medical care, the effect of that factor would be overestimated.

For example, a study of alcohol in emergency room patients compared those injured to those who appeared for illnesses (Wechsler et al., 1969). Since we do not know the effect of the mix of illnesses seen in such clinics on alcohol use or the effect of alcohol use on seeking medical care for injury or illness, the extent of over- or underestimation of alcohol's effect on injury is uncertain from such a comparison. If alcohol contributes to the problem presented by the control patients or to the probability of seeking medical attention, the difference in alcohol measured between cases and controls could be less than if persons exposed to the circumstances of injury who had no reason to seek medical attention were chosen as controls. If the medical condition were such that the control patient would not have been engaged in activities similar to that of the injured person, the effect of aspects of those activities would be overestimated.

One study used people who died of other causes as controls to emphasize the overinvolvement of people in certain occupations in motor vehicle deaths (Loomis, 1991). Since the controls are just as dead as the cases, the usefulness of such a study for preventing death is ephemeral.

Even worse is a survey of people who were involved in motor vehicle crashes and a random sample of licensed drivers not involved in crashes as to frequency of use of cellular phones (Violanti and Marshall, 1996). No determination was made of whether the phone was in use when the driver crashed, much less cellular phone use at the same times and places. A later study that more precisely specified phone use in proximity to the time of the crash from records of phone calls suggested an increased risk of motor vehicle crashes related to phone use in cars (Redelmeier and Tibshirani, 1997).

The fundamental issue in selection of cases and controls is what should be allowed to vary as the hypothesized cause, or causes in stratified samples, and what should be held constant. If the variables to be held constant can be other than randomly distributed between cases and controls, the purpose of the design is defeated. If the factor or factors treated as potential causes are not directly connected to injury or are unchangeable, the study is a waste of limited resources for research.

Collection of retrospective data on cases and controls also presents numerous problems. In assault cases, it may not be possible to identify the assailant, or if identified, the assailant may be noncooperative or falsify information. If a person is injured in a neighborhood, controls that have knowledge of the injury may give misleading information because of denial of personal vulnerability or other psychological factors. Even if data can be obtained by observation, such as by watching children engaging in the activity involved in the case, knowledge of the injury may change who participates or how they participate.

The human host or vector (assaulted person, driver) has been the unit of analysis in most case–control studies, to the neglect of factors that may be more subject to change for injury control. Case–control designs can also provide strong evidence regarding vehicle and environmental factors.

For example, advocates of the use of tractor-trailer trucks with more than one trailer argued that the risk was less because the crash rates per vehicle were similar, but fewer trucks were used because of more cargo per trip. A case–control study of trucks in crashes and trucks observed at the same time of day, on the same roads, moving in the same direction, revealed that two-trailer trucks were two to three times more likely to crash in the same environment, more than offsetting the advantage of carrying increased cargo (Stein and Jones, 1988).

In a study of environmental factors in motor vehicle crashes, the driver and vehicle can serve as their own controls. For example, the characteristics of crash sites where occupants of vehicles died striking fixed objects along the roadside were compared to sites one mile away in the direction from which the vehicle traveled. Since the driver and vehicle factors presumably did not change in a mile, those factors were virtually constant at the case and comparison sites. The substantial differences in road curvature and gradient of the road, coupled with no difference in number of potential objects along the road, indicated that environmental modifications would greatly reduce the severity of fixed-object crashes at sites with the identified characteristics (Wright and Robertson, 1976).

Subsequent research using this study design found excess involvement of similar road characteristics in off-road rollover fatalities (Zador et al., 1987), vehicles running into water leading to occupant drowning (Wintemute et al., 1990), and multiple-vehicle crashes at other than intersections (Fulgham et al., 1989). Since two vehicles were involved in the latter study, two control sites were studied for each case, one mile in the direction from which each vehicle traveled.

The power of case–control designs is sometimes poorly understood by those in a position to disseminate the results. For, example, federal road authorities ignore the specification of curvature and grade characteristics as road conditions that can be used to target sites for modification. The magazine *Public Roads* is a Federal Highway Administration publication that circulates to the officials who decide where, when, and how roads are to be built or modified. Articles on a decision-making system called the Interactive Highway Safety Design Model (Regan, 1994; Lum and Regan, 1995) contained no information on curvature and grade criteria established by the mentioned case–control studies. When the editor of *Public Roads* was informed of this in 1996, he refused to publish material on the issue.

RETROSPECTIVE COHORT STUDIES

The more removed in time of data gathered retrospectively, the greater the problems in measurement. Occasionally, one may be able to use extant records, such as school records, arrest records, motor vehicle records, and the like, to obtain direct or proxy measures of certain variables. The most common source of data in retrospective studies is interview or questionnaire, but the steepness of the forget curve and the tendency for people to recreate their histories to foster a more favorable image severely limit the validity of recalled information. For example, in a study of people in motor vehicle crashes involving injury that was reported to police, persons involved were interviewed at different time periods following the incident. The percentage of interviewees who reported the injury declined from 97 percent in the first three months to 73 percent 9–12 months after the crash (National Center for Health Statistics, 1972). More frequent but less severe injuries may be thought too trivial to mention or may be forgotten. Comparison of weekly fall reports among the elderly and recall at the end of the year indicated significant under-reporting at year's end (Cummings et al., 1988).

Where specific measures of variables worthy of study have been obtained in a cohort in the past, and it is possible to obtain data on subsequent injury, a retrospective cohort study may be less costly than a prospective study. For example, a cohort of children was studied at the time they were shedding their baby teeth. Concentration of lead in the teeth was measured as well as academic achievement, reaction times, and several other aspects of psychomotor performance. Also, teachers' behavioral ratings of various behaviors (distractable, hyperactive, impulsive) that might increase risk of injury were obtained (Needleman et al., 1979). If the subsequent clinical records of these children could be identified, the extent of the correlation of relevant factors to subsequent injuries might be studied. Such a study would require tracing those that had moved, and reliability checks on reported clinical facilities used.

PROSPECTIVE COHORT STUDIES

The likelihood of collecting reliable and valid data is much greater when data are collected prospectively in a cohort of relevant units of analysis and the cohort is followed to measure the incidence and severity of the outcomes of interest. A major disadvantage of this design is that very large samples and a long period of data collection are required to obtain statistical power when the outcome is relatively rare.

For example, in the United States, the annual hospitalized or fatal injury rate from motor vehicles is about 300 per 100,000 population for males and less than 200 per 100,000 population for females. If one could obtain data on hypothesized causes in a cohort of 100,000 people representative of the population, it would take nearly four years of data collection to obtain data on 1,000 injury cases. Controlling statistically for several factors would spread the cases very thinly among the various combinations of factors. The numbers of cases identified would be increased if less severe injuries were included, but as noted previously, the causes of less severe injuries are often different from causes of more severe injuries. In the case of motor vehicles, for example, the causes of low-speed "fender benders," which occur more often during the day in congested traffic, are often different from the causes of severe and fatal injuries, which occur disproportionately at night, at higher speeds, and in little, often no, traffic.

A prospective cohort design may be efficient for study of certain age groups with higher injury rates. For example, about one in five newly licensed 16-year-old drivers will have a motor vehicle crash resulting in injury or more than $400 in property damage within two years. If reliable and valid data on the behavioral factors and abilities in figure 8-1 could be obtained from 16-year-olds in several high schools, and their licensure, vehicle use, and crash experience measured in a subsequent two-year period, the data might provide better specification of the magnitude of the hypothesized paths in the model for that age group. In communities with a substantial dropout rate before age 16, however, the usefulness of the findings would be limited. Also, follow-up of those students who leave home or whose families move would be difficult.

An interesting example of a prospective cohort study involved the extent to which people who used tranquilizers (benzodiazepines) were treated for injury. Using claims from a health insurance plan, researchers compared the injury claims for 4,554 persons younger than 65 years who had a pharmacy claim for tranquilizers during a nine-month period, but not during the preceding three months, compared to a sample of persons who did not have a claim for tranquilizer use and were unrelated to the users. Three nonusers were matched to each user by age, gender, and calendar month when tranquilizer use began.

One obvious question is whether any difference in injury rates is the result of factors that precipitated the perceived need for tranquilizers rather than the possible effect of the drugs. Also, the use of the drugs could at least partly be the result of postinjury anxiety. The researchers found that injury claims were substantially higher in the user group in the three months prior to prescription of the drug. Therefore, comparison of the rate of injury while the users were using the drug was controlled statistically for preuse injury rate, as well as general care seeking and use of mental health services. The relative risk of hospitalization for injury to those who had no injury in the three months prior to prescription of the drug was higher than for the total study group (Oster et al., 1990). Apparently, neither prior injury nor discretionary use of medical services totally accounted for the higher injury rates of tranquilizer users.

CROSS-SECTIONAL STUDIES

A cross-sectional study involves measurement of relevant variables in a sample of appropriate units of analysis during a specified time period. The effect of a given factor is estimated by the direction and degree of its correlation to the outcome of interest. The validity of the inference of causation depends on assumptions about the time order of the variables and the extent and pattern of covariation among the factor of interest and other factors.

Suppose that a researcher obtained measures of some or all of the behavioral factors in figure 8-1 in a series of drivers hospitalized for injury and correlated them to relevant circumstances of the injury. The data indicate that attention spans are shorter and impulsiveness is more frequent among drivers that ran off the road and hit fixed objects than among drivers that were struck from behind. Since the presence of subclinical brain injuries may be different in the two sets of drivers, and such injuries could affect attention spans or impulsiveness, the inference that these factors were present in the degree measured prior to the crashes would be questionable.

Cross-sectional studies also do not provide definitive evidence of causation when there is covariation among hypothesized causal factors. If A is correlated to B, but X is also correlated to A and B, there are several possibilities. A could cause X, which causes B. X could cause A, which causes B. The three variables could be intertwined in a feedback system. Also, the correlation could be spurious. This happens when X causes A and B independently and there is no causal relationship between A and B. Again, that is what epidemiologists call "confounding."

Some of these possibilities can be ruled out by reasonable assumptions about the time sequence of the factors, or whether the X factor can reasonably be expected to play a causal role. For example, when researchers examined the rollover rates of certain utility vehicles (Jeeps, Broncos, Blazers), they inferred from physics that the higher rollover rates of these vehicles relative to cars was the result of differences in stability—the g force to overturn the vehicle—calculated by the width between the center of the tires divided by twice the height of center of gravity (Snyder et al., 1980). Road tests of the least stable vehicle, the Jeep CJ-5, driven by remote control indicated that it would roll over in low-speed turns (Insurance Institute for Highway Safety, 1980). A critic of the research claimed that the higher rollover rates of lower stability vehicles could have occurred because of differences in mileage or use by higher risk drivers or in higher risk environments (Joksch, 1983).

Since the rollover rates of the least stable utility vehicles were 3–20 times those of cars, the argument that mileage could account for the difference was unreasonable—for that to be true, the least stable vehicles would have to be driven more miles in a year than most vehicles are driven in their average 10 years of use (Robertson and Kelley, 1989). Also, other risk factors would contribute to all types of crashes—hitting trees and poles, hitting other vehicles—yet the stability factor was strongly correlated with rollover rates but hardly at all with nonrollover rates.

Since miles of use by particular drivers in particular environments was unknown, it was not possible to calculate milage-based rates of rollover and other types of crashes correlated with driver and environmental factors. Using a mathematical model of the potential relationship of proportional mortality of higher and lower risk drivers and environments, however, it was possible to rule out other factors as an explanation of the correlation of stability and rollover.

If stability were correlated with different use of the vehicles by low- and high-risk drivers or in low- and high-risk environments, the ratio of rollover crashes under low-risk conditions to those under high-risk conditions would be a function of the ratio of mileage in low- and high-risk conditions and therefore should be correlated to stability. Stated mathematically:

$$c\,\frac{L}{H} = \frac{\text{RL}}{\text{RH}} = b(S)$$

where

L = low exposure to a risk factor
H = high exposure to a risk factor
c = constant ratio of risk from low- to high-risk factor
RL = fatal rollovers in low-risk-factor situations
RH = fatal rollovers in high-risk-factor situations
b = slope of the correlation
S = stability value for a given vehicle

Using data from the Fatality Analysis Reporting System (FARS) for several years, RL/RH was not significantly correlated with vehicle stability for any of the major driver or environmental risk factors, except whether or not the vehicle rolled over on or off the road. The ratio of on-road to off-road rollovers was higher, the less stable the vehicle. This suggests that the side force of turning contributed more often to those rollovers, since ramping or going over embankments would usually occur off the road (Robertson, 1989). This methodology was also employed in the study in appendix 9-1.

Although data on every possible risk factor are not included in FARS, there are none excluded that could be correlated to stability, and exclusively to rollover crashes, strongly enough to render the strong correlation of stability and rollover spurious. Furthermore, the correlation of stability and rollover has causal plausibility. It is predicted from well-known physics.

Where major variables are unmeasured or are intercorrelated without a clear indication of time sequence, a cross-sectional study cannot be definitive in specifying causal chains. One useful function of cross-sectional studies is to indicate maximum magnitude of a given correlation. If the correlation of a hypothesized causal factor and the type, severity, or risk of injury is weak or nonexistent in a cross-sectional study, it is unlikely to be found a major factor in a study with a more powerful design unless the cross-sectional study includes invalid or biased measurement.

Using logical assumptions about the time sequence of variables in a causal model, it may be possible to analyze cross-sectional data in ways that enhance confidence in the degree of contribution of particular hypothesized causal chains. Social scientists have developed methods for such analyses of what they call causal paths using regression for quantitative variables (Blalock, 1964) and comparison of proportions and log-linear techniques for categorical data (Hellevik, 1984). These models are highly sensitive to assumptions of direction of causation and variable specification, however.

An example of misuse of "causal path analysis" is an attempt to discredit the studies of vehicle stability and rollover using police reports from Michigan and Florida. Unable to find behavioral and environmental factors that explained the variance attributable to stability, the authors of the study included "single-vehicle accident" as a "cause" in the model (Donelson et al., 1994). Since the majority of rollovers of lower stability vehicles occur when the vehicle rolls rather than slides to the side, collisions with other vehicles are less frequent than in nonrollovers. Also, "single-vehicle accident" does not mean that no other vehicle was involved. In some instances, the driver is making a sharp turn to avoid a collision with another vehicle. In multiple-vehicle crashes, it is not possible to specify which vehicle rolled from the Florida data. Therefore, the vehicles may have been misclassified, as well.

Attribution of lack of collision with another vehicle as a cause of the rollover should have been obviously absurd to the authors and those who reviewed the paper prior to publication. The lack of reference in the paper to any of the previous research on rollover should have been a signal of ethical lapse and bias, as well.

ECOLOGICAL STUDIES

Frequently one can easily obtain data on injuries in geographical areas and correlate the rates to other characteristics of those geographical areas obtained from other sources. For example, one might correlate injury rates per population in states or counties to census data on incomes, housing characteristics, and other factors in those counties. The correlations obtained are called ecological correlations.

A major problem with causal inferences from ecological correlations is that the hypothesized causal factor, or the factors that are controlled statistically, may not have occurred in the same unit of analysis as the effect (Robinson, 1950). If motor vehicle occupant injuries were found to be higher in low-income areas, that does not necessarily mean that persons with low income are any more likely to be the persons in severe crashes in those areas. The roads in low-income areas could be more hazardous because of lack of funds to maintain them, upgrade them, or remove hazards. They may be equally hazardous to all vehicle occupants irrespective of individual income.

The usefulness of such correlations depends on the interpretation. If the correlation were used as justification to modify the roads in the lower income areas, the injury rate may be reduced if the modifications chosen are effective. If the data are used to argue against action on the grounds that poverty is intractable, they are a hindrance to action.

Almost as silly as correlating motorcycle crash rates over time with number of robins in the environment over time is work on correlations of unemployment and fatal crash rates by statisticians at the National Highway Traffic Safety Administration (NHTSA). Fluctuations in total number of deaths were found almost perfectly correlated inversely with fluctuations in unemployment or in the nonlabor force, corrected for the 1974 oil boycott (e.g., Hedlund, 1984). Stress theories would predict greater risk per mile driven among the unemployed. Indeed, when rural mileage is entered into a multivariate equation with unemployment and fatalities per population, the inverse correlation between unemployment and the fatal rate reverses; that is, there is a higher fatality rate per population when the unemployment rate is high (Leigh and Waldon, 1991). Even if the NHTSA study held up under scrutiny, at the individual level unemployment is likely to account for only a small proportion of fatal crashes, and few would advocate increased unemployment as a policy to reduce motor vehicle injuries.

The statistical technique (regression) used by NHTSA finds the line or curve that best describes the extent to which one factor predicts another. Regression coefficients indicate the increase (or decrease if minus) in a unit of the outcome variable per unit of the predictor variable. Correlation is how closely the data fit the line or curve: 1 if the fit is perfect, and 0 if the relationship between the variables is random scatter.

Correlation of aggregated data, such as injury rates and the economy, gives falsely high correlations. Year-to-year fluctuations in aggregated rates vary narrowly compared to the magnitude of the total rate above zero. The correlation is based not on the range of possible rates given combinations of driver, vehicle, and environmental factors, but on the marginal fluctuation of rates that fluctuate with the economy not accounting for the base rate maintained by the presence of the other factors. A regression equation with greater disaggregation of these factors is discussed in chapter 13.

Ecological studies can be used to estimate the effects of changes in factors that affect a set of ecological units as a whole, such as changes in laws among states or other legal jurisdictions. In such studies, the researcher must be able to specify that the change in law or other factor applied to the particular units of analysis associated with the injuries for the results to be valid. As noted in chapter 12, cross-sectional studies using ecological data have been especially misleading in that regard. Ecological studies are more convincing when a change in injury rates over time is shown to occur coincident with a change in law or other factor during a period in which other factors did not change appreciably.

MIXED DESIGNS

Many studies do not fit into a neat classification of study designs. The efficacy of a study design is not whether it can be easily classified, but whether it reveals usable information without substantial bias. It is better to describe the study procedure and the efforts made to account for bias rather than state that the study followed some design classification that may not be totally accurate in its implication for the procedures followed (Cummings et al., 1990).

DATA ANALYSIS

The types of variables involved and the study design substantially determine the analysis of data from a research project. Familiarity with the use and interpretation of various statistics appropriate to particular types of data and study designs is essential for data analysis and report preparation. Students and researchers in epidemiology should be familiar with statistical procedures (e.g., Armitage, 1971; Fleiss, 1981; Hellevik, 1984; Riegelman, 1981), and those who are not should consult a statistician in the design stage of a research project. The best statistician in the world cannot produce some magical statistical trick to rescue what the study design has ignored or biased. Here, a few basic principles and comparisons of analytical methods are reviewed as a basis for consideration of issues that commonly arise.

One consideration that is often ignored is the requirement of a given journal. Some journals require confidence intervals on estimates of percentages, rates, regression coefficients, rate ratios, and odds ratios, rather than probabilities (p values) that an estimate could be the result of chance fluctuation in samples. Deciding, before data analysis and writing the report, where the report will be submitted and checking out the requirements and style of the target publication can save time and trouble.

Another consideration is the potential use of the results. Table 9-1 presents several measures used in summarizing the correlation of categorical data with two categories of each variable (partly from Abramson, 1985). There are obviously more potential measures of association of numbers in the table than there are numbers in the table. The statistic(s) to be used depends on the potential uses of the data.

If the results have potential for use in screening persons, vehicles, or environments for some intervention to reduce injury, the issue of statistical significance is much less relevant than the sensitivity and specificity of the factor as a basis for screening. Sensitivity is the proportion of persons injured that had the screening

Table 9-1. Common Measures of Association of Categorical Data

	Injured	Not Injured	Total
Factor present	a	b	$a + b$
Factor absent	c	d	$c + d$
Total	$a + c$	$b + d$	$N = a + b + c + d$

Sensitivity = $a/(a + c)$
Specificity = $d/(b + d)$
Odds ratio = ad/bc
Rate ratio = $[a/(a + b)]/[c/(c + d)]$
Assuming a risk factor:
    Rate difference = $[a/(a + b)] - [c/(c + d)]$
    Population excess risk = $[(a + c)/N] - [c/(c + d)]$
    Attributable risk = $[a/(a + b) - c/(c + d)]/[a/(a + b)]$
    Attributable fraction in population = $[(a + c)/N - c/(c + d)]/[(a + c)/N]$
Assuming a protective factor:
    Excess risk if unprotected = $c/[(c + d) - a(a + b)]$
    Population excess risk = $(a + c)/[N - a(a + b)]$
    Preventable fraction of the unprotected = $[c/(c + d) - a(a + b)]/[c/(c + d)]$
    Prevented fraction in the population = $[c/(c + d) - (a + c)/N]/[c/(c + d)]$
    Preventable fraction in the population = $[(a + c)/N - a/(a + b)]/[(a + c)/N]$

factor present prior to injury. Specificity is the proportion of persons not injured for whom the screening factor was absent. Assuming that the sample is not biased, if sensitivity is near 1.00, the factor will identify most of the people who would be injured. If specificity is near 1.00, the factor will not misidentify many people who would not be injured. From the public health standpoint, it is desirable that sensitivity be high. From the economic standpoint, if the intervention costs money, it is desirable that specificity be high. Too many missed cases (false negatives) greatly dilute the potential effect of the countermeasure, and too many cases included that would not be injured (false positives) make the application of the countermeasure more expensive.

Notice in table 9-1 that, if the factor is a necessary condition for injury, c would be zero and the odds ratio and rate ratio would each be infinite. The rate difference would be 1.00 only if the factor were a necessary and sufficient condition and could be small if the proportion injured of the population where the factor was present were small. The population excess risk would be even smaller if the latter were true. The attributable risk and attributable fraction in the population, however, would each be 1.00, indicating that all of the injuries could be eliminated by eliminating the risk factor. Yet the latter two statistics are seldom reported in analyses of injury data. If the researcher presents the data and the data are population based, however, they can be calculated.

The advantage of the odds ratio is that studies with different designs can be compared. Rate ratio, rate difference, population excess risk, attributable risk, and attributable fraction in the population are not comparable among studies unless the data are population based, or are adjusted for the sampling fraction if based on a sample.

The use of the statistics measuring effects of a protective factor (table 9-1) assumes that the protection examined is randomly distributed in the population at risk. If those at higher or lower risk are more or less likely to use the protection, the statistics will vary depending on the proportion of the population using the protection. In chapters 11 and 12, the effects of differential use of seat belts by those at higher and lower risk of severe crashes, and the estimates of seat belt effectiveness with and without belt use laws, are discussed in this regard.

In this and the preceding chapters, mention is made of "regression" and percentage of variation explained. Unfortunately, these statistical techniques are often left out of introductory biostatistics courses. The calculations are complicated, but the concept is straightforward. Figure 9-1 shows a regression line fitted to the plot of fatal, rollover rates of popular utility vehicles in the 1980s, where rollover was the first event that did harm to the vehicle or occupants, as a function of $T/2H$ (track width divided by twice the center of gravity height). The computer program that fits the line minimizes the deviations of each observation from the line and gives the result in the form of an equation, in this case:

$$\text{Rollover Rate} = 106 - 86(T/2H)$$

If you know the $T/2H$ for a vehicle, you can put it in the equation and get the expected rollover rate. The scatter around the line occurs because of other factors. The number in parentheses by each vehicle is the wheelbase, the distance from front to rear axle. Notice that the two vehicles substantially below the regression line (Bronco and SBlazer) have longer wheelbases than those near the line at that $T/2H$, and the outlier on the high side, the Jeep CJ5, has a very short wheelbase. In Appendix 15-1, an equation that includes $T/2H$, wheelbase, and nonrollover for a larger sample of vehicles is discussed.

Wheelbase "explains" some of the variation not predicted by $T/2H$. Percent variation explained, called R^2, is 1 minus the ratio of squared deviations from the

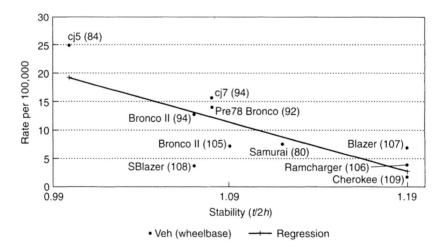

Figure 9-1. First-Harmful-Event Rollovers per 100,000 Vehicles in Use per Year. Numbers in Parentheses Are Wheelbases.

line to the total squared deviations from the average of the predicted variable, in this case rollover rates. If all the data points were on the line, the variation explained would be $1 - 0 = 1$, or 100 percent. If the scatter is totally random, the line would have no slope and the variation explained would be $1 - 1 = 0$, or 0 percent.

Notice also in figure 9-1 that the line will cross zero at $0 = 105 - 86(T/2H)$, or $T/2H = 1.22$. Since passenger cars have $T/2H$ up to 1.62, it is obvious that a straight-line regression will not fit the data if cars are included. In that case, a regression model that estimates two lines, one less than 1.2 and one at 1.2 or greater, can be used (Robertson and Maloney, 1997). There are also regression programs that fit curves rather than straight lines.

A variation on the concept of regression is logistic regression. The predicted outcome in a logistic regression is the logarithm of the odds of an outcome such as rollover. The equation that predicts back to the rate is not a straight line and is a little more complicated (appendix 9-1), but the basic idea is to predict a particular outcome by knowing one or more risk factors. Other things being equal, if those "other things" have been adequately controlled, it is then possible to say how much difference changing the risk factor will make in the outcome.

META-ANALYSIS

Statistical techniques are also available to examine various studies simultaneously to obtain a consensus estimate of the effect of a given factor or the effect of an intervention. Selection of studies for such analyses is problematic because studies that produce results that are not statistically significant are often not published (Bunn et al., 2001). Also, many study reports do not include adequate detail on the results and how the data were obtained to weight the attributes and liabilities of including the study in a meta-analysis.

A wide-ranging set of meta-analyses of human, vehicle, and environmental factors to reduce motor vehicle injuries is available (Elvik and Vaa, 2004). The adequacy of each should be judged based on the quality of the research included.

APPENDIX 9-1

An Example of Ruling Out Alternative Explanations: The Effect of Vehicle Weight, Size, Crashworthiness, and Stability on Fatalities and Fuel Economy

The energy of a moving vehicle is its mass multiplied by the square of its velocity, divided by 2. In other words, at equal speeds, the more the weight of vehicles (indicative of mass) and their contents, the more the energy that must be managed in crashes. Since more weight decreases fuel economy and increases braking distance, it would appear that weight reduction would decrease both injuries and fuel consumption. However, weight is an advantage to the occupants of the heavier vehicle in a two-vehicle collision, and in single-vehicle impacts, more weight may bend or break relatively fixed objects, such as smaller trees, that would otherwise compromise the integrity of passenger compartments. Two-car crash tests show far greater forces from reversed deceleration on the occupants of the lighter vehicle, i.e., the vehicle goes from forward to reverse movement in milliseconds.

Vehicle size provides space for air bags and seat belts to restrain occupants who move at precrash speed in a crash unless restrained. If the weight differential in the two-vehicle crash is large enough, the passenger compartment of the lighter vehicle may be penetrated, neutralizing the advantage of space (Insurance Institute for Highway Safety, 1972). In the past, most studies of weight and size used wheelbase—the distance from the front to rear axles of passenger vehicles—as the indicator of space (e.g., Robertson and Baker, 1976).

Vehicle wheelbase and weight are correlated—those with longer wheelbases tend to be heavier. Analysts in the 1970s noted that manufacturers could reduce fuel use without comprising safety by using materials that reduce vehicle weight without reducing size (O'Neill et al., 1974). Nevertheless, most of the vehicle manufacturers developed heavier sport utility vehicles (SUVs), promoted them as safer, and sold them at premium prices. Researchers have noted the severe consequences to occupants of cars (Gabler and Hollowell, 1998) and other road users struck by these heavier vehicles (Wenzel and Ross, 2005). Also, the weight of many of these vehicles is distributed higher from the ground than in passenger cars without compensating increase in distance between the centers of the tires (track width), increasing rollover death rates for occupants (Robertson, 1989). Risk to vehicle occupants in crashes is also related to crashworthiness—the extent to which the vehicle absorbs energy outside the passenger compartment and minimizes forces on vehicle occupants, particularly to the face and chest, where most fatal injuries occur.

The analysis reported here estimated the effects on fatalities of each of these factors controlling statistically for the effect of the others. The subject vehicles were 1999–2002 model passenger vehicles, including vans and SUVs, but excluding pickup trucks, during their first years of use through 2004. Pickup trucks were excluded as subject vehicles because of lack of data on sales by the substantial variation in weight and wheelbase within the same make and model. Driver deaths and all road user deaths that involved these vehicles were analyzed separately. All road users include drivers and other occupants of the subject vehicles and those in collisions with them. Pedestrians, bicyclists, and motorcyclists who died in collisions with the subject vehicles are also included because their risk may be increased by the longer stopping distances of heavier vehicles.

Fatalities throughout the United States that occurred within 30 days of a crash were obtained from FARS. Included in FARS are data on curb weight and wheelbase of the passenger vehicles as well as environmental conditions, and driver data such as age, gender, blood alcohol, and prior crash and violation records. Included were 1999–2000 model passenger vehicles in use during 2000–2004 used more than 200,000 years, collectively, during that period and for which data on stability were available (Walz, 2005). Collisions involving more than two vehicles were eliminated to minimize double counting. In two-vehicle collisions, deaths were assigned only to the vehicle in which they occurred. Pickup trucks were excluded as subject vehicles because of lack of data on sales by the substantial variation in weight and wheelbase within the same make-model. Where the subject vehicles collided with a truck and one or more occupants of either vehicle died, the cases were included. The data were available for 67 make-model combinations.

Years of use were calculated by multiplying the sales of a given make-model in a given month (Ward's Automotive Yearbook, 2000–2004) by the number of months remaining through 2004 and dividing the total by 12. A total of 14,438 deaths occurred to people as occupants or other road users in collisions of these vehicles during 104,970,000 years of use. There were 7,263 driver deaths in the vehicles, 50 percent of total deaths and 66 percent of deaths to occupants of the subject vehicles.

Lateral distance needed for a 180-degree turn, examined as an indicator of vehicle size, was less correlated with weight than was wheelbase (table 9-2, see http://www.internetautoguide.com, accessed August 2006, for vehicle parameters). The frontal, offset crash tests conducted by the Insurance Institute for Highway Safety (IIHS) were used to construct an index of crashworthiness. These tests are done at 40 miles per hour with a 40 percent overlap of the front of the vehicle in a crash with a fixed barrier (see http://www.hwysafety.org, accessed August 2006). The tests are thought to better simulate a common type of severe crash than the full-front barrier crashes at 35 miles per hour conducted by the U.S. government. The institute rates the vehicles on a 4-point scale on several factors. This study employed the scores on life-threatening factors: structural integrity, forces on the head and, separately, the chest of a test dummy, and performance of the restraint systems (seat belts and air bags) in restricting movement of the dummy. A summary measure was obtained by averaging the ratings (good = 1, acceptable = 2, marginal = 3, and poor = 4) among the four factors on each vehicle.

The correlations of the factors potentially predictive of fatalities and fuel economy are presented in table 9-2. Although squaring a correlation to get an accurate indicator of covariance cannot produce a negative number, the original sign on the correlation is indicated here to show direction of the correlation. The strongest correlation in the table is between weight and fuel economy. A multiple regression including the other factors indicated that weight is the only factor with a significant effect on fuel economy. Turn distance was strongly correlated with wheelbase but was less correlated with weight. Therefore, wheelbase was

Table 9-2. R^2 Among Potential Predictors of Fatalities

	Weight	Wheelbase	Turn Distance	T/2H	Crash Test	Van	SUV
Wheelbase	0.51						
Turn distance	0.43	0.50					
T/2H	0.16	0.01	0.01				
Crash test	0.01	0.01	0.00	0.18			
Van	0.12	0.18	0.07	0.00	0.02		
SUV	0.13	−0.06	−0.01	0.13	0.04	0.00	
Fuel economy	−0.68	−0.18	−0.18	0.31	−0.03	0.08	−0.33

eliminated from the analysis to minimize the effects of colinearity. None of the other correlations are worrisome in that regard.

The coefficients on log odds of driver deaths and all deaths in which given make-models were involved are shown in table 9-3, along with standard errors of the estimates (SEs). Because vans and SUVs are thought to be driven by less risky drivers, they each have their own coefficient in the analysis. Coefficients on passenger cars exclusive of sports car, vans, and SUVs are shown separately to illustrate that the effects are not the result of special characteristics of vans and SUVs, such as larger engines or four-wheel drive.

Increased vehicle weight is advantageous to the survival of drivers but adverse to other road users, as indicated by the negative coefficient for all road users. The coefficient on weight for drivers of passenger cars is not significant. Risk is lowered by higher stability ratios, longer turn distance, and "good" ratings on all four elements of crashworthiness. Vans and SUVs are less involved in fatalities when the other factors are controlled statistically. Notice that the coefficients on size, stability, crashworthiness, and type vehicle are higher for drivers' deaths than for all deaths, indicative of occupant protection, while weight contributes to deaths to other road users in collisions with heavier vehicles.

Least squares regression was used to estimate the potential for confounded effects. For example, if younger drivers more often drive smaller vehicles, some or all of the correlation of vehicle size and odds of death should be attributed to the factors that produce higher risk in driving by younger drivers. Since there are no data on the use of specific makes and models of vehicles in high- or low-risk environments or by high- or low-risk drivers, it is necessary to assess the potential for confounding indirectly from the crash data (Robertson and Kelley, 1989). If there is confounding of the effect of vehicle weight by age of driver, the ratio of older to younger drivers among the makes and models must be negatively correlated with the vehicles' weights. Therefore, the ratio of low to high risk of

Table 9-3. Log Odds of Driver Deaths and All Deaths in Relation to Vehicle Parameters

| | Cars, Vans, SUVs | | | | Passenger Cars | | | |
| | Driver | | All Deaths | | Driver | | All Deaths | |
	Effect	SE	Effect	SE	Effect	SE	Effect	SE
Intercept	−5.503	0.924	−7.763	0.615	−9.593	0.243	−9.613	0.177
Weight (100 lbs)	−0.013	0.004	0.012	0.003	0.001	0.004	0.023	0.003
Turn distance (ft)	−0.014	0.008	−0.011	0.005	−0.022	0.009	−0.019	0.006
Crash test	0.452	0.021	0.380	0.015	0.524	0.025	0.475	0.019
Average T/2H <1.2, else 1.2	−3.174	0.761	−1.410	0.504				
Van	−0.884	0.067	−0.644	0.040				
SUV	−0.455	0.061	−0.365	0.041				

Table 9-4. R^2 (R sign retained) of Vehicle Factors in Relation to Low to High Ratios of Other Risk Factors

	Curb Weight	Turn Distance	Stability (T/2H)	Crash Test Average	Van	SUV
Environmental						
Urban/rural	0.03	0.04	0.03	0.00	0.02	0.00
Interstate/other	0.01	0.03	–0.10	–0.07	0.00	0.01
On road/off road	0.06	0.06	0.01	–0.03	0.01	–0.07
3+ lanes/2-lane	0.00	–0.02	–0.02	0.00	0.01	0.00
Speed limit <55/55+	–0.01	0.12	0.00	0.00	0.06	–0.01
Straight/curve	0.11	0.00	–0.01	–0.06	0.06	0.00
Level/grade	0.03	0.07	0.04	0.06	0.27	–0.08
Concrete/blacktop	0.00	0.00	0.00	0.00	0.00	0.00
Dry/wet	0.06	0.22	–0.01	0.00	0.18	–0.01
Daylight/other	0.06	–0.03	0.00	0.00	0.00	0.03
Drivers						
Valid Lic./other	0.09	0.04	0.02	0.00	0.10	0.00
No prior crash/1+	0.09	0.04	0.03	–0.03	0.04	0.01
No suspension/1+	0.11	0.06	0.02	–0.02	0.08	0.00
No prior DWI/1+	0.00	0.00	0.02	0.02	0.00	0.01
No prior speed/1+	0.05	0.10	0.00	0.00	0.03	0.00
No conviction/1+	0.01	0.01	0.03	–0.02	0.05	0.00
No BAC/BAC	0.04	0.11	0.00	0.00	0.31	–0.06
No illegal alcohol/0.08+	0.00	0.00	0.00	0.00	0.00	0.00
25+/<25 years old	0.12	0.14	0.00	0.00	0.04	–0.01
Women/men	–0.09	–0.06	0.05	0.00	0.03	0.01

BAC, blood alcohol concentration; DWI, driving while impaired conviction.

10 major environmental factors and 10 major driver factors per vehicle was correlated to parameters of the vehicles to rule in or out the potential for confounding (table 9-4).

In most instances, there was no significant correlation among the ratio of low to high risk of the environmental and behavioral factors in relation to vehicle characteristics. Most of the few modest correlations of any significance were in the opposite direction from any indication of higher risk among the vehicles with higher risk characteristics. Higher risk among drivers of heavier and larger vehicles was indicated only by their more frequent use by male drivers. In the aggregate, the low correlations, and the reverse direction of most of the significant ones, suggest no confounding factor that would negate the findings that weight, size, stability, and crashworthiness are primary factors in vehicle mortality rates.

So, given the lack of confounding and the spiffy logistic regression coefficients in table 9-3, how does one estimate the percentage difference that could be accomplished by changing vehicle factors? If the parameters in the equation are changed, one at a time, to the parameter achieved by the best vehicles and the difference summed across vehicles, the number of fatalities that would have survived can be estimated. Consider the correlation of weight and turn distance in figure 9-2. The weights of vehicles increase approximately 156 pounds per foot

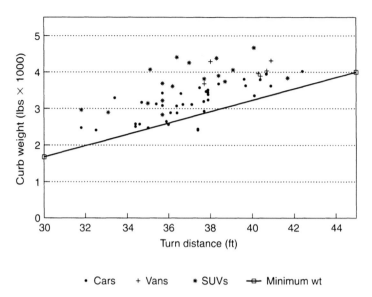

Cars   + Vans   * SUVs   —□— Minimum wt

Figure 9-2. Vehicle Weight by Turn Distance

increase in turn distance. A line drawn through the points along the bottom edge of the data indicates the minimum weight achieved by those vehicles at a given turn distance, described by the equation (156 × turn distance in feet) – 3000. Using the equation predicting odds of all deaths in table 9-3, the expected lives lost if weight was minimized was subtracted from the actual lives lost for each make-model combination, given the extant curb weight for each vehicle.

The equation $1/(1 + e^{-x})$, where x is the regression equation in table 9-3 [–7.7635 + 0.0124(weight) + 0.11(turn distance) – 0.38(crash worthiness) – 1.41($T/2H$) + 0.644(van) + 0.3652(SUV)] gives the predicted fatality rate for a given vehicle model. Multiplication of the rate times the years of use gives expected lives lost. If the minimum weight achievable, (56 × turn distance) – 3000, is substituted in the equation for weight, the expected lives lost at the minimum weight is estimated. The sum of the differences across vehicle models between actual deaths and expected deaths at minimum weight is 4,032, indicating that about 28 percent of the persons killed in collisions involving these vehicles during the years studied would have survived if the vehicles were at minimum weight for their turn radius. Of course, the total deaths over the life of these vehicles will be much larger.

Substitution of 1 for crashworthiness in the equation and calculating the differences due to that factor yields 3,604 (25 percent) of the deaths that would have been prevented if all of the vehicles received the top crashworthiness rating, based on the IIHS crash tests of these vehicles. Similarly, using the difference in gasoline mileage between actual and minimum weight achieved at a given turn distance, assuming 12,000 miles per vehicle per year, resulted in an estimated 16 percent reduction in fuel use, if the manufacturers had minimized weight per vehicle turn distance. Contrary to claims that more vehicle weight is safer, increased vehicle weight contributes to more deaths and more fuel use.

Substituting 1.2 for *T/2H* in the equation yields 415 (3 percent) deaths that would have been prevented if those vehicles with stabilities less than 1.2 had been 1.2 or above. The sum of the percentages of deaths that could have been prevented with decreased weight (25 percent), improved crashworthiness (28 percent), and better stability (3 percent) is 56 percent, substantially more than half. Not included in the study is electronic stability control technology that detects driver loss of control of vehicles and automatically corrects braking and steering. It has been shown repeatedly to reduce severe crashes substantially. One study of specific make-models of vehicles sold in the United States found a 42 percent reduction in fatal crashes of vehicles that had the equipment installed but no other major changes in the vehicles' characteristics (Farmer, 2006).

Size rather than weight may be the factor in certain off-road fatalities that are not counted in FARS. Research in the State of Washington found that more than a third of deaths where a child was killed when the vehicle backed over them occurred off the road, mainly backed over in driveways and parking lots. In about 76 percent of such cases, the vehicle was a truck, utility vehicle, or van, but in on-road pedestrian fatalities to children, the vast majority of the vehicles were cars (Brison et al., 1988). While the exact risk is not calculable from such a comparison, it is doubtful that children's exposure to vehicles being operated in reverse in driveways is substantially different between cars and trucks, vans, or utility vehicles in use on the road. It makes sense that the increased height of these vehicles decreases the ability of the drivers to see the area behind the vehicle when backing up. A subsequent case–control study of children struck in driveways falsely claimed that no studies of driveway injury had been done and ignored vehicles factors (Roberts et al., 1995). The study did note that a shared driveway among households increases the risk and that removal of play areas from driveways reduces the risk. A study of nonfatal as well as fatal injury found that severity of injury was greater when a child was backed over by a minivan, SUV, or pickup than by a car (Pinkney et al., 2006).

NOTE

A short version of this appendix was previously published in Robertson LS (2006) Blood and oil: vehicle characteristics in relation to fatality risk and fuel economy. *Am J Public Health*. 96:1906–1909.

References

Abramson JH (1985) Cross-sectional studies. In Holland WW, Detels R, and Knox G (eds.), *Oxford Textbook of Public Health. Vol. 3. Investigative Methods in Public Health.* Oxford, UK: Oxford University Press.

Armitage P (1971) *Statistical Methods in Medical Research.* New York, NY: John Wiley and Sons.

Blalock HM Jr (1964) *Causal Inferences in Nonexperimental Research.* Chapel Hill, NC: University of North Carolina Press.

Brison RJ, Wicklund K, and Mueller BA (1988) Fatal pedestrian injuries to young children: a different pattern of injury. *Am J Public Health*. 78:793–795.

Bunn F, DiGuiseppi CG, and Roberts I (2001) Systematic review of injury studies. In Rivara F, et al., (eds.), *Injury Control: A Guide to Research and Program Evaluation*. Cambridge, UK: Cambridge University Press.

Cummings SR, Kelsey JL, and Nevitt MC (1990) Methodologic issues in the study of frequent and recurrent health problems. *Ann Epidemiol.* 1:49–56.

Cummings SR, Nevitt MC, and Kidd S (1988) Forgetting falls. The limited accuracy of recall in the elderly. *J Am Geriatr Soc.* 36:613–616.

Donelson AC, Menich RP, Ray RM, and McCarthy RL (1994) Statistical analysis of vehicle rollover: causal modeling. *38th Annual Proceedings of the Association for the Advancement of Automotive Medicine*. Barrington, IL: Association for the Advancement of Automotive Medicine.

Elvik R, and Vaa T (2004) *The Handbook of Road Safety Measures*. Amsterdam: Elsevier.

Farmer CM (2006) Effects of Electronic Stability Control: An Update. *Traffic Injury Prevention.* 7:319–324.

Fleiss JL (1981) *Statistical Methods for Rates and Proportions*. 2nd ed. New York, NY: Wiley.

Fulgham R, et al. (1989) *A Case-Control Study of Road Features in Multiple-Vehicle Fatal Crashes* [mimeo]. Gallup, NM: Indian Health Service Hospital.

Gabler HC, and Hollowell WT (1998) *The Aggressivity of Light Trucks and Vans in Traffic Crashes*. Paper No. 980908. Warrendale, PA: Society of Automotive Engineers.

Goodman RA, Mercy JA, Layde PM, and Thacker SB (1988) Case–control studies: design issues for criminological applications. *J Quant Criminol.* 4:71–84.

Haddon W Jr, Valien P, McCarroll JR, and Umberger CJ (1961) A controlled investigation of adult pedestrians fatally injured by motor vehicles in Manhatten. *J Chronic Dis.* 14:655–678.

Hedlund JH (1984) Recent U.S. traffic fatality trends. In Evans L, and Schwing RC (eds.), *Human Behavior and Traffic Safety*. New York, NY: Plenum.

Hellevik O (1984) *Introduction to Causal Analysis*. London: George Allen and Unwin.

Insurance Institute for Highway Safety (1972) *Small Cars and Crashes* [film]. New York, NY: Harvest A-V.

Insurance Institute for Highway Safety (2006) Minicars. Status Report. 41:1–3, December 19.

Insurance Institute for Highway Safety (1980) Serious rollover problems found in Jeep CJ-5 utility vehicles. *Status Rep.* 15:1–4, December 22.

Joksch H (1983) Comments on the paper 'Rollovers and serious driver injury differences among various utility vehicles, pickup trucks, and passenger car groups.' *Q J Am Assoc Auto Med.* 5:35–43.

Kellerman AL, Rivara FP, Rushforth NB, Banton JG, Reay DT, Francisco JT, Locci AB, Prodzinski J, Hackman BB, and Somes G (1993) Gun ownership as a risk factor for homicide in the home. *New Engl J Med.* 329:1084–1119.

Leigh JP, and Waldon HM (1991) Unemployment and highway fatalities. *J Health Politics Policy Law.* 16:135–156.

Loomis DP (1991) Occupation, industry, and fatal motor vehicle crashes in 20 states, 1986–1987. *Am J Public Health.* 81:733–735.

Loomis TA, and West TC (1958) The influence of alcohol on automobile driving ability. *Q J Stud Alcohol.* 19:30–46.

Lum H, and Regan JA (1995) Interactive highway safety design model: accident predictive module. *Public Roads.* 58:14–17.

Lundquist EF (1953) *Design and Analysis of Experiments in Psychology and Education*. Boston, MA: Houghton Mifflin.

McCarroll JR, and Haddon W Jr (1962) A controlled study of fatal automobile accidents in New York City. *J Chronic Dis.* 15:811–826.

McGough H, and Wolf ME (2001) Ethical issues. In Rivara FP, et al. (eds.), *Injury Control: A Guide to Research and Program Evaluation*. Cambridge, UK: Cambridge University Press.

National Center for Health Statistics (1972) *Optimum Recall Period for Reporting Persons Injured in Motor Vehicle Accidents*. Rockville, MD: U.S. Department of Health, Education and Welfare.

Needleman HL, Gunnoe C, Leviton A, Reed R, Peresie H, Maher C, and Barrett P (1979) Deficits in psychologic and classroom performance of children with elevated dentine lead levels. *New Engl J Med*. 300:689–732.

O'Neill B, Joksch H, and Haddon W Jr (1974) Relationship between car size, car weight, and crash injuries in car-to-car crashes. In *Proceedings of the Third International Conference on Automotive Safety*. Washington, DC: U.S. Government Printing Office.

Oster G, Huse DM, Adams SF, Imbimbo J, and Russell MW (1990) Benzodiazepine tranquilizers and the risk of accidental injury. *Am J Public Health*. 80:1467–1470.

Pinkney KA, Smith A, Mann NC, Gary D, Davis A, and Dean JM (2006) Risk of pediatric back-over injuries in residential driveways by vehicle type. *Pediatr Emerg Care*. 22:402–407.

Redelmeier DA, and Tibshirani RJ (1997) Association between cellular-telephone calls and motor vehicle collisions. *New Engl J Med*. 336:453–458.

Regan JA (1994) The interactive highway safety design model: designing for safety by analyzing road geometrics. *Public Roads*. 58:17–43.

Riegelman RK (1981) *Studying a Study and Testing a Test*. Boston, MA: Little, Brown.

Roberts I, Norton R, and Jackson R (1995) Driveway-related child pedestrian injuries: a case–control study. *Pediatrics*. 95:405–408.

Robertson LS (1989) Risk of fatal rollover in utility vehicles relative to static stability. *Am J Public Health*. 79:300–303.

Robertson LS (2006) Blood and oil: vehicle characteristics in relation to fatality risk and fuel economy. *Am J Public Health*.96:1906–1909.

Robertson LS, and Baker SP (1976) Motor vehicle sizes in 1440 fatal crashes. *Accid Anal Prev*. 8:167–175.

Robertson LS, and Kelley AB (1989) Static stability as a predictor of overturn in fatal motor vehicle crashes. *J Trauma*. 29:313–319.

Robertson LS, and Maloney A (1997) Motor vehicle rollover and static stability: an exposure study. *Am J Public Health*. 87:839–841.

Robinson WS (1950) Ecological correlation and the behavior of individuals. *Am Soc Rev*. 15:351–357.

Snyder RG, McDole TL, Ladd WM, and Minahan DJ (1980) *On-Road Crash Experience of Utility Vehicles*. Ann Arbor, MI: University of Michigan Highway Safety Research Institute.

Stein HS, and Jones IS (1988) Crash involvement of large trucks by configuration: a case–control study. *Am J Public Health*. 78:491–498.

Violanti JM, and Marshall JR (1996) Cellular phones and traffic accidents: an epidemiological approach. *Accid Anal Prev*. 28:265–270.

Walz MC (2005) *Trends in the Static Stability Factor of Passenger Cars, Light Trucks, and Vans*. Washington, DC: National Highway Traffic Safety Administration.

Ward's Automotive Yearbook (2000–2004) Southfield, MI: Ward's Communications.

Wechsler H, Kasey EH, Thum D, and Demone HW Jr (1969) Alcohol level and home accidents. *Public Health Rep*. 84:1043–1050.

Wenzel T, and Ross M (2005) The effects of vehicle model and driver behavior on risk. *Accid Anal Prev*. 37:479–494.

Wintemute GJ, Kraus JF, Teret SP, and Wright M (1990) Death resulting from motor vehicle immersions: the nature of the injuries, personal and environmental contributing factors, and potential interventions. *Am J Public Health.* 80:1068–1070.

Wright PH, and Robertson LS (1976) Priorities for roadside hazard modification: a study of 300 fatal roadside object crashes. *Traffic Eng.* 46:24–30.

Zador PL, Stein HS, Hall JW, and Wright PH (1987) Relationships between vertical and horizontal roadway alignments and the incidence of fatal rollover crashes in New Mexico and Georgia. *Transport Res Rec.* 1111:27–42.

10

Human Factors

Most people who are injured are doing something at the time—driving, riding in a vehicle, walking, working, or playing. So are people who are infected by micro-organisms, but those who study injury place more emphasis on behavior than do those who study most infectious diseases. Notable exceptions are infectious diseases transmitted by sex. Ironically, sexual behavior in moving vehicles has been neglected as a topic for research.

Historically, manufacturers of injurious products emphasized behavior of the injured to divert attention from the products (Eastman, 1984). Despite the evidence that changes in vehicle crashworthiness accounted for most of the major reductions in car occupant fatalities per mile during the last third of the twentieth century (chapter 13), employees of General Motors have continued to argue that the major emphasis in injury control should be on behavior (Evans, 1996, 2004; Evans and Schwing, 1985). In the mid 1990s, the head of the National Highway Traffic Safety Administration (NHTSA), who has legal responsibility for vehicle safety, joined the industry chorus (Frame, 1996).

The argument for behavioral causation is convenient for the industry and its apologists, particularly when industry negligence is alleged (appendix 10-1). Despite the claims of industry spin doctors and their apologists in government, injury control has never been a simple choice of changing agents and vehicles of injury versus changing behavior. The issue is what factors can be changed to reduce harm, and how much injury reduction can be achieved by deliberate attempts at changing the factors. Certainly not all injuries are preventable by vehicle or environmental modifications, and behavioral change can be accomplished to some extent. To do so will require a better scientific understanding of behaviors that are modifiable.

BEHAVIORAL THEORIES

Behavior change strategies would be easier to construct if behavioral and social scientists could agree on human behaviors that are changeable. For example, historical arguments regarding the best approaches to crime prevention turned on the issue of the extent to which behavior is modifiable at what stages of development (Tremblay and Craig, 1995).

The operant conditioning model prevalent among experimental psychologists portrays human beings as trainable by reward and punishment to do virtually anything, and often ignores biological limitations, as well as cognitions that intervene between the input of rewards and punishments and the output in behavior. The neoclassic economic model, and that of some cognitive psychologists, views human beings as rational "utility" (goal) optimizers. There is also little room for human physical or psychological limitations in this model, but rather than being mainly responsive to external stimuli as in the operant conditioning model, each person weighs each option for behavior as to its probability for accomplishing or experiencing a utility, and discounts the cost in terms of the time between the immediate situation and the ultimate goal. The origin of the "utilities" is often obscure in such theories.

Many sociologists view behavior as largely determined by the internalized cultural and social environment, including learned social customs and mores, socioeconomic status, and peer pressure. Socio- and psychobiologists emphasize the effects of genetics on the biological factors that contribute to motivations such as rivalry, emotions such as rage, cognitive limitations, and neuronal-motor function. Certain psychologists and psychiatrists look for the major motivations for behavior in the unconscious mind, largely determined by relationships with parents or guardians in infancy and early childhood.

Devotees to any one of these approaches may object to the oversimplification in a one-sentence description of what are often very complex and detailed theories. Also, the list is by no means exhaustive. There are numerous eclectic mixtures.

Each of the theories may have some merit for subsets of a population engaged in a given activity at a given time. Human beings are very complicated, and at any one time in the course of a lifetime, several of the factors emphasized by the various schools of thought may influence the behavior of the moment. Therefore, it is not surprising that behavioral and social scientists who have attempted to apply their disparate theories to behaviors that increase or decrease probability of injury have found one or more of their hypotheses supported to some degree by data. In many such instances, the hypothesis has some predictive value, but in others the research "results" are artifacts of research design or invalid assumptions about the data or its interpretation. The usefulness of the valid biological, psychological, economic, and social predictors of injury depends on the strength of the correlations and the extent to which the factors are subject to change by intervention.

DEVELOPMENTAL STAGES IN CHILDHOOD

Not only do the causal models of different schools of thought look quite different, but also the relative strength of a given causal path in any causal model of injury must differ dramatically depending on the stage of development of the individual (Kane, 1985). Age is a proxy for a mix of the factors emphasized in behavioral theories as well as differential vulnerability of tissue to energy insults, and the probability of being in situations where energy exchanges are more or less likely.

During 1976–1977 in the United States, the motor-vehicle-occupant death rate per population of infants younger than one year was twice that of 1-year-olds but less than that of 2-year-olds. The rate declined as children grew older, until age 6, where it leveled, and the rate among 6- to 12-year-olds was about a third that of infants (Baker, 1979). Does this mean that parents were conditioned to love their children more and take better care of them as they grew? Do children increase in utility as they develop? Are the social and economic pressures on new parents so severe that their driving ability deteriorates enormously? Do some new parents have a subconscious hate for their newborn that manifests in driving behavior, endangering themselves as well as the infant?

Perhaps a few of the behavioral and social scientists extremely dedicated to their respective theories would view such hypotheses as worthy of research, but scientists aware of anatomy and physics considered other hypotheses. The tissues of infants are less tolerant of energy insults, and certain positions in the vehicles increase the mechanical forces on them in crashes. Using formula 2.1 describing kinetic energy, it can be shown that an unrestrained 10-pound baby becomes a 300-pound flying object in a 30-mph crash. Furthermore, when placed in the lap of an adult, an infant in a frontal crash will be crushed between the interior front structures of the vehicle and the similarly multiplied weight of an unrestrained adult attempting to hold the infant.

Social and behavioral factors undoubtedly affect the transportation of children in particular types of vehicles, their seating arrangement in the vehicles, and whether or not they are restrained. Children may also distract drivers, but probably no more at 1 than at 6 years of age. The relative effects of these factors on injury rates have not been studied in sufficient detail to weight them as contributors to injury.

During 1980–1984 in the United States, vehicle occupant death rates of children younger than 1 year declined 37 percent, and those of 1- to 4-year-olds declined 25 percent, as child restraint use laws were adopted (Robertson, 1989). These reductions were associated with increases in observed child restraint use in urban environments, which increased from less than 10 percent (Williams, 1976) to 49 percent (National Highway Traffic Safety Administration, 1989). Children seated in the front seat in vehicles in fatal crashes declined from 42 to 31 percent in the 1990s in association with publicized warnings regarding the danger of passenger airbags to out-of-position children in front seats (Wittenberg et al., 2001).

Child development may be modified by brain damage associated with low birth weight, in-utero alcohol and drug exposure, serotonin deficiency, or head trauma in childhood. Such factors have been associated with later violent behavior that led a National Research Council panel on violence to recommend longitudinal studies to better delineate their potential effects (Reiss and Roth, 1993). Assaults on children are strongly correlated with the presence of adults other than biological parents in the household (Reading, 2006).

As children develop motor skills, they become more active. For a time, the motor skills develop more rapidly than do perceptual and cognitive skills. Children's injuries reflect the hazards in the environments in which they are placed or find themselves, and the behaviors that expose them to energy exchanges, as well as changing tissue vulnerabilities (Rivara, 1982a). They roll, and later crawl, off beds and other elevated surfaces. Their heads are larger than their bodies, and hanging sometimes asphyxiates those that squeeze their bodies between crib slats. Children attempt to swallow foods and other objects that are of a size to block respiration when lodged in the trachea. Toxic chemicals and plants are also swallowed. They wander into swimming pools, hot tubs, and spas. They touch hot surfaces, pull over containers of hot liquids, and are placed in, or turn on, overheated water.

At given points in development, children apparently learn to largely avoid certain hazards to which they remain exposed in their environments. Head injuries associated with stairs and window or door glass decline by half from age 2 to 3, and those associated with furniture and other household fixtures decline rapidly after ages 6–7 (Rivara, 1982b). At ages 4–9, children playing with matches and lighters start fires, disproportionate to their numbers in the population at that age (Cole et al., 1986). As they develop the ability to run, climb, and operate vehicles such as tricycles, bicycles, guns, skateboards, and motorized vehicles, children's involvement in injuries associated with these activities increase.

A variety of research questions have been raised by these injury distributions (Rivara, 1982a). To what extent does differential understanding of developmental stages by parents account for their children's exposure to hazards? If there are differences in knowledge, does giving information to the less informed result in reduced exposures and injuries? What are the capabilities of children relative to proposed countermeasures? For example, if fencing is the option chosen to reduce children's access to swimming pools, what types of fences can children breach (Rabinovich et al., 1994)? To know how to modify firearms to prevent child use, what is the limit of children's ability to pull the trigger of extant firearms (Naureckas et al., 1995)?

The age differences in injuries vary by gender in some cases and not in others. Are the differences in males and females learned, biological, or some combination of the two? What other characteristics of children, if any, are predictive of injury given similar exposure to hazards? Are such characteristics short-lived, or do they persist through several developmental stages? How does one distinguish cases of unintentional injury and child abuse (Kemp et al., 1994)? Are any of the predictive characteristics modifiable, and do attempts at modification result in reduced injury? One review of attempts to reduce antisocial behavior in children indicates that early interventions with prospective and new parents are more effective than later school-based approaches (Tremblay and Craig, 1995). Nevertheless, school and afterschool programs have been shown experimentally to reduce aggressive behavior as rated by teachers and parents (Hudley, 2003).

Less often considered are questions regarding stimuli generated outside the home. What influence does advertising have on decisions to purchase hazardous products? How much of such influence is exerted through programs and commercials directed at children? How many hazardous products are received as gifts and from whom? How often do the injuries associated with hazardous products occur from products that belong to neighbors, friends, relatives, and others outside the home?

The references cited above indicate that epidemiologists and others interested in children's injuries have attempted to answer a few of the questions using a variety of methodological approaches. This is not the place for an exhaustive literature review, which should be undertaken before attempting new research.

ADOLESCENTS AND YOUNG ADULTS

The most severe injuries to teenagers and young adults occur in motor vehicles and assaults, particularly assaults on self or others with guns in the United States (Baker et al., 1992). Males are substantially more involved than females as drivers and assailants, and whites are more often killed in motor vehicles and suicides, while blacks are more often killed in assaults. Females are often involved as "straw purchasers" of guns for males with criminal records, and dealers are willing to sell, in some cases even if they know the eventual recipient cannot legally own the gun (Sorenson and Vittes, 2003).

Again, behavioral theories contain all sorts of hypotheses as potential explanations, but the research in support of many of them is inadequate or nonexistent. Adolescence and young adulthood are periods of accelerated separation from parental influence, sexual maturity and establishment of sexual relationships, struggle for economic independence, and adaptation to changing expectations from peers and adults (Gilula and Daniels, 1969). Terms such as inexperience, risk taking, sensation seeking, impulsiveness, and alcohol and drug "abuse" are used to describe the behaviors of adolescents and young adults that may contribute to injury.

One study in Canada found that motor vehicle crash rates of newly licensed drivers at ages 17, 18, and 19 were similar to those of drivers of the same age who had been licensed one, two, or three years (Pierce, 1977). Therefore, driving experience did not seem to be a major factor in the substantial decline in crash rates from age 16 to 19. A study of Michigan drivers found the opposite among 18- to 20-year-olds. Those with two years of driving experience had lower crash rates than did those with one year of experience, but the age effect persisted in addition to experience. Younger teenage drivers with the same experience as older drivers had higher crash rates (Eby, 1995). In such studies of nonfatal crashes based on police reports, differences in reporting crashes to police, which can be a function of insurance rating and other factors, may bias the results. A study of prior driver experience of licensed drivers in fatal crashes compared to a sample of same-age licensed drivers would be more convincing. A case–control study of motorcyclists where the cases were identified from hospital emergency department cases and coroners indicated little effect of riding experience, but familiarity with the motorcycle made some difference (Mullin et al., 2000).

The term "risk taker" implies that the person knows the risk and deliberately behaves in such a way as to increase risk to self. Certainly some suicide attempts and assaults are the result of deliberate choices, but the extent to which perception of risk is actually associated with various types of risky behavior is unknown. The involvement of alcohol, other drugs, and mental illness in many cases of presumed deliberate assaults on self and others raises doubt about the preinjury state of mind of the persons affected by these factors (Graham, 2003). The hypothesis that risk denial or belief in personal invulnerability is a factor is at least as plausible as the "risk-taker" hypothesis. Studies of perceived risk in motor vehicles indicate that younger drivers more often think their peers at higher risk than themselves, compared to such perceptions among older drivers (Bragg and Finn, 1982; Matthews and Moran, 1986), yet the authors of those studies persisted in calling the risk-denying young drivers "risk takers."

Motor vehicle injuries are common enough in the adolescent years such that prospective cohort studies could be undertaken to measure the extent to which knowledge of risk, beliefs about personal vulnerability; impulsiveness; mental illness; conflicts with parents, lovers, or peers; challenges from peers; and economic difficulties are predictive of being a driver in a crash-causing injury. Becoming the assailant or the injured in an assault may be subject to study by similar methods, although identification of cases not reported to police would be difficult given the potential for reluctance to report involvement.

Unwarranted conclusions have been drawn from the examination of patients after injury and inference of preinjury psychopathology. For example, one study of patients in a trauma center, excluding two-thirds (those with a Glasgow Coma Score less than 15 as well as children younger than 18 and those receiving narcotics for pain), claimed that the patients had higher than normal "preinjury psychopathology." The measure of "psychopathology" consisted of a questionnaire with items such as "I feel isolated" and "I have low/very low spirits" (Whetsall et al., 1989). The questionnaire was administered to people in a hospital after trauma who were unlikely to be in high spirits, so it should have been obvious to the researchers that these are not necessarily measures of prehospital states of mind. No attempt was made to correlate the responses to the behavior of the respondents at the time of injury, that is, whether the respondents' behavior contributed to the injury. Prospective studies of questionnaire measures of psychological traits and car crashes do not indicate a correlation (e.g., Schuster and Guilford, 1964), but temporary psychological states are not captured by such methods (Robertson, 1983).

The literature on assaults and homicides is limited mainly to descriptive studies. Some correlations among relationship of assailant and victim, weapon if any, and biological, psychological, social, and demographic characteristics have been reported, but there is substantial disagreement regarding causation, partly resulting from numerous methodological issues (Rosenberg et al., 1986). Characteristics of assailants and interactions among couples in domestic assaults have been described (Shupe et al., 1987), but no data were collected on couples not involved, so whether the alleged causal factors were less prevalent in those who do not have such problems is not known.

Race is emphasized in many studies of homicide because of the very high rates among young black males. Studies of domestic homicide indicate, however, that the correlation with race disappears when household crowding is controlled statistically (Centerwell, 1995). When mostly black juveniles with single parents are moved from poverty neighborhoods to more middle-class environments in random housing assignments, their assault and other crime rates plunge (Ludwig et al., 2001). It is the socioeconomic consequences of the way races have been treated historically and the criminal cultures that have historically accompanied poverty among a variety of ethnic groups that explains the differences in violence, not the genetics of race. In some cases, poverty is mitigated by cultural factors. It has been claimed that recent Mexican immigrants to the United States have substantially lower involvement in violence than would be expected from their economic status (Sampson et al., 2005), but the claims are based on self-reports, which are less reliable than counts of fatal cases. Some immigrants to the United States apparently adapt to the gun culture quickly. Although suicide rates are lower, homicides rates are higher among many immigrant groups than among their native counterparts of similar ethnic origin (Sorenson and Shen, 1999).

Aggression has been studied extensively in controlled laboratory experiments under a wide variety of experimental conditions (Mattson, 2003; Siegel, 2005). The relevance of these studies to assaults in homes, streets, and bars, or to aggressive driving, is open to debate. One well-designed study of alcohol and aggression in college students, for example, randomly divided the students into four groups: (1) alcohol and threatened, (2) alcohol and not threatened, (3) placebo and threatened, and (4) placebo and not threatened. Strong flavoring masked the alcohol and placebo. The subjects were placed in a situation where they were supposedly competing with a person in another room on a reaction-time task in which each subject could deliver an electric shock to the other. The situation was presumed as threatening, but those in the "nonthreatened" condition heard their "opponent" object to hurting someone. There was no difference in intensity of shock delivered to "opponents" between those with and without alcohol in the nonthreatened groups. Those in the threatened group delivered more intense shocks to their "opponents" and, if they had also consumed alcohol, they delivered very strong shocks to their "opponents" (Taylor et al., 1976).

Given knowledge of such results, an injury epidemiologist wants to know how much of the variation in assaults can be explained by alcohol and threatening situations. How does a researcher obtain unbiased samples of assailants and potential assailants in which alcohol can be measured? What constitutes a threat? Is there a relatively small set of threats that can be identified in large numbers of assault cases? Is the assault directed toward someone perceived as threatening or a scapegoat such as a child, spouse, or lover?

If the set of factors that are threatening to persons who are potential assailants were limited to a few, such as unemployment or fear of unemployment, harassment by peers, and degradation of self-esteem by spouses or lovers, then it may be possible to find ways to help people cope with such threats. If the threats are so diverse that none accounts for a substantial part of the problem, then the probable success of changing threats to reduce assault is diminished.

Among the most publicized claims about causation of spouse and child battering is that the batterer was abused as a child. While being abused as a child may increase the risk of becoming an abusing adult, the majority of abusers were not abused as children (Rosenberg et al., 1986). Therefore, as desirable as reduction in child abuse would be, it would not reduce battering in the next generation as much as the publicized claims would have us believe.

Intimate partner homicide is substantially related to mental illness (Farooque et al., 2005). One way of studying these issues in a population would be to identify from police records a sample of households that had one or more domestic disputes reported within the past year. Controls for comparison could be selected by identifying residents of other households in the same block and randomly choosing one or more that had no domestic disputes reported to police in the past year. Interviews with family members, preferably augmented by validity checks where possible, such as employment history, might reveal a set of threats, mental illness, or other factors that, separately or in combination with alcohol, are amenable to change. Self-reports of violent sexual aggression did not involve alcohol use disproportionately but did involve refusal to use alcohol by the victim (Racket et al., 2004).

The advantage of using police-reported cases is the potential for obtaining objective data on alcohol. A small pilot study could be undertaken to see whether cases and controls would cooperate with a request for breath alcohol, with the controls tested at the same time of day and day of week as the dispute was reported in the cases.

The study design would be subject to criticism because it would not identify the set of battered women and children that do not come to the attention of police. Protocols for identifying such cases have been developed (Stark et al., 1981), and researchers with clinical affiliations should be able to identify many such cases in that setting, but objective measurement of alcohol in the batterer in those circumstances probably would not be feasible. Great care must be exercised in such research to avoid placing the battered person at greater jeopardy for having revealed the batterer, however inadvertently.

Descriptive studies of suicides of teenagers and young adults indicate clusters of types of problems (legal, interpersonal, history of mental illness), method used (firearm, hanging, drugs, gas), and age group (Gerberich et al., 1985). Case–control studies, such as the Houston study described by Silverman and Simon (2001), are needed to determine which from among the identified factors are risk factors or can be used to identify persons at higher risk. One such finding from the Houston study is that attempters had changed residence more often than controls within the last 12 months. Another design would select cases from each cluster and controls with similar problems to reveal the extent to which suicides within a given cluster are correlated to the misfit of personality and social environment, availability of method used, and other variables in theories of suicide.

Little research has been conducted on attempts to change exposure to potential injury hazards by offering programs to youth that keep them from hazardous environments. In the United States, programs to open schools and other facilities for "midnight basketball" for low-income youth were treated as a joke by political opponents of any government involvement, rather than taken seriously as a program to be studied. Claims of success based on simple trends in crime rates in cities that have the programs are inadequate. Controls on changes in other factors, such as influx of Mexican immigrants, are needed to rule out those factors as explanations. In Brazil, some 370 programs to engage so-called "street children" in productive activities were initiated, but the effect on injuries and other problems of these children has apparently not been evaluated (Berger and Mohan, 1996).

A neglected area of research in adolescent and young adult injuries is the extent of recruitment to danger. To what extent is the use of cars and guns in hazardous ways a function of nightly doses of television portrayals of such behavior? To what extent do organized clubs for hazardous activities recruit new participants? What is the involvement of the industries that sell equipment for hazardous activities (e.g., hang gliding, scuba diving, sky diving, motorcycling, gun use, fast cars) involved in promoting the activity through clubs and magazines? How many of the injured were led to the activity by such promotion?

ADULTHOOD

In the middle years of life, injury rates are lower for most types of injuries. Injuries to workers in certain occupations are major exceptions (Baker et al., 1992). The generally lower injuries in the middle years of life could result partly from greater knowledge of risks and partly from changes in exposure, such as reduced driving at night and reduced "partying" on weekends.

The effect of knowledge seems limited. Denial of risks is not confined to teenagers and young adults. After presenting the risks of gassing, hand burns, and child poisonings from household cleansers to a sample of consumers, they were asked how much more or less likely than average such injuries were in their homes. Only 2–3 percent said more likely, and 40–65 percent said less likely (Viscusi and Magat, 1987). These results are similar to those obtained when a random sample of new-car buyers were asked whether their chances of being injured or killed in a car crash were greater than, the same as, or less than "people like yourself." Six percent said greater and 40 percent said less (Robertson, 1977). Whether the less extreme deniers are at more or less actual risk than the more extreme deniers has apparently not been studied.

Race and gender differences that persist in particular types of injury rates during middle age are often cited, but race and gender are no more modifiable than age. They are of interest only as identifiers of groups in which causal factors differ in kind or magnitude or as identifiers for targeting programs to modify risk factors.

Too often, conclusions about race and gender are based on stereotypes. When the author told colleagues he was reviewing the literature on injuries to Native Americans in the 1980s, virtually every one stated with conviction that alcohol accounted for the higher injury rates in that population.

The literature indicated that, while alcohol is a problem among several Native American groups, it probably does not account for nearly the variation in injury rates that stereotypical thinking suggests. The only study found in which blood alcohol was measured among injured Native Americans indicated that more Native Americans were tested in the same jurisdiction relative to whites, 63 percent versus 45 percent (Westermeyer and Brantner, 1972). Therefore, the involvement of alcohol measured objectively was not available in a sample without potential selection bias. A study of Native Americans and others in fatal motor vehicle crashes in Arizona relied on invalid police reports for the majority of assessments of alcohol in Native Americans (Campos-Outcalt et al., 1997). Although the article claimed that there was no difference in the proportion chemically tested for alcohol concentration, recalculation of the numbers in the article indicates that 33 percent of Native Americans were tested and 56 percent of others were tested. If the police were more oriented to expecting alcohol in Native Americans, the estimate of alcohol involvement would be biased.

Comparison of different groups of Native Americans in Oklahoma found that the rate of deaths attributed to "alcoholism," cirrhosis, or alcohol poisoning was 29 times higher in the group with the highest rates relative to the group with the lowest rates. (Stratton et al., 1978). Age-adjusted alcoholism death rates among Native Americans declined about 40 percent in the early 1980s (Howard et al., 2000). Self-reported total abstinence from alcohol is twice as high among Native Americans as among whites. In groups where intoxication is frowned upon, drinking is done alone and in secret. In groups with a tradition of the seeking of visions and endurance dancing, heavy alcohol consumption in public is more acceptable, particularly among young males (Levy and Kunitz, 1974; Kunitz, 1976; May, 1982). The stereotype apparently evolved from historical accounts of "Indians and firewater" and the very noticeable public drinking in certain groups, particularly in towns near reservations.

The social factors that influence if, when, and where drinking occurs undoubtedly influence the risk of particular types of injuries, such as the high rate of deaths from cold and exposure among Native Americans in New Mexico (Sewell et al., 1989). Prior to declines associated with injury control programs for Native Americans (Smith and Robertson, 2000), Native Americans had more than twice the injury death rates of the U.S. population as a whole. If one compares total injury death rates of Native Americans with those of rural isolated populations generally, however, the differences were small (Robertson, 1985).

Among U.S. Navy personnel, Native Americans were hospitalized for "alcoholism" three time more often per capita than whites or blacks, yet their hospitalizations for injury per capita were 13 percent less than those for whites and blacks (Hoiberg et al., 1981). Injury rates are similar among races whose living and working conditions are similar. The major explanations for racial differences in injury rates are more likely to be found in the vehicles and environments to which they are exposed rather than in biological and personality theories, or racial stereotypes.

The extent to which gender differences in injury rates can be attributed to biological factors, social factors, or interaction among biological and social factors probably differs by type of injury. Women are usually at less risk of most types of injuries as teenagers and adults, but there are exceptions. In domestic violence that does not involve weapons, women often strike men as well as vice versa, but the severe injuries from violence in homes are most often to women and children (Rosenberg et al., 1986), probably because men are physically stronger, on average, than women and children. Most of the studies of dominance behavior, hormones, alcohol, and other potential factors in aggressive behavior have not included women (Mazur and Robertson, 1972).

Combat veterans have higher injury rates than do other military veterans. Various hypotheses have been advanced to explain this finding, but none have been tested adequately (Bell et al., 2001).

GROWING OLD

Severe injury rates tend to increase among the elderly for several types of injury (Rice and MacKenzie, 1989). Although some exposures are decreased among the elderly (e.g., miles driven, driving at night), and injury incidence is lower, when injury does occur, the consequences in length of hospital stays and mortality are more severe. Decreases in visual acuity, hearing, and mental alertness, as well as multiple prescription drug use, probably increase risk of incidence, but reduced exposure to driving, industrial machines, and farm equipment probably results in lower incidence. Certain exposures, such as use of stairs or walking on other surfaces that are conducive to falls, are not changed or may even increase after retirement. The elderly have particularly high injury rates from falls. In social environments where the young prey on or abuse the elderly, they are the victims of assault, and some resort to suicide to escape social circumstances or physical debilitation that they are no longer willing to tolerate.

Elderly people suffer various types of losses, including friends, spouse, occasionally a child, job, status, income, power, self-esteem, self-confidence, hearing, sight, other aspects of personal control or competence, and health, all of which are thought to contribute to suicide (Osgood, 1985). In a case–control study in Sweden, suicide risk was substantially higher in persons with visual impairment, neurological disorders, and malignancies (Waern et al., 2002). Many among the elderly support the availability of physician-assisted suicide for the terminally ill, such as that allowed by law in Oregon. Combined homicide–suicide among the elderly, where the involvement of guns predominates, has also been studied by case–control methods (Malphurs and Cohen, 2005).

The exact contribution of exposure to energy exchanges by degree of energy generated versus tissue vulnerability to particular types of injury among the elderly has not been specified. Certainly the elderly person injured with the same degree of severity as a younger person is more likely to die than the younger person (Baker et al., 1974).

Attention to risk of falls in the elderly has increased. Among the factors related to falls potentially amenable to change are leg extension strength and gait (Graafmans et al., 1996; Tinetti et al., 1995a) and modifiable environmental factors, such as characteristics of stairs (Tinetti et al., 1995b), which have been found markedly different between the homes of fallers and controls (Locklear, 1991). Studies of falls refer to relative strong correlates (multiple pharmaceutical use, visual acuity, and fear of falling) as "predictors" (Delbaere et al., 2006) but do not consider how many false positives and false negatives occur in such predictions. That information is important to apply countermeasures efficiently.

POSTTRAUMA BEHAVIOR

A much neglected area of research is the effect of trauma on subsequent behavior. Obviously, the lives of persons with noncorrected disabilities are changed—drastically in the case of severe spinal cord and brain injury. Documentation of the extent of these effects is important to understand the total, often nonquantifiable, costs of injury.

Other effects of injury may be subtler or not appear immediately. How many people change their behavior as a result of injury? What is the effect on subsequent fear and anxiety of trauma to oneself or to relatives and friends? To what extent does neighborhood violence change the behavior patterns of people in the neighborhood? Does fear of falling result in less mobility among the elderly (Tinetti et al., 1994), further contributing to the risk? Does subtle brain injury contribute to intellectual or emotional deficits, or increase risk of brain diseases such as Alzheimer's disease and epilepsy?

Some of these questions raise thorny methodological issues. To the extent that the hypothesized effect of trauma could also contribute to the incidence, posttrauma measurement may overstate the effect of trauma. For example, one research project measured intelligence quotients of persons who had been injured and correlated them to the injured persons' scores on the Glascow Coma Scale and the Injury Severity Score. Persons who were more severely injured had lower IQs (Gensemer et al., 1989). However, if lower IQ contributes to the probability of severe injury, the inference of a causal effect of trauma on IQ would be overstated. A correlation of lower precrash IQs (measured at army induction) and fatal motor vehicle injury has been found (O'Toole, 1990).

Where preinjury measures are available, such as IQ scores from school, military, or other records, researchers interested in posttrauma effects should attempt to obtain the records. Where such measures are not available, the IQ of a sample of siblings or childhood friends of the injured could be used for comparison. To the extent that IQ is predictive, the issue of limits to modifiability of IQ is relevant to prevention.

Case–control studies of Alzheimer's disease consistently find a history of head trauma more frequent in persons with the disease—24 percent of cases and 8 percent of genetically unrelated relatives and friends matched by gender and approximate age in one study (Graves et al., 1990). The odds ratios were higher for those whose head injury did not result in loss of consciousness and among those with more recent head trauma. Although there are reasonable biological explanations for head trauma contributing to the disease, and although the average period between the head trauma and onset of symptoms minus one year was long—21.3 years for cases—it is not possible to exclude the disease or some correlate of the disease as a precursor to trauma rather than exclusively a posttrauma effect. It would be useful to compare cases in which the behavior of the person did or did not contribute to the injury, but recall of spouses or others regarding long past incidents is a major methodological problem.

APPENDIX 10-1

Truck Fires—Behavior and Vehicle Factors

In its 1973–1987 C/K pickup trucks, General Motors chose to place fuel tanks on the sides outside the frame of the vehicle next to external sheet metal to increase fuel capacity relative to competitive trucks. Other manufacturers placed the tank within the frame. The issue of risk of fire in GM pickups was publicized in 1992 when a family whose son died in a GM truck fire sued GM and demanded a trial rather than accept a private settlement from the company (Applebome, 1993).

The Center for Auto Safety petitioned the NHTSA to recall the vehicles based in part on data indicating higher fatal fire rates in GM pickups compared to similar-sized Ford pickups during 1981–1986. General Motors hired a consulting firm that claimed the GM trucks posed no unreasonable risk because some small cars and trucks had a higher fire risk, although its data clearly indicated a higher fatal fire rate in GM pickups compared to similar-sized pickups (Lange et al., 1992). General Motors later retracted the claim that its pickups had a lower overall fatality rate than Ford's pickups—admitting that the total occupant fatality rate in GM C/K pickups was actually higher than Ford's of similar size (Meier, 1992).

Then GM turned that argument on its head. In a submission to NHTSA, GM argued that its trucks have higher fatal fire rates because "more aggressive" drivers drove them (General Motors Corporation, 1993). In 1988, GM introduced a redesigned pickup truck with the gasoline tank inside the frame. Comparison of GM and Ford full-sized pickups (table 10-1) indicates that, when all fatal crashes, not

Table 10-1. Fatal Crash per Million per Year of 1981–1991 GM and Ford Pickup Trucks in Calendar Years 1981–1992

	Model Years							
	1981–1987				1988–1991			
	GM		Ford		GM		Ford	
	N	Rate	N	Rate	N	Rate	N	Rate
Fire most harm								
Vehicles	139	5.1	85	3.4	23	3.2	26	4.2
Occupant deaths	164	6.0	104	4.2	29	4.1	32	5.2
All fires								
Vehicles	389	14.2	265	10.6	66	9.3	66	10.8
Occupant deaths	400	14.6	245	9.8	71	10.0	76	12.4
Nonfire								
Vehicles	9,209	336.1	8,376	336.0	2,831	398.7	2,241	65.8
Occupant deaths	4,699	171.5	3,595	144.2	1,468	206.8	892	145.6

Table 10-2. Fatal Fire Rates in Side Impacts per Million per Year of 1981–1991 GM and Ford
Pickup Trucks in Calendar Years 1981–1992

	Model Years							
	1981–1987				1988–1991			
	GM		Ford		GM		Ford	
	N	Rate	N	Rate	N	Rate	N	Rate
Fire most harm								
Vehicles	36	1.3	11	0.4	2	0.3	2	0.3
Occupant deaths	41	1.5	11	0.4	3	0.4	2	0.3
All fires								
Vehicles	72	2.6	30	1.1	7	1.0	6	1.0
Occupant deaths	84	3.1	31	1.1	7	1.0	6	1.0

just those fatal to occupants, are considered, pre-1988 GM trucks were no more
involved than Ford trucks, contrary to the "aggressive" driver hypothesis. The fire
rates in the pre-1988 GM trucks were substantially higher than in the Ford trucks,
but the difference disappeared in the 1988 and subsequent models that had tanks
inside the frames. The differences in the pre-1988 vehicles are more remarkable
when the data are limited to side impacts—clock positions 8–10 o'clock and
2–4 o'clock (table 10-2).

General Motors also constructed an "Aggressive Driver Demographic Factors
Index" by adding the percentage of 21 factors available in the Fatality Analysis
Reporting System (FARS) to support its claim that drivers of its pickups were
more aggressive. Some of these factors were driver characteristics, and some,
such as number of vehicles in the crash, whether the vehicle ran off the road,
and posted speed 55 mph or greater, were not. Several of the factors are highly
correlated (29 years of age or younger, police indicates "driving too fast," one or
more speeding convictions, vehicle speed 55 mph or greater). Posted speed is
obviously not indicative of aggressive driving, and the speed-related factors are obviously not additive. The summation of several indicators of the same phenomenon is
methodologically indefensible. Also, data on actual vehicle speeds in the crashes
are missing on more than half the cases in FARS. It was the behavior of GM, when
its executives decided to place the gas tanks outside the frame, and not the drivers
of its trucks that accounted for excess fire deaths.

References

Applebome P (1993) GM is held liable over fuel tanks in pickup trucks. *New York Times*,
    April 5, p. 1.
Baker SP (1979) Motor vehicle occupant deaths in young children. *Pediatrics.* 64:860–861.
Baker SP, O'Neill B, Haddon W Jr, and Long WB (1974) The injury severity score: a method
    of describing patients with multiple injuries and evaluating emergency care. *J Trauma.*
    14:187.

Baker SP, O'Neill B, Ginsburg M, and Li G (1992) *The Injury Fact Book*. 2nd ed. New York, NY: Oxford University Press.

Bell NS, Amoroso PJ, Wegman DH, and Senier L (2001) Proposed explanations for excess injury among veterans of the Persian Gulf War and a call for greater attention from policymakers and researchers. *Inj Prev*. 7:4–9.

Berger LR, and Mohan D (1996) *Injury Control: A Global View*. Delhi, India: Oxford University Press.

Bragg WE, and Finn P (1982) *Young Driver Risk-Taking Research: Technical Report of Experimental Study*. Washington, DC: National Highway Traffic Safety Administration.

Campos-Outcalt D, Prybylski D, Watkins AJ, Rothfus D, and Dellapena A (1997) Motor-vehicle crash fatalities among American Indians and non-Indians in Arizona, 1970 through 1988. *Am J Public Health*. 87:282–285.

Centerwell BS (1995) Race, socioeconomic status and domestic homicide. *JAMA*. 273:1755–1758.

Cole RE, Grolnick WS, Laurenitis LR, McAndrews MM, and Matkoski KM (1986) *Children and Fire*. Albany, NY: New York Department of State.

Delbaere K, Van den Noortgate N, Bourgois J, Vanderstraeten G, Tine W, and Cambier D (2006) The Physical Performance Test as a predictor of frequent fallers: a prospective community-based cohort study. *Clin Rehabil*. 20:83–90.

Eastman JW (1984) *Styling Versus Safety*. Lanham, MD: University Press of America. Available at: http://www.autohazardsinfo.org/. Accessed September 2006.

Eby DW (1995) *An Analysis of Michigan Crash Likelihood: Age Versus Driving Experience*. Ann Arbor, MI: University of Michigan Transportation Research Center.

Evans L (1996) Comment: the dominant role of driver behavior in traffic safety. *Am J Public Health*. 86:784–786.

Evans L (2004) *Traffic Safety*. Bloomfield Hills, MI: Science Serving Society.

Evans L, and Schwing RC (eds.) (1985) *Human Behavior and Traffic Safety*. New York, NY: Plenum.

Farooque RS, Stout RG, and Ernst FA (2005) Heterosexual intimate partner homicide: review of ten years of clinical experience *J Forensic Sci*. 50:648–651.

Frame P (1996) Has Martinez dropped the ball at NHTSA? *Automotive News*, June 24, p. 1.

General Motors Corporation (1993) *Evaluation of GM 1973–87 C/K Pickup Trucks, Part III: Analysis of FARS Fire Rates in Side Collisions for Fullsize Pickups and Supplemental Statistical Presentations*. Submission to the National Highway Traffic Safety Administration, August 10.

Gensemer IB, Walker JC, McMurry FG, and Brotman SJ (1989) IQ levels following trauma. *J Trauma*. 29:1616–1619.

Gerberich, SG, Hays M, Mandel J, Gibson R, and Van der Heide C (1985) Analyses of suicides in adolescents and young adults. In Laaser, U, Senault R, and Viehaus H (eds.), *Primary Health Care in the Making, Proceedings: International Congress of Preventive Medicine, Heidelberg, Germany, September 1983*. Heidelberg: Springer-Verlag.

Gilula MF, and Daniels DN (1969) Violence and man's struggle to adapt. *Science*. 164:396–405.

Graafmans WC, Ooms ME, Hofstee HM, Bezemer PD, Bouter LM, and Lips P (1996) Falls in the elderly: prospective study of risk factors and risk profiles. *Am J Epidemiol*. 143:1129–1136.

Graham K (2003) Social drinking and aggression. In Mattson MP (ed.), *Neurobiology of Aggression*. Totowa, NJ: Humana Press.

Graves AB, White E, Koepsell TD, Reifler BV, van Belle G, Larson GB, and Raskind M (1990) The association between head trauma and Alzheimer's disease. *Am J Epidemiol.* 131:491–501.

Hoiberg A, Bernard SP, and Ernst J (1981) Racial differences in hospitalization rates among navy enlisted men. *Public Health Rep.* 96:121–127.

Howard MO, Walker RD, Walker PS, and Rhodes ER (2000) Alcoholism and substance abuse. In Rhodes ER (ed.), *American Indian Health.* Baltimore, MD: Johns Hopkins Press.

Hudley C (2003) Cognitive-behavioral intervention for childhood aggression. In Mattson MP (ed.), *Neurobiology of Aggression.* Totowa, NJ: Humana Press.

Kane DN (1985) *Environmental Hazards to Young Children.* Phoenix, AZ: Oryx Press.

Kemp AM, Mott AM, and Sibert JR (1994) Accidents and child abuse in bathtub submersions. *Arch Dis Child.* 70:435–438.

Kunitz SJ (1976) Fertility, mortality, and social organization. *Hum Biol.* 48:361–377.

Lange RC, Ray RM, and McCarthy RM (1992) *Analysis of Light-Duty Motor Vehicle Collision-Fire Rates.* Menlo Park, CA: Failure Analysis Associates.

Levy JE, and Kunitz SJ (1974) *Indian Drinking: Navajo Practices and Anglo-American Theories.* New York, NY: John Wiley and Sons.

Locklear G (1991) *A Retrospective Case-Control Study of Porch Step Falls Occurring on the Ft. Apache Indian Reservation, 1987 to 1989* [mimeo]. Phoenix, AZ: Environmental Health Services Branch, Indian Health Service.

Ludwig J, Duncan GJ, and Hirschfield P (2001) Urban poverty and juvenile crime: evidence from a randomized housing mobility experiment. *Q J Econ.* 115:655–679.

Malphurs JE, and Cohen D (2005) A state-wide case-control study of spousal homicide-suicide in older persons. *Am J Geriatr Psychiatry.* 13:211–217.

Matthews ML, and Moran AR (1986) Age differences in male drivers' perception of accident risk: the role of perceived driving ability. *Accid Anal Prev.* 18:299–313.

Mattson MP (ed.) (2003) *Neurobiology of Aggression.* Totowa, NJ: Humana Press.

May P (1982) Substance abuse and American Indians: prevalence and susceptibility. *Int J Addict.* 17:1185–1209.

Mazur A, and Robertson LS (1972) *Biology and Social Behavior.* New York, NY: Free Press.

Meier B (1992) GM retreats on claims about fatal truck fires. *New York Times,* December 2, p. A20.

Mullin B, Jackson R, Langley J, and Norton R (2000) Increasing age and experience: are both protective against motorcycle injury? A case-control study. *Inj Prev.* 6:32–35.

National Highway Traffic Safety Administration (1989) *Restraint System Use in the Traffic Population: 1988 Annual Report.* Washington, DC: U.S. Department of Transportation.

Naureckas SM, Galanter C, Naureckas ET, and Christoffel KK (1995) Children's and women's ability to fire handguns. *Arch Pediatr Adolesc Med.* 149:1318–1322.

Osgood NJ (1985) *Suicide in the Elderly.* Rockville, MD: Aspen.

O'Toole BI (1990) Intelligence and behavior and motor vehicle and motor vehicle accident mortality. *Accid Anal Prev.* 22:211–221.

Pierce JA (1977) *Drivers First Licensed in Ontario, October 1969 to October 1975.* Toronto: Ontario Ministry of Transportation and Communication.

Rabinovich BA, Lerner ND, and Huey RW (1994) Young children's ability to climb fences. *Hum Factors.* 36:733–744.

Racket VI, Wireman CM, Vaughan RD, and White JW (2004) Rates and risk factors for sexual violence among an ethnically diverse sample of adolescents. *Arch Pediatr Adolesc Med.* 158:1132–1139.

Reading R (2006) Child deaths resulting from inflicted injuries: household risk factors and perpetrator characteristics. *Child Care Health Dev.* 32:253–256.

Reiss AJ, and Roth JA (1993) *Understanding and Preventing Violence.* Washington, DC: National Academy Press.

Rice DP, and MacKenzie EJ (1989) *Cost of Injury in the United States: A Report to Congress, 1989.* San Francisco, CA, and Baltimore, MD: Institute for Health and Aging, University of California, and Injury Prevention Center, Johns Hopkins University.

Rivara FP (1982a) Epidemiology of childhood injuries: review of current research and presentation of conceptual framework. *Am J Dis Child.* 136:399–405.

Rivara FP (1982b) Epidemiology of childhood injuries. In Bergman AB (ed.), *Preventing Childhood Injuries.* Columbus, OH: Ross Laboratories.

Robertson LS (1977) Car crashes: perceived vulnerability and willingness to pay for crash protection. *J Community Health.* 3:136–141.

Robertson LS (1983) *Injuries: Causes, Control Strategies and Public Policy.* Lexington, MA: DC Heath.

Robertson LS (1985) *Epidemiological Assessment of the Contributing Factors of Injury Mortality and Morbidity Among Native Americans.* Springfield, VA: National Technical Information Service.

Robertson LS (1989) Childhood injury prevention: some lessons learned. In Haller JA (ed.), *Emergency Medical Services for Children.* Columbus, OH: Ross Laboratories.

Rosenberg ML, Stark E, and Zahn MA (1986) Interpersonal violence: homicide and spouse abuse. In Last JM (ed.), *Public Health and Preventive Medicine.* New York, NY: Appleton Century Croft.

Sampson RJ, Morenoff JD, and Raudenbush S (2005) Social anatomy of racial and ethnic disparities in violence. *Am J Public Health.* 95:224–232.

Schuster DH and Guilford JP (1964) The psychometric prediction of problem drivers. *Hum Factors.* 6:393–421.

Sewell CM, Becker TM, Wiggins CL, Key CR, Hull HF, and Samet JM (1989) Injury mortality in New Mexico's American Indians, Hispanics, and non-Hispanic whites, 1958 to 1982. *West J Med.* 150:708–713.

Shupe A, Stacey WA, and Hazelwood LR (1987) *Violent Men, Violent Couples.* Lexington, MA: DC Heath.

Siegel A (2005) *The Neurobiology of Aggression and Rage.* Boca Raton, FL: CRC Press.

Silverman MM, and Simon TR (eds.) (2001) The Houston case-control study of nearly lethal suicide attempts. *Suicide Life Threat Behav.* 32(suppl):1–48.

Smith RJ, and Robertson LS (2000) Unintentional injuries and trauma. In Rhoades ER (ed.), *American Indian Health.* Baltimore, MD: Johns Hopkins University Press.

Sorenson SB, and Shen H (1999) Mortality among young immigrants to California: injury compared to disease deaths. *J Immigr Health.* 1:41–47.

Sorenson SB, and Vittes KA (2003) Buying a handgun for someone else: firearm dealer willingness to sell. *Inj Prev.* 9:147–150.

Stark E, Flitcraft A, and Zuckerman D (1981) *Wife Abuse in the Medical Setting: An Introduction for Health Personnel.* Monograph no. 7. Washington, DC: Office of Domestic Violence.

Stratton R, Zeiner A, and Paredes A (1978) Tribal affiliation and prevalence of alcohol problems. *J Stud Alcohol.* 39:1166–1177.

Taylor SP, Gammon CB, and Capasso DR (1976) Aggression as a function of the interaction of alcohol and threat. *J Pers Soc Psychol.* 34:938–941.

Tinetti ME, Doucette J, Claus E, and Marttoli R (1995a) Risk factors for serious injury during falls by older persons in the community. *J Am Geriatr Soc.* 43:1214–1221.

Tinetti ME, Doucette JT, and Claus EB (1995b) The contribution of predisposing and situational risk factors to serious fall injuries. *J Am Geriatr Soc.* 43:1207–1213.

Tinetti ME, Mendes de Leon CF, Doucette JT, and Baker DI (1994) Fear of falling and fall-related efficacy in relationship to functioning among community-living elders. *J Gerontol.* 49:M140–M170.

Tremblay RE, and Craig WM (1995) Developmental crime prevention. In Tonry M, and Farrington DP (eds.), *Building a Safer Society: Strategic Approaches to Crime Prevention.* Chicago, IL: University of Chicago Press.

Viscusi WK, and Magat WA (1987) *Learning About Risk: Consumer and Worker Responses to Hazard Information.* Cambridge, MA: Harvard University Press.

Waern M, Rubenowitz E, Runeson B, Skoog I, Wilhelmson K, and Alleback P (2002) Burden of illness and suicide in elderly people: case-control study. *BMJ.* 324:1355.

Westermeyer J, and Brantner J (1972) Violent death and alcohol use among the Chippewa in Minnesota. *Minn Med.* 55:749–752.

Whetsall LA, Patterson CM, Young DH, and Shiller WR (1989) Preinjury psychopathology in trauma patients. *J Trauma.* 29:1158–1162.

Williams AF (1976) Observed child restraint use in automobiles. *Am J Dis Child.* 130:1311–1317.

Wittenberg E, Goldie SJ, and Graham JD (2001) Predictors of hazardous child seating behavior in fatal motor vehicle crashes: 1990 to 1998. *Pediatrics.* 108:438–442.

11

Evaluation of Programs to Change Human Factors Voluntarily

Programs aimed at changing human factors without resort to law are of three types: (1) attempts to change abilities, such as driving skills among drivers and strength and gait among the elderly; (2) attempts to change behaviors that are presumed or known to contribute to risk, such as storage of materials hazardous to children, violent responses to peer challenges, speeding, and alcohol use; and (3) attempts to increase use of protection, such as child restraints, seat belts, motorcycle and bicycle helmets, and certain sports equipment. Various techniques are used to promote behavioral change—information and motivation by education in schools and media campaigns, outreach programs for children and the elderly, behavior modification using incentives or punishments, and enhancement of perception.

Among the issues to be considered in attempting to modify behavior relative to children's injuries are the seriousness of the injuries; whether to focus on the parents' or guardians' behavior, the children's behavior, or the behavior of others; and the variety of injuries on which to focus in any one attempt to modify behavior. If a program can be demonstrated to reduce injuries, another major consideration is the means of implementation. If there is no societal organization or institution to implement the program among those who would benefit, demonstration of effectiveness is irrelevant.

CONTROLLED EXPERIMENTS

One great advantage to evaluation of behavior change programs is that many can be researched in a controlled experiment, the most definitive of study designs. One project that had an exemplary research design is questionable regarding its focus. In a prepaid medical plan serving an upper middle-class clientele, parents who brought children in for medical visits (excluding those with very acute illnesses or chronic conditions) were randomly assigned to experimental and control groups.

Parents in the experimental group were counseled regarding a variety of hazards to children in the home and were given a booklet emphasizing 10 such hazards and a packet of electrical outlet covers. In a follow-up telephone call, the parents in the experimental group were asked whether they had changed given hazards, and those who said no were encouraged to do so. In an unannounced home visit, the numbers of hazards observed were recorded in both experimental and control groups (Dershewitz and Williamson, 1977).

Two aspects of the research design are excellent: (1) the random assignment of experimental and control groups should equalize the potential effects of factors other than the counseling between the two groups, and (2) actual observation of certain targeted hazards rules out the potential biases of self-reporting. Such biases were indeed noted by comparing the results of the telephone interview and the observed hazards. While differences in the experimental and control group were obtained in the telephone interviews, there were no differences between the two groups in hazards actually observed in the homes.

The problem with the approach is the lack of focus on one or a few hazards likely to result in severe injury. The types of hazards included cleaning agents, prescription drugs, waxes and polishes, nonprescription drugs, coins, jewelry, watches, keys, appliances on countertops, matches, pins, needles, kitchen knives, and hazards on the floor. These differ substantially in associated injuries and severity. The lack of focus on one or a few of the most important may have defeated the purpose of the counseling.

Projects with a similar research design, but focused exclusively on a single problem, have found favorable effects of counseling parents. A 40 percent reduction in injuries from falls among infants was found relative to a control group after counseling in the experimental group (Kravitz, 1973). Counseling and demonstration of use of child restraints in two studies, and counseling regarding smoke detectors in another, found increased use in the counseled group when actually observed (Berger et al., 1984; Miller et al., 1982; Reisinger et al., 1981). A review of randomized trials of the effects of home visiting programs on injuries indicates some effectiveness (Roberts et al., 1996). Nevertheless, the extent of use of this approach is apparently unusual. For example, only 4.1 percent of pediatricians report counseling regarding drowning hazards, and only 17 percent of those with training in such hazards did so (O'Flaherty and Pirie, 1997).

In a randomized trial among primary care practices in England, a variety of checklists and information were given to the parents in the experimental group. They also received free equipment such as stair guards and smoke alarms. There was no significant difference in subsequent injury-related clinic visits among children in the experimental and control groups. Also, only 55 of 162 practices agreed to be in the study at the outset (Kendrick et al., 1999).

These results raise other research questions. How many behaviors can be influenced at any one time by counseling? Given the demonstration of the effectiveness of counseling regarding certain behaviors, how many physicians actually use the information? If many do not, how can the behavior of physicians be changed?

Attempts at influencing children's behavior directly have also had some success. For example, based on research that indicated "dart-out" as the most important type of child pedestrian injuries up to age 9, a program directed at that specific behavior in that age group was developed. A cartoon character called "Willy Whistle," as well as older children portrayed as role models, was shown in films, television spots, and posters in mid block and intersection situations. The characters in these media demonstrated to children that they should always stop at the edge of curbs and the edge of parked cars.

The materials were used by television stations and in the schools in three communities. Data were collected on children's knowledge, and observers at selected sites recorded child behaviors, before and after the campaign. Also, police reports of pedestrian injuries were compared for the two periods. Knowledge increases were substantial, and correct behaviors observed among children on the streets increased somewhat. Mid block dart and dash injuries declined among 3- to 7-year-olds, but those at other locations did not change appreciably (Blomberg et al., 1983).

There are two problems with this approach, one methodological and one regarding implementation. Without a comparison to control cities, it is not possible to estimate precisely how much of the observed injury reduction can be attributed to the campaign. Without continued implementation in these and other cities, the campaign is useful only to demonstrate a principle. An attempt to find out where the campaign was used some six years subsequent to the study found only one city in which it had been systematically implemented afterward.

A number of controlled trials of pedestrian education have been implemented with mixed results regarding road-crossing behavior. The studies did not follow up to see if pedestrian injuries were reduced in those instances where crossing behavior changed (Duperrex et al., 2002). Several controlled trials have shown reductions in sports injuries related to behavior and the use of protective equipment (Parkkari et al., 2001).

In a controlled trial aimed at the reduction of violence, violent offenders in the experimental group met the parents of victims of violent trauma, were shown the clinical consequences to trauma patients, and were given mental health referrals. The authors found an 85 percent reduction in repeat offenses among the experimental group compared to the control group. The researchers were lucky that the observed effect was large because the numbers of offenders in the two groups (38 each) were too small to detect a smaller but important difference (Scott et al., 2002). The study should be repeated on a larger sample to gain confidence that the reductions are as large as the small study found. The disadvantage of a program based on repeat offenses is that the original offense is not prevented.

A double-blind trial of the effect of diet on violent behavior found that consuming certain vitamins, minerals, and essential fatty acids for two weeks produced a 35 percent reduction in offenses among prisoners compared to a control group given placebos. Although the subjects were incarcerated, there is no reason to believe that the results cannot be generalized, albeit at a less frequent baseline rate (Gesch et al., 2002). Students in schools randomly assigned to receive instruction in "Safe Dates" reported fewer instances of violence on dates than those in control schools (Foshee et al., 2004).

Many educational and other behavioral change programs are not subjected to such careful study before being adopted. Seldom considered is the possibility that a program could be ineffective at best or potentially harmful. Driver education was introduced in the public schools without research on its effects, based on the premise that driving skills were a primary factor in the probability of a crash and that those skills could be improved by training.

Decades later, the first controlled experiment indicated that high school driver training did not reduce individual drivers' crashes per mile driven, but increased the number of drivers licensed at an earlier age such that the risk per population was increased (Shaoul, 1975). The adverse effect was found to be widespread in an ecological study of teenage licensure and involvement in fatal crashes in 27 U.S. states during a period when driver education was increased by federal funding supplements (Robertson and Zador, 1978). A comparative study of driver licensure and crash records of teenagers in schools that dropped the courses, compared to those in schools that retained the courses, found large reductions in months licensed before age 18 and parallel reductions in crashes among those in schools that dropped the courses (Robertson, 1980). Nevertheless, decades later, in many communities, teenagers continue to receive driver training in high schools.

Several principles are illustrated by this experience. The value of a program intended to reduce injuries is not necessarily a function of the good intentions of the program's proponents. Skill or behavior change programs can have unintended harmful effects, and those effects are often found only by well-designed research. This is particularly true of programs that have the potential to increase exposure to hazards. Once a program becomes institutionalized, it is difficult to remove it no matter how ineffective or harmful its consequences.

A major barrier to the scientific evaluation of programs is the reluctance of those who develop, advocate, or profit from programs to have them evaluated objectively. In some cases, their investment in the programs is only psychological, but in others it is economic. Authors of textbooks used in driver education courses and an insurance company that sold driving simulators to schools were among the most adamant critics of the high school driver education studies. They pointed to old studies of differences in driving records of students who had the course and those who did not as indicative of efficacy. However, those studies did not account for selection of the courses by students, or their parents, who were different in other ways that accounted for the differences in driving records (McGuire and Kersh, 1969).

Although experimental-control studies of ensconced programs may be difficult to initiate, clever researchers can sometimes find ways to design studies that reveal biases in other types of evaluations. For example, the "defensive driving" course that is sold widely by the National Safety Council has apparently never been subjected to an experimental-control study. The effect of self-selection in the course was controlled in one evaluation, but in a situation where everyone who selected the course could not be enrolled. Comparison of the driving records of those who took the course at one point and those who took it later showed no difference in crashes in the interim period (Mulhern, 1977). Therefore, when self-selection was constant, the course had no apparent effect. At its Web site regarding a virtual version of the Defensive Driving Course, the National Safety Council (2006) says, "Over 40 years and 50 million drivers later, no other driver improvement course has a higher rate of success in reducing the number and severity of collisions for its participants." Of course, that is technically true if the defensive driving program has no effect and no other program does either. A meta-analysis of 21 controlled experiments of postlicense driver training found no evidence of effectiveness (Ker et al., 2004).

The variety of programs attempting to reduce driving while intoxicated among young drivers is large. One survey in the 1980s identified 248. These are most commonly single sessions or short segments in the curricula of senior high schools. The programs vary in focus, and some are multifocused. About 83 percent of surveyed programs emphasize personal knowledge and skills regarding decisions to drink and drive, and 48 percent include emphasis on resistance to peer pressure. Virtually none of these programs had been evaluated as to effectiveness in actually reducing injuries by strict scientific standards, although some data are available on pre- and postprogram knowledge, attitudes, and self-reported behavior (Vegega and Klitzner, 1988). Such data are known to be misleading (see chapter 7).

Virtually all of the attempts to reduce alcohol-related injuries are directed at driving while intoxicated. There seems to have been little notice that drunk walking, drunk arguing, and even drunk sleeping, given fire/smoke hazards, are also dangerous. If the anti-alcohol-driving programs were successful in reducing driving while intoxicated without reducing intoxication, it is no certainty that the overall severe injury rate would be reduced, given the possibility that the intoxicated would engage in other activities in which risk is increased by intoxication. Not only does the lack of program evaluation suggest the need for research, but also the research should examine the effects on the total severe injury rate, not just that in motor vehicles.

Much of injury control in industry is oriented to worker education, but research on the effects of corporate programs is seldom published. Claims have been made that so-called "back schools" have reduced incidence, lost days, and workers' compensation costs from back pain and strain, but details on how the research was conducted was not indicated (Isernhagen, 1988). Since diagnosis of pain and strain is largely subjective, and willingness to work with back strain or pain has been shown to decrease substantially as a function of amount of workers compensation increases, adjusted for inflation (Robertson and Keeve, 1983), attention to measurement issues and what is actually affecting the changes observed is needed.

In the case of low back pain, the emphasis prevalent in this book on the physics of energy exchanges may not be as applicable. Low back pain is only slightly correlated to heavy lifting. While 47 percent of workers doing heavy lifting in a division of one company during a 10-year period reported such pain, 35 percent of those doing light or sedentary work also reported low back pain (Rowe, 1983). Indeed, there is little evidence of any ameliorative benefit of a wide variety of remedies for prevention or treatment of lower back pain (U.S. Preventive Services Task Force, 2004).

Therefore, carefully controlled experiments should be conducted to find to what extent any changes in claimed pain or strain related to "back schools" or other programs is a result of workers' gratitude for increased attention to their problems by management versus actual changes in lifting behavior related to the educational content of a given program (Snook and White, 1984). In this case, two control groups would be advisable—one in which management without specific ameliorative instruction shows increased concern, and one in which there is neither a program nor management attention to workers' back injuries.

Some successes of educational programs in industry have been reported. For example, participation in an 18- to 24-hour intensive course on emergency preparedness is associated with fewer drowning and hypothermia deaths among commercial fishermen in Alaska (Perkins, 1995). Miners were successfully trained in proficient use of gas masks, but performance deteriorated rapidly after three months without repeated practice (Vaught et al., 1993).

Since the vast majority of the population views television, it is a potential media for behavior change. Two types of use of television to change behavior have been attempted: public service advertising (e.g., "buckle up for safety") and integration of messages in dramatic programs (e.g., showing the consequences of drunk driving in dramatic series). Documentaries on television "magazine" shows (e.g., *Dateline NBC, 60 Minutes, 20/20*) and self-administered knowledge tests (e.g., the National Driving Test) may also change behavior but are not primarily intended for that purpose.

While the ad-type messages are short and can be inserted relatively frequently in breaks in programming if the time is donated or a sponsor is found, the integrated messages in dramatic programs and documentaries are likely to be seen infrequently. The effects of ads and other programs could be studied experimentally in communities with split-cable television systems that advertisers use to study product advertising. When the outcome behavior is frequent and easily observable, such as seat belt use, the effects of the program can be measured unobtrusively (e.g., Robertson et al., 1974). The effects on behaviors such as alcohol use would require stopping a sample of drivers and obtaining breath tests, which could be done with police department cooperation, but the author is unaware of any such study related to television ad campaigns.

A rather large body of research has been conducted on attempts to persuade people to use seat belts, but very little on other important behaviors, such as type of vehicle purchased and purchase of smoke detectors. In contrast to the failure to increase belt use appreciably by advertising, various lottery-like incentive systems and direct warnings, for example, a sticker on the dash saying, "Belt use required in this vehicle," have been found to increase belt use, in some cases substantially (Geller, 1988).

Despite the demonstrated success of the latter approaches, they have not been adopted for widespread use. The adoption of this approach to reduce health care and absentee costs in corporations should be attractive to their executives, but the number of industries with belt use or other incentive systems for injury-related behaviors is unknown. At the community level, governments have not undertaken such programs, and apparently private organizations have not used such programs on a large scale.

There is a substantial literature indicating that if the behavior to reduce risk is needed frequently, it is more difficult to persuade people to do it than in cases where the behavior is required only once (Robertson, 1975). Therefore, one would expect that persuading people to use seat belts consistently would be more difficult than persuading them to purchase a relatively safer vehicle. Yet much research and program effort has been directed at belt use and virtually none at vehicle purchase behavior.

A great dissertation project could be undertaken to distribute the results of the Insurance Institute's 45-mph crash tests to an experimental group and compare their subsequent vehicle purchases to a control group to see to what degree, if any, the experimental group was more likely to purchase the more crashworthy vehicles. (To look up the test results by make and model, see http://www.iihs. org/ratings/default.aspx, accessed August 2006.)

The effect of various therapies and exercise on agility and tissue vulnerability of the elderly is under active investigation. The emphasis in studies of falls among the elderly is often on perceptual and motor abilities, changes in blood pressure, and so-called "drop attack" in which the person collapses for no apparent reason. Multiple drug use and poor vision are primary risk factors (Delbaere et al., 2006).

Several experimental trials of various approaches such as exercise and balance programs and modifications of multiple drug prescriptions indicate fewer falls among those in the programs (Ory et al., 1993; Tinetti et al., 1993; Buchner et al., 1993; Robitaille et al., 2005). Staff education in nursing facilities was unsuccessful, as was staff assessment of patients followed by prevention efforts (Ray et al., 2005; Kerse et al., 2004). Other approaches, such as use of energy-absorbing protective garments in subacute hospital care and nursing home facilities, are effective (Haines et al., 2004; Meyer et al., 2005).

SCREENING ON HUMAN FACTORS

To the extent that measurable human factors are predictive of injury, these factors could be used to refuse employment or select people for some sort of injury reduction program. For example, among the 10 percent of applicants for positions in the postal service who had urine tests positive for marijuana (7.8 percent) or cocaine (2.2 percent), injury rates on the job were 85 percent higher than for those negative for the drugs, controlling for several other factors (Zwerling et al., 1990). If persons who tested positive for the drugs had not been hired, the postal service would have experienced fewer injuries. However, the net benefit for society is more questionable. If those persons refused employment became employed in a more hazardous environment or were engaged in more hazardous activities if they remained unemployed, the net effect could be worse. Research on the subsequent injuries of persons refused employment on the basis of drug screens or other factors would be interesting and perhaps useful.

If, on the basis of screening, those at higher risk were placed in behavior change programs that reduce injuries, the screening could have a net benefit. If the screening is not sensitive or if the program is ineffective, the usefulness of such programs can be very limited or even harmful. Children with burn scars in Ghana were found to have repeated burns at a rate less, not more, than expected from the prevalent rate (Forjuoh, 1996). Therefore, prior burns are not sensitive in identifying new cases. The author examined the Fatality Analysis Reporting System data in counties in which more than 90 percent of fatally injured drivers were tested for alcohol and noted that about 80 percent of fatally injured drivers with illegal blood alcohol had no prior convictions for driving while intoxicated. Therefore, screening those with such convictions for treatment programs will have a maximum 20 percent effect even if the programs were perfectly effective. Persons assigned to an education-rehabilitation program rather than the usual court procedure in one county had a higher subsequent crash record, probably because license suspension is more effective than education-rehabilitation (Preusser et al., 1976). Evaluation of attempts to improve screening for commercial drivers' licenses found no effect (Hagge and Romanowicz, 1996).

Authors of a study of suicide rates subsequent to emergency department visits for a variety of conditions cleverly included text searches of clinical narratives to detect mention of suicide attempts, suicide ideation, self-harm, or overdose. On the basis of the relatively higher subsequent suicide rates among those so detected, they recommended psychiatric referral and treatment, if appropriate, for persons identified as potentially suicidal using these criteria (Crandall et al., 2006). Such a recommendation raises two issues. First, since 98 percent of people who met the criteria did not commit suicide (false positives), the process would be expensive. Second, the efficacy of the treatment would have to be high given that most of those referred are not really at risk.

MULTIPLE COMMUNITY CHANGES

Some experiments have adopted a more communitywide approach directed toward either one goal, such as reduction of injuries from fireworks or increased bicycle helmet use, or multiple goals, such as reductions in several injury rates simultaneously.

Study of fireworks injuries associated with New Year celebrations in Naples, Italy, showed that 60 percent of injuries occurred from illegal fireworks and that children's injuries often occurred while attempting to relight unexploded fireworks or from powder assembled from partially exploded fireworks. A community program to reduce the injuries in the holiday season at the end of 1993 included police seizure of 12.5 million illegal fireworks, street sweeping to remove partially and unexploded fireworks, and an increased public information program relative to previous years. During that holiday season, 48 percent fewer injuries from fireworks were treated in 18 surveyed emergency departments compared to the holiday season in the previous year (D'Argenio et al., 1996).

In Harstad, Norway, distribution to the local population of information on pedestrian injury, including locations where they occurred and stories of individual cases, was accompanied by a substantial reduction in hospitalization for child pedestrian and bicycle injury (Ytterstad, 1995). Unfortunately, neither the Naples nor the Harstad study looked at other communities without programs to assess the possibility that other factors were reducing the injuries studied. Several studies that employed such comparisons found little or no effect of communitywide efforts to control a variety of injuries (Spinks et al., 2004).

A case–control study of head injuries to helmeted and nonhelmeted bicyclists— showing 85 percent effectiveness of helmets (Thompson et al., 1989)—encouraged researchers to launch a study of a campaign to promote helmet use. A control community was included to measure the trend in bicycle helmet use where there was no campaign. The campaign was directed at both parents and children and had several features in addition to television spots and a program in elementary schools. Tags urging helmet purchase were hung on bicycles for sale. Coupons for free french fries at fast-food outlets and free tickets for baseball games were distributed to helmet users, and coupons for discounts of $25 toward helmet purchases were distributed at various organizations and events. Helmet use by bicyclists, observed at a sample of sites in the community, increased from 5.5 percent to 15.7 percent, compared to an increase of only 2.6 percentage points in the control community that had no special effort to promote bicycle helmet use (DiGuiseppi et al., 1989). A study of such a program in Quebec found a similar effect overall but a much greater effect in middle-class and wealthy communities than in those less wealthy (Farley et al., 1996).

That is not to say that underprivileged communities cannot benefit from injury control programs if the programs are tailored to the needs of the children and their families. Based on surveillance of injuries in central Harlem, a neighborhood including some 28,000 children in 1990, a program aimed at the most severe injuries to children 5–16 years old was initiated (Davidson et al., 1994). The targeted injuries included those from motor vehicles, falls, assaults, and firearms (intentional or not). Such injuries to same-age children in a comparison neighborhood, Washington Heights, that had no program were examined to rule out trends not related to the program. The program included renovation of playgrounds, increased child supervision including involvement in skill training (dance, art, sports, horticulture, and carpentry), education in prevention of injury and violence, and lowered costs of bicycle helmets. An appealing aspect of the program is that many of the activities have intrinsic value even if they have no discernible impact on injuries.

Although the results were not entirely unambiguous, there was apparently a reduction in some of the targeted injuries. Since injuries also declined in the comparison community, other factors may have accounted for some of the observed reductions. The major evidence for efficacy of the program was that targeted injuries except falls declined in Harlem, but nontargeted injuries did not, while all injuries declined in Washington Heights. It also makes sense that children diverted from street activities would have decreases in motor vehicle and assault injuries without changes in fall injuries that occur in sports.

Particularly encouraging was the decline in assault and gun injuries, which decreased in Harlem while increasing in the comparison neighborhood during the intervention period (Durkin et al., 1996). This is likely due to diversion of children from the street culture rather than training in conflict resolution. Students in seventh-grade classes who had such training were compared to those from other classes without training. Contrary to the intended effect, the students with training reported an increase in aggression and delinquency relative to the comparison group (Colyer et al., 1996). Because of the questionable validity of self-reports, more definitive data on injuries related to training in conflict resolution are needed.

Various communities have developed coalitions, ad campaigns, school programs, and clinical interventions aimed at reducing violence, but there is precious little effort to evaluate their effects. One volume published in 1996 in which such efforts are described (Hampton et al., 1996) contains no reference to a study of 10 communities where peer mediation in potentially violent situations was studied and found ineffective (Spiro and DeJong, 1991). There was also no reference to the aforementioned success of alternative activities in Harlem.

The World Health Organization has promoted the concept of "Safe Communities," and various communities have qualified based on several criteria for infrastructure and community involvement. Research in Sweden, comparing injury hospitalization trends in the designated communities with similar communities not seeking "Safe Community" designation, found higher injury rates more often than not in the designated communities. While there may be some selection bias in communities applying for the designation, the results are not sanguine (Nilsen, et al., 2007). There is no indication that the approach outlined in chapter 7 to target specific injuries and pair them with countermeasures was used in the "Safe Communities".

GROUP BEHAVIOR

This chapter has noted several instances in which programs such as increasing supervision and alternative activities for children and adolescents, behavior-change counseling, and incentive systems resulted in reduced injuries or behavior that would reduce risk. Some behavioral scientists have been defensive about the emphasis by epidemiologists on the agents, vehicles, and physical environmental factors that cause or contribute to injury, pointing to the noted studies as evidence that behavioral factors can also be changed. No one denies the latter, but as noted for some of the known effective behavior-change approaches, effective ones are not being used and harmful ones remain in use. Perhaps behavioral scientists that emphasize the efficacy of a behavioral approach could design research that demonstrates how to remove barriers to the use of effective programs, whether oriented to behavior, agents, vehicles, or environments.

People behave differently in groups than they would as individuals. One interesting group phenomenon is "pluralistic ignorance" (Thibault and Kelley, 1965). In groups (corporations, governments, injury control coalitions), people will agree to action or inaction to which they would not personally commit in the absence of the group because they falsely believe the others in the group (or its constituency) support the action. One fascinating area for research is the extent to which revelation of pluralistic ignorance changes action.

An example occurred in White River, Arizona, where horses in the road were frequently struck by motor vehicles. The White Mountain Apache Tribal Council had years earlier adopted a law prohibiting horses in the road, but there were no provisions for enforcement. When a health educator became concerned about the issue, he found that the injury surveillance system had identified the problem as a priority (Rothfus and Akin, 1988).

He talked with members of the council, but they were not convinced that other council members or the population would favor having to pay fines for their stray animals. He then conducted a community survey to see if there was support for removing horses from the road. The survey revealed overwhelming community desire for action. When the council was shown the survey, a wrangler was appointed to search for and round up stray animals daily, and the owners were fined. The incidence of vehicle collisions with domestic livestock was greatly reduced (Anderson, 1995).

ENVIRONMENT AND BEHAVIOR

The extent to which physical and social environments can be modified to reduce violence is an important area for research. Apparently, night lighting of high-crime areas reduces fear far more than incidence (Murray, 1996). Numerous approaches have been proposed, and some employed, such as various types of barriers (e.g., bullet-proof windows in cash windows of service stations and other establishments), bus stop placement, and street closures (Clarke, 1992). Two or more clerks in convenience stores reduce robberies, as do signs indicating limited cash, access control, and location of stores in areas of high traffic (Hunter and Jeffery, 1992).

Although some researchers claim that the vast majority of motor vehicle crashes are the result of "driver error" (e.g., Treat, 1977), they do not specify the extent to which the "error" is enhanced by vehicle characteristics or environmental conditions. Perception of speed by vehicle occupants is more related to sound than to vision (Evans, 1971). Yet some vehicle manufacturers attempt to minimize sound and maximize speed capability. What, if any, is the difference in crash rates between vehicles that filter out varying degrees of noise, controlling for radio use and other factors?

The crashes of drivers turning left across the paths of motorcycles are 10 times more frequent than crashes of motorcyclists turning left in front of cars (Griffin, 1974), perhaps because of misperception of speeds of smaller vehicles.

Several studies indicate that vehicle and environmental changes to enhance perception can be effective. Experiments in which vehicles in corporate and government fleets were equipped with a variety of rear brake-light configurations found that a high-mounted, center light substantially reduced rear-end crashes while braking (e.g., Reilly et al., 1980). Similar research is needed on the effect of the so-called heads-up display of the speedometer—that is, display of the speed of the vehicle nearer the driver's line of sight.

Crash rates of vehicles at intersections are related to the length of the amber phase of traffic control lights (Zador et al., 1984). Controlled experiments specify the extent to which incidence and severity of injury are affected by changes in light timing. In one such study, pedestrian/bicyclist collisions were reduced 37 percent at intersections where signals were changed to conform to Institute of Transportation Engineers proposed standards (Retting et al., 2002). Separate tracks for walking and bicycling, cycle lanes through intersections, and grade-separated crossing points reduce injury to pedestrians and bicyclists. Various other changes in roads that moderate speeds or alter traffic patterns (rumble strips, speed bumps, bypasses, roundabouts, interchanges, limited access roads, road alignment, sight distance, one-way traffic, limited parking) have been shown to reduce injuries to vehicle occupants, as well (Elvik and Vaa, 2004).

Evidence that road lighting greatly reduces crashes where they cluster at night is noted in chapter 7. Lines painted across the road at exponentially decreased intervals reduces speed of drivers crossing them and, when studied at sites in England, resulted in substantially reduced crashes at certain sites (Denton, 1980). Various road markings at curves have a differential effect on speed, depending on type of vehicle (cars vs. trucks), and deserve further study of their effect on crash incidence and severity (Shinar et al., 1980). Crashes of aircraft on runways also raise the issue of the extent to which runway versus taxiway markings are clear.

References

Anderson HS (1995) *An Evaluation of the Livestock Control Project on the Fort Apache Indian Reservation.* White River, AZ: White Mountain Apache Health Education Department.

Berger LR, Saunders S, Armitage K, and Schauer L (1984) Promoting the use of car safety devices for infants: an intensive health education approach. *Pediatrics.* 74:16–19.

Blomberg RD, Preusser DF, Hale A, and Leaf WA (1983) *Experimental Field Test of Proposed Pedestrian Safety Messages.* Washington, DC: National Highway Traffic Safety Administration.

Buchner DM, Cress ME, Wagner EH, de Lateur BJ, Price R, and Abrass IB (1993) The Seattle FICSIT/MoveIt study: the effect of exercise on gait and balance in older adults. *J Am Geriatr Soc.* 41:321–325.

Clarke RV (ed.) (1992) *Situational Crime Prevention: Successful Case Studies.* New York, NY: Harrow and Heston.

Colyer E, Thompkins T, Durkin M, and Barlow B (1996) Can conflict resolution training increase aggressive behavior in young adolescents? *Am J Public Health.* 86:1028.

Crandall C, Fullerton-Gleason L, Aguero R, and LaValley J (2006) Subsequent suicide mortality among emergency department patients seen for suicidal behavior. *Acad Emerg Med.* 13:435–442.

D'Argenio P, Cafaro L, Santonastasi F, Taggi F, and Binkin N (1996) Capodanno Senza Danno: the effects of an intervention program on fireworks injuries in Naples. *Am J Public Health.* 86:84–86.

Davidson LL, Durkin MS, Kuhn L, O'Connor P, Barlow B, and Heagarty MC (1994) The impact of the Safe Kids/Healthy Neighborhoods Injury Prevention Program in Harlem, 1988 through 1991. *Am J Public Health.* 84:580–586.

Delbaere K, Van den Noortgate N, Bourgois J, Vanderstraeten G, Tine W, and Cambier D (2006) The Physical Performance Test as a predictor of frequent fallers: a prospective community-based cohort study. *Clin Rehabil.* 20:83–90.

Denton GG (1980) The influence of visual pattern on perceived speed. *Perception.* 9:393–402.

Dershewitz RA, and Williamson JW (1977) Prevention of childhood household injuries: a controlled clinical trial. *Am J Public Health.* 67:1148–1153.

DiGuiseppi CG, Rivara FP, Koepsell TD, and Polissar L (1989) Bicycle helmet use by children: evaluation of a community-wide helmet campaign. *JAMA.* 262:2256–2261.

Duperrex O, Bunn F, and Roberts I (2002) Safety education of pedestrians for injury prevention: a systematic review of randomised controlled trials. *BMJ.* 324:1129.

Durkin MS, Kuhn L, Davidson LL, Laraque D, and Barlow B (1996) Epidemiology and prevention of severe assault and gun injuries to children in an urban community. *J Trauma.* 41:667–673.

Elvik R, and Vaa T (2004) *The Handbook of Road Safety Measures.* New York, NY: Elsevier.

Evans L (1971) Speed estimation from a moving automobile. *Hum Factors.* 13:23–27.

Farley C, Haddad S, and Brown B (1996) The effects of a 4-year program promoting bicycle helmet use among children in Quebec. *Am J Public Health.* 86:46–51.

Forjuoh SN (1996) Burn repetitions in Ghanaian children: prevalence, epidemiological characteristics and socioenvironmental factors. *Burns.* 22:539–542.

Foshee VA, Bauman KE, Ennett ST, Linder GF, Benefield T, and Suchindran C (2004) Assessing the long-term effects of the Safe Dates Program and a booster in preventing and reducing adolescent dating violence victimization and perpetration. *Am J Public Health.* 94:619–624.

Geller ES (1988) A behavioral approach to transportation safety. *Bull N Y Acad Med.* 64:632–661.

Gesch CB, Hammond SM, Hampson SE, and Eves E (2002) Influence of supplementary vitamins, minerals and essential fatty acids on the antisocial behaviour of young adult prisoners: randomised, placebo controlled trial. *Br J Psychiatry.* 181:22–28.

Griffin LI III (1974) *Motorcycle Accidents: Who When, Where, and Why.* Chapel Hill, NC: North Carolina Highway Safety Research Center.

Hagge RA, Romanowicz PA (1996) Evaluation of California's commercial driver license program. *Acc Analysis and Prevention.* 28:547–559.

Haines TP, Bennell KL, Osborne RH, and Hill KD (2004) Effectiveness of targeted falls prevention programme in subacute hospital setting: randomised controlled trial. *BMJ.* 328:676–679.

Hampton RL, Jenkins P, and Gullotta TP (1996) *Preventing Violence in America.* Thousand Oaks, CA: Sage Publications.

Hunter RD, and Jeffery CR (1992) Preventing convenience store robbery through environmental design. In Clarke RV (ed.), *Situational Crime Prevention: Successful Case Studies.* New York, NY: Harrow and Heston.

Isernhagen SJ (1988) *Work Injury: Management and Prevention.* Rockville, MD: Aspen.

Kendrick D, Marsh P, Fielding K, and Miller P (1999) Preventing injuries in children: cluster randomised controlled trial in primary care. *BMJ.* 318:980–983.

Ker K, Roberts I, Collierb T, Beyer F, Bunn F, and Frost C (2004) Post-licence driver education for the prevention of road traffic crashes: a systematic review of randomised controlled trials. *Accid Anal Prev.* 37:305–313.

Kerse N, Butler M, Robinson E, and Todd M (2004) Fall prevention in residential care: a cluster, randomized, controlled trial. *J Am Geriatr Soc.* 52:524–531.

Kravitz H (1973) Prevention of falls in infancy by counseling mothers. *Ill Med J.* 144:570–573.

McGuire FL, and Kersh RC (1969) *An Evaluation of Driver Education.* Berkeley, CA: University of California Press.

Meyer G, Wegscheider K, Kersten J, Icks A, and Mühlhauser I (2005) Increased use of hip protectors in nursing homes: economic analysis of a cluster randomized, controlled trial. *J Am Geriatr Soc.* 53:2153–2158.

Miller RE, Reisinger KS, Blatter MM, and Wucher F (1982) Pediatric counseling and the subsequent use of smoke detectors. *Am J Public Health.* 72:392–393.

Mulhern T (1977) *The National Safety Council's Defensive Driving Course as an Accident and Violation Countermeasure.* Unpublished doctoral dissertation. College Station, TX: Texas A&M University.

Murray C (1996) The physical environment. In Wilson JQ, and Petersilia J (eds.), *Crime.* San Francisco, CA: Institute for Contemporary Studies.

National Safety Council (2006) Virtual Defensive Driving Course™. Available at: http://www.nsc.org/train/ddc/virtualddc/. Accessed August 2006.

Nilsen P, Ekman R, Ekman DS, Ryen L, and Linqvist K (2007) Effectiveness of community-based injury prevention Long-term injury rate levels, changes, and trends for 14 Swedish WHO-designated Safe Communities. *Accid Anal Prev.* 39:267–273.

O'Flaherty JE, and Pirie PL (1997) Prevention of pediatric drowning and near drowning: a survey of members of the American Academy of Pediatrics. *Pediatrics.* 99:169–174.

Ory MG, Schechtman KB, Miller JP, Hadley EC, Fiatarone MA, Province MA, Arfken CL, Morgan D, Weiss S, and Kaplan M (1993) Frailty and injuries in later life: the FICSIT trails. *J Am Geriatr Soc.* 41:283–296.

Parkkari Y, Kujala JM, and Kannu P (2001) Is it possible to prevent sports injuries? Review of controlled clinical trials and recommendations for future work. *Sports Med.* 31:985–995.

Perkins R (1995) Evaluation of an Alaskan marine safety training program. *Public Health Rep.* 110:701–702.

Preusser DF, Ulmer RG, and Adams JR (1976) Driver record evaluation of a drinking driver rehabilitation program. *J Saf Res.* 8:98–105.

Ray WA, Taylor JA, Brown AK, Gideon P, Hall K, Arbogast P, and Meredith S (2005) Prevention of fall-related injuries in long-term care: a randomized controlled trial of staff education. *Arch Intern Med.* 165:2293–2298.

Reilly RE, Kurke DS, and Bukenmaier CC (1980) *Validation of the Reduction of Rear-End Collisions by a High-Mounted Auxiliary Stoplamp.* Washington, DC: National Highway Traffic Safety Administration.

Reisinger KS, Williams AL, Wells JAK, John CE, Roberts TR, and Pogainy HJ (1981) The effect of pediatricians' counselling on infant restraint use. *Pediatrics.* 67:201–206.

Retting AR, Chapline JF, and Williams AF (2002) Changes in crash risk following retiming of traffic signal change intervals. *Accid Anal Prev.* 34:215–220.

Roberts I, Kramer MS, and Suissa S (1996) Does home visiting prevent childhood injury? A systematic review of randomised controlled trials. *BMJ.* 312:29–33.

Robertson LS (1975) Behavioral research and strategies in public health: a demur. *Soc Sci Med.* 9:165–170.

Robertson LS (1980) Crash involvement of teenaged drivers when driver education is eliminated from high school. *Am J Public Health.* 70:599–603.

Robertson LS, Kelley AB, O'Neill B, Wixon CW, Eiswirth RS, and Haddon W Jr (1974) A controlled study of the effect of television messages on safety belt use. *Am J Public Health.* 64:1071–1080.

Robertson LS, and Keeve JP (1983) Worker injuries: the effects of workers' compensation and OSHA inspections. *J Health Polit Policy Law.* 8:581–597.

Robertson LS, and Zador PL (1978) Driver education and crash involvement of teenaged drivers. *Am J Public Health.* 68:959–965.

Robitaille Y, Laforest S, Fournier M, Gauvin L, Parisien M, Corriveau H, Trickey F, and Damestoy N (2005) Moving forward in fall prevention: an intervention to improve balance among older adults in real-world settings. *Am J Public Health.* 95:2049–2057.

Rothfus GL, and Akin DP (1988) *A Study of Motor Vehicle Crashes: White Apache Reservation, 1985–86.* Phoenix, AZ: Indian Health Service.

Rowe ML (1983) *Backache at Work.* Fairport, NY: Perinton Press.

Scott KK, Tepas JJ III, Frykberg E, Taylor PM, and Plotkin AJ (2002) Turning point: rethinking violence-evaluation of program efficacy in reducing adolescent violent crime recidivism. *J Trauma Inj Infect Crit Care.* 53:21–27.

Shaoul J (1975) *The Use of Accidents and Traffic Offenses as Criteria for Evaluating Courses in Driver Education.* Salford, UK: University of Salford.

Shinar D, Rockwell TH, and Malecki JA (1980) The effects of changes in driver perception on rural curve negotiation. *Ergonomics.* 23:263–275.

Snook SH, and White AH (1984) Education and Training. In Pope MH, Frymoyer JW, and Andersson G (eds.), *Occupational Low Back Pain.* New York, NY: Praeger.

Spinks A, Turner C, McClure R, and Nixon J (2004) Community based prevention programs targeting all injuries for children. *Inj Prev.* 10:180–185.

Spiro A, and DeJong W (1991) *Preventing Interpersonal Violence Among Teens.* Final Report on National Institute of Justice Grant 87-IJ-CX, 009. Washington, DC: National Institute of Justice.

Thibault JW, and Kelley HH (1965) *The Social Psychology of Groups.* New York, NY: John Wiley and Sons.

Thompson RS, Rivara FP, and Thompson DC (1989) A case-control study of the effectiveness of bicycle safety helmets *New Engl J Med.* 320:1361–1367.

Tinetti ME, Baker DI, Garrett PA, Gottschalk M, Koch ML, and Horwitz RI (1993) Yale FICSIT: risk factor abatement strategy for fall prevention. *J Am Geriat Soc.* 41:315–320.

Treat JR (1977) Tri-level study of the causes of traffic accidents: an overview of final results. In *21st Proceedings of the Association for the Advancement of Automotive Medicine.* Barrington, IL: Association for the Advancement of Automotive Medicine.

U.S. Preventive Services Task Force (2004) *Primary Care Interventions to Prevent Low Back Pain: Brief Evidence Update.* Rockville, MD: Agency for Healthcare Research and Quality. Available at: http://www.ahrq.gov/clinic/3rduspstf/lowback/lowbackup. htm. Accessed September 2006.

Vaught C, Brnich MJ, Wiehagen WJ, Cole HP, and Kellner HJ (1993) *An Overview of Research on Self-Contained Self-Rescuer Training.* Bulletin 695. Pittsburgh, PA: U.S. Department of the Interior Bureau of Mines.

Vegega ME, and Klitzner MD (1988) What have we learned about youth anti-drinking-driving programs? *Eval Prog Plan.* 11:203–217.

Ytterstad B (1995) The Harstad injury prevention study: hospital based injury recording used for outcome evaluation of community-based prevention of bicyclist and pedestrian injury. *Scand J Prim Health Care.* 13:141–149.

Zador PL, Stein H, Shapiro S, and Tarnoff P (1984) *Effect of Signal Timing on Traffic Flow and Crashes at Signalized Intersections.* Washington, DC: Insurance Institute for Highway Safety.

Zwerling C, Ryan J, and Orav EJ (1990) The efficacy of preemployment drug screening for marijuana and cocaine in predicting employment outcome. *JAMA.* 264:2639–2643.

12

Evaluation of Laws and Rules
Directed at Individual Behavior

Governments sometimes impose laws applicable to the public or segments of the public in an attempt to change behavior to reduce injuries. Also, in organizations such as corporations, sports leagues, and summer camps, there are often formal rules that proscribe or require particular behaviors thought to be related to injury risk. For example, changing certain rules for sports events has been found to strongly reduce injury rates (Roberts et al., 1996). This chapter focuses primarily on the use of epidemiological data in evaluating the effects of laws and their enforcement on injury incidence or severity.

Epidemiological data may provide lawmakers and administrators with information to justify, change, or repeal laws or rules (Bergman, 1992). For example, the high infant and toddler mortality rates in motor vehicles during the 1970s were used to persuade legislators to enact laws requiring restraint use among younger children. Postenactment analysis identified gaps in coverage of child-restraint laws, indicating that 39 percent of children 0–5 years old killed as occupants were exempted from the laws, and thus demonstrated a need for legislators to consider filling the gaps (Teret et al., 1986). A study of the laws effects among the 50 states indicated a reduction of about 4.8 percent in the fatality rate for each additional year of age from 1 to 6 in which child restraint use is required (Houston et al., 2001).

To simplify discussion, the word "law" is used here to refer to laws and administrative rules directed at individual behavior. Two types of laws have been adopted in attempts to reduce injuries: those that proscribe behavior thought to increase risk and those that require behavior thought to increase protection. Examples of proscribed behaviors are drunk driving and exceeding posted speed limits in motor vehicles. Protective laws include required use of hardhats at work-sites, required use of helmets by motorcyclists, and required use of seat belts or child restraints by vehicle occupants.

The theoretical models regarding the effect of law on proscribed behaviors are called deterrence theories (e.g., Ross, 1982). Such theories focus on several factors that may affect the behavior in question: probability of detection of the proscribed behavior by the enforcement authority, probability of conviction for the offense, time from detection to conviction, and severity of punishment if convicted.

Two types of deterrence are possible: specific deterrence of repetition of the proscribed behavior (recidivism) by those detected, and general deterrence, which includes reduction in the proscribed behavior of those not detected. Research on detected recidivism is relatively easy using police, court, or medical records, but the inferences of the effects of law on general deterrence are more difficult to support with scientific evidence.

The "public health" and "criminal justice" approaches have been falsely characterized as a difference between prevention of first offenses versus reduction of recidivism (Moore, 1995). Most theoretical criminologists have long recognized the possible general deterrent effects of laws and their enforcement. The "public health" approach may help lawmakers and law enforcers recognize that the effects of laws are influenced by factors in addition to incapacitation and punishment.

Required protective behaviors not only include use of protective equipment, such as seat belts in motor vehicles, but may also include procedures to be followed, such as the checklists of airline pilots. Although there is less theory regarding the effects of such laws than that regarding deterrence, a body of research does suggest some generalizations whereby the probable success of the laws can be estimated. It can be argued that deterrence theory applies to protective laws, as well, but coercing someone into doing something that they would not ordinarily do is not necessarily the same thing as deterring someone from doing something that he or she is wont to do.

The premises of deterrence theory at least partly depend on the question of the extent of intent in human behavior related to injury. If all homicides or assaults were well planned by people weighing the costs and benefits, as economic theories of "crime" would have us believe (e.g., Becker, 1968), then enough increase in the cost to the offenders should deter potential offenders from the acts. To the extent that assault is momentarily impulsive or reactive behavior without rational deliberation, or the result of mental illness, weighing of the potential consequences by the assailant may be inconsequential (Smith and Warren, 1978). Similarly, to the extent that alcohol use, seat belt use, or whatever behavior is the result of psychological, social, or cultural factors that preclude or override concerns about detection or punishment, the effect of protective laws and their enforcement will be diminished. In some instances, the effects of laws may be diminished because people are exempted for reasons of religion or custom. For example, Sikhs in India and Great Britain are exempted from laws requiring helmet use on motorcycles because the turbans required by their religion do not accommodate commercially available helmets (Berger and Mohan, 1996). Turbans provide some protection but are not as effective as helmets (Sood, 1988).

Most drivers deliberately or inadvertently violate traffic laws daily, and the discretion of the police in enforcement often looks arbitrary and sometimes capricious (Ross, 1960). How much this leads to disrespect for law and police beyond the road environment is unknown, but it is likely that frequent observation of law violations increases the probability of such behavior. Police may discriminate by race, gender, and socioeconomic status with impunity (Cressey, 1975) unless the incident escalates into violence, as several publicized cases have in recent years in the United States, further increasing the disrespect among those in identifiable groups who feel singled out.

RESEARCH QUESTIONS AND STUDY DESIGNS

Most of the research on laws focuses on the effects of enforcement or punishment. Little attention has been paid to how laws aimed at injury reduction are enacted. No one familiar with the strong antigovernment sentiment in Tennessee politics would have expected that state to be the first to enact a law requiring children to be restrained in cars. Nevertheless, persistent lobbying by pediatricians and other groups of citizens was successful (Sanders, 1982). All U.S. states subsequently followed Tennessee's lead, albeit with significant gaps in the coverage. While the United States for years lagged behind most of the wealthier countries in the enactment of belt use laws, those countries were just as slow to enact child-restraint laws.

Laws are seldom uniformly adopted among states of the United States, and some have been difficult to retain once enacted, such as motorcycle helmet use laws. Although hypotheses regarding the social and political processes that lead to enactment or resistance to laws by legislators may not be viewed by epidemiologists as within their purview, those with backgrounds in sociology and political science may find the subject of interest.

One question that has been little explored is the origin and sustenance of the lobbying in opposition to laws to reduce injury. No doubt many of the opponents are sincerely concerned that their rights or economic interests are at stake, but there may be a more cynical element. Some of the lobbyists, or magazine and newsletter publishers, may care little or nothing about the issue in question but use it to enrich themselves by continuously stirring up opposition with claims that the rights of whatever group (gun owners, motorcyclists) are being violated. Collection of dues, subscriptions to magazines and newsletters, and sale of other propaganda can be very profitable. Of course, proponents of laws can be exploited in a similar manner.

Once a law is enacted, the simplest question regarding a law is whether it reduces injuries. The simplest, but sometimes misleading, research design to answer the question is to compare injury rates before and after the law. If other factors are changing that would have increased or reduced injuries during the same period of time, the change in injuries can be falsely attributed to the law.

For example, when a supervising judge in Chicago required seven-day jail sentences for drunk driving during a period in 1970–1971, the death rate in the city declined and the rule was declared a success. Aware of the threats to validity in before–after comparisons (Campbell, 1969), researchers designed a quasi-experimental study to examine the effect of Chicago's judicial policy. Comparison of the death rates in Chicago and the nearby city of Milwaukee during the same period indicated that a similar decline occurred at the same time in Milwaukee, which did not have a policy of mandatory jail sentences (Robertson et al., 1973). The reduction in fatality rates was likely the result of recession in the economy or changes in weather patterns that happened to coincide with the judge's sentencing policy.

Most laws applied to individual behavior in the United States are enacted in state and local jurisdictions. While this is disadvantageous in obtaining the uniform application of laws of known efficacy, it gives the researcher an opportunity to study the effect of laws of unknown or questionable efficacy in jurisdictions that introduce them relative to those that do not. Evaluation of the effect of enactment of laws that were in effect before data systems on relevant injuries were initiated is not possible, although the waxing and waning of enforcement may provide opportunities for study.

One of the threats to valid conclusions in before–after research designs without comparison jurisdictions, particularly in smaller jurisdictions where numbers fluctuate substantially in short periods of time, is so-called regression to the mean (Campbell, 1969). That is, if a new law or increased enforcement is initiated in areas based on a high injury rate in a short period, the rate would be expected to trend toward the average in a subsequent period irrespective of the change in policy. For example, the National Highway Traffic Safety Administration allocated $10 million in grants to states in 1973 for intensified law enforcement based on research indicating a reduction in fatalities after such enforcement in six counties. The counties were selected primarily on the basis of unusually high fatality rates. Using data from counties chosen on the basis of similar criteria in the same and another state, subsequent research showed that similar reductions in fatalities occurred in counties comparably chosen but without special enforcement (Williams and Robertson, 1975).

Therefore, the reduction in the counties with special enforcement probably occurred because of return to normal from an unusual increase prior to the program, not because of special enforcement. While it makes sense to target efforts at areas where injuries are the most acute, claims of the effectiveness of a law or other injury control effort based on application in areas with unusually high rates prior to implementation is highly suspect. Effectiveness should be studied in areas that have no inordinate rates. If effectiveness is established, then efficient application dictates that the countermeasure with known effectiveness be targeted at areas with the higher rates.

When the law applies to a country as a whole, there may not be another country for comparison nearby that has comparable weather or other factors that could affect changes in injury rates. A research methodology that has been employed to evaluate the effect of laws in that circumstance is the interrupted time series (Campbell, 1969; Hoff, 1983). If one can obtain data on injury rates for an extended period of time before and after a law change, an abrupt and substantial change in the rates coincident with the change in law, enforcement, or punishment is usually indicative of the effect of the change in policy, particularly if such abrupt changes have not occurred in the rates in the past.

Sometimes gradual change in injury trends from before to after a change in law or enforcement is attributed to the law, but such inferences are highly questionable without replication in other jurisdictions and times. A trend may change for all sorts of reasons, and a continuation of a previous trend may occur for a reason different from the trend to that point. Lack of a change in trend may mask the effect of an efficacious policy if other factors are changing to offset it. For example, if the rural to urban migration of populations (which is usually accompanied by a downward trend in motor vehicle death rates, due to congestion and lower speeds in urban areas) slows about the time that an effective alcohol countermeasure is introduced, the effect of the alcohol countermeasure could be underestimated unless most of the drivers' blood alcohols are available for analysis.

Both from the scientific and practical points of view, replication of research results is very important. Replication refers to finding a similar result when a study is repeated in a different study population. Particularly when there is no reasonable comparison or control group, replication is needed to assure that change in injuries at a time of change in law, enforcement, or punishment was not for reasons other than the legal effect. In the case of the effect of "crackdowns" on alcohol and driving, interrupted time series in several jurisdictions indicate that a publicized increase in police activity results in a temporary reduction in vehicle-related injuries, the time of the effect varying from a few months to a few years (Ross, 1982).

Most police crackdowns are locally determined, and there is little research on why some communities undertake such efforts and others do not. Stimulation of community efforts by grant programs can have an effect, but many communities do not even apply for the funds. In Massachusetts, for example, communities were offered $70,000 per year for five years to initiate police enforcement and community activities to reduce drunk driving and alcohol use. Thirty responded and six were funded, resulting in reductions in motor vehicle injuries in those six compared to others who applied but were not funded (Hingson et al., 1996). Dozens of communities did not apply. It would be worthwhile to know why.

Perception of increased probability of arrest often has a deterrent effect, but changes in severity of punishment do not have much if any effect (Ross, 1982, 1992; Ross and Klette, 1995). The practical implication of the replicated findings is that "crackdowns" that increase the probability of arrest, or at least the perception of increased probability of arrest, will reduce the injury rate for a time, even in countries with somewhat differing cultures and legal traditions. The results leave open questions of how long such "crackdowns" can be maintained in terms of publicity and actual police activity, how often they can be repeated in the same population with the same effect, and whether a long-term change in behavior can be achieved with repetition (Hingson et al., 1988).

A decline in the proportion of fatally injured drivers with illegal blood alcohol was observed during the late 1980s and early 1990s in the United States (National Highway Traffic Safety Administration, 1995), partly due to the reenactment of laws changing the legal drinking age to 21 years in several states (Robertson, 1989) and partly due to other laws and enforcement (Zador et al., 1988). Increased public attention to dieting and the marketing of beverages with less alcohol per volume may have also contributed to the reduction, but evaluation of the effect of such factors is difficult because of the lack of disaggregated data regarding these factors in drivers in crashes relative to those exposed to the same road and other conditions.

A more complex variation of time-series analysis is the multivariate analysis of the fluctuation of injury rates during a period of time in one or more ecological units (country, provinces, states, cities) relative to fluctuations in factors thought to affect those rates, including laws or aspects of law enforcement. In addition to the fact that ecological-level data do not necessarily reflect the characteristics of the individuals injured (or assailants and drivers in crashes), as noted in chapter 8 (the ecological fallacy), the specification of the statistical models and the intercorrelation of factors at the ecological level render the estimates of effects from such analyses highly problematic. These problems have long been recognized in the analysis of economic data (Orcutt et al., 1968; Leamer, 1983), but economists particularly persist in performing such questionable analyses.

The effects of police manpower and police expenditures per capita have been studied with such models, and the results vary remarkably depending on the ecological units used, the assumed causal variables controlled, and the types of outcomes measured. The unit of analysis and the type of crime analyzed may be more or less sensitive to the ecological fallacy or the direction and degree of effect. Use of smaller jurisdictions, such as cities, narrows the variation in factors such as poverty, concentration of minority populations, and other socioeconomic factors. If the increased enforcement merely moved the criminal activity to the suburbs, however, the estimate of effect would be overstated. The latter would not be true if the analysis were confined to domestic violence or crimes of passion, but in the noted studies, these are usually lumped together with all murders and police-reported assaults, or felonies generally. Use of larger ecological units, such as metropolitan areas or states, might give better estimates of the overall effect, but these estimates might be confounded in different ways by the variation of other factors, as well as large differences in concentration of enforcement within smaller segments of such ecological units.

On the assumption that allocations of budgets for police and equipment are in response to crime, as well as possibly having an effect on crime, the regression equations on the time series are sometimes estimated in two or more stages. One review of 11 such studies noted effects on various crimes varying from estimates of substantial effect of police manpower or expenditures, to no effect, to adverse effects (O'Connor and Gilman, 1978). The latter could occur, for example, if the police and certain criminals, or minorities who fear police as much or more than criminals, engaged in an arms race.

One of the more controversial issues that has been subjected to a variety of analyses is gun legislation. Gun-related deaths and injuries are rare in most countries where the ownership of guns is prohibited for most people, or tightly controlled. The population rate of all assaults in a region of Denmark in a year was about 75 percent of those in the Northeastern Ohio Trauma Study, but the Danish homicide rate was only 20 percent of that in the Ohio study. The difference in homicide rates is mainly the result of greater gun involvement in assaults in Ohio. Private ownership of guns is allowed in Denmark only for hunting (Baker, 1985).

Even countries that have substantial social and political unrest have lower gun deaths per capita than many cities in the United States. Detroit, Michigan, had more gun-related deaths in 1973 than Northern Ireland, with a similar-sized population, during 5.5 years of renewed "troubles" in Northern Ireland in 1969–1974 (Zimring and Hawkins, 1987). Long-term comparisons of trends in violent crime as various countries imposed strict gun control indicate substantial effectiveness of such laws, but the weaker types of such laws typical in the United States had no discernible effects (Podell and Archer, 1994). Also, the effects of laws vary among U.S. states. For example, laws regarding child access to guns were found to reduce gun involvement in child deaths in one state but not several others (Webster and Starnes, 2000).

Opponents of gun control laws point to low gun death rates in Israel and Switzerland where substantial numbers of citizens keep guns as part of the reserve defense forces. Important questions for research are: What criteria do these countries use to screen recruits to the defense reserves? How is the screening implemented? How many people are not allowed to have guns on the basis of the screening? Do the citizen-soldiers have loaded guns or are there conditions for the issuance of ammunition? Does the recipient of ammunition have to account for its whereabouts and use? The answers might provide guidance for more effective gun regulation in countries where guns are ubiquitous and where gun death rates are high.

The effects of new gun laws in the United States are limited by the prelaw prevalence of gun ownership, and the effects of extant state and local laws are tempered by the movement of guns from jurisdictions with few restrictions to those with more strict laws. The results of studies of gun laws in the United States are in substantial conflict, less so in the case of effects on suicide than in effects on homicide.

Using an index of strictness of combinations of various types of laws, comparisons of jurisdictions found gun-related deaths lower in jurisdictions with stricter gun laws, and particularly where there is licensure of dealers, licensure by owners, and a waiting period between sale and delivery (Geisel et al., 1969). As indicated further below, when persons in the community other than police augment enforcement, in this case dealers, laws tend to be more effective.

The argument against studies showing a lower gun death rate related to gun control laws is: "You didn't control for X." For example, other researchers found that when the region of the country is controlled statistically, the correlation of the gun strictness index and gun death rate is no longer statistically significant. This was interpreted as demonstration of a spurious correlation; that is, gun death rates were said to be the result of the "frontier culture" of the South and Southwest rather than gun control laws, which are more prevalent in the North and East (Magaddino and Medoff, 1984). Since no one has attempted to measure "frontier culture," that is a dubious interpretation. For example, in Texas, a state that has been stereotyped as having a "frontier culture," Dallas and Houston had the highest seat belt use in response to law, more than 15 percentage points higher than the highest use in 17 cities in other states (Goryl and Bowman, 1987). That hardly seems the manifestation of a "frontier culture" thumbing its nose at laws.

The effect of gun legislation on suicide rates is less controversial. Researchers who have questioned the effect on homicide rates found that suicide rates are substantially lower in areas with stricter gun laws (Medoff and Magaddino, 1983).

Studies of severity of punishment of those who use guns have been limited. There is some evidence that a mandatory sentence for possession of a firearm during various crimes reduces homicides from firearms. Comparison of trends in percentage of homicides and suicides from firearms in New Jersey relative to the remainder of the United States before and after a mandatory sentencing law in 1981 indicates a substantial reduction in gun involvement in homicides but not suicides (Fife and Abrams, 1989). Since New Jersey had relatively strict gun laws prior to the mandatory sentencing law (Geisel et al., 1969), the results may not be generalized to states without such combinations of laws.

Almost all of the studies of gun laws are of aggregated data. It would be useful to compare individual level data on homicides and suicides with guns in jurisdictions with different gun laws regarding such factors as the age of the gun. Was the gun legally or illegally possessed? How was the gun obtained? What was the history of the gun (e.g., a gun possessed illegally where the death occurred but purchased legally elsewhere)?

The augmentation of law enforcement by persons other than police in the community is probably a substantial factor in the effect of several laws known to reduce injuries. Examples are laws that prohibit driving by 16-year-olds after a certain time in the evening. Since the police cannot easily see drivers at night, much less make a judgment regarding their ages, it is unlikely that arrest activity by police is effective in enforcement of such curfews. Yet a comparison of matched states with and without the laws indicates 25–62 percent reductions in crashes of 16-year-old drivers during the curfew hours (Preusser et al., 1984). A comparison of 47 cities with curfews for teenagers and 77 cities without curfews indicates a 23 percent reduction in motor vehicle deaths among 13- to 17-year-olds (Preusser et al., 1993). It is likely that many parents enforce the law by requiring their youngsters to be home during the hours that the curfew is in effect. A comparison of other types of fatalities would be useful to assess what effect, if any, curfews have on deaths other than those related to motor vehicles.

Several states have adopted "provisional licenses" or "graduated licenses," the latter based on demonstrated effectiveness of such laws in a few states and other countries (see http://www.iihs.org/laws/state_laws/grad_license.html, accessed September 2006). Comparison of teenage driver involvement in fatalities among the states found that reductions were associated with the stronger laws (Li-Hui et al., 2006; Morrisey et al., 2006).

Other jurisdictional comparisons have also suggested effectiveness of laws related to risks other than assaults and motor vehicles. Drowning of children in swimming pools was 65 percent less frequent in Honolulu, where pool fencing is required, than in Brisbane, Australia, with no requirement. The two cities had similar weather and pool-to-household ratios (Pearn et al., 1979). Comparison of adjacent affluent counties in Maryland and Virginia, with and without require-ments for household smoke detectors, found 25 percent fewer deaths in house fires where smoke detectors were required (McLoughlin et al., 1985).

Since most legislative bodies are unlikely to enact a law for research purposes, the enactment of laws is not necessarily random, and research must be designed to account for prelaw differences and changing conditions among jurisdictions. The use of rules in corporate settings could be studied in randomized experimental-control studies, but if such are conducted, they usually are not reported in the literature. Attempts have been made to study the effects of differing sanctions by having judges randomly assign sentences, but in some cases, many judges would not cooperate, preferring to retain their discretion (Ross and Blumenthal, 1975).

Police departments have been somewhat more amenable to the use of randomized experimental designs in an attempt to find out if resources can be more effectively allocated or if certain procedures are more effective. For example, during more than a year, 15 police districts in Kansas City were divided into three groups of five each: one set had the usual preventive patrol activity of a patrol car per district; a second had double to triple the usual patrol; and a third had no preventive patrol—the police responded only when called regarding a problem. Comparison of various crime rates and motor vehicle crashes among the areas, including victimization surveys, as well as those reported to police, indicated no differences in assaults and motor vehicle crashes. The three comparisons that were statistically significant—sex crimes other than rape, home burglaries, and community vandalism—did not consistently support a case for more intensive patrols (Kelling et al., 1974).

Several subsequent experimental studies were undertaken in an attempt to define aspects of police procedure and response that might make a difference, but more recent efforts are focused on first defining the dimensions of the variety of problems that the police encounter and developing tailored prevention programs or responses (Goldstein, 1990). This is no less than the use of epidemiological surveillance and analysis of relatively homogeneous subsets of the problem noted in chapters 6 and 7. This approach requires a reorientation of policing from treating each incident as a case to be investigated and resolved to a search for patterns that can guide targeted efforts. The research evidence indicates that concentration of police activity in "hot spots" of crime, particularly in unpredictable sequences for limited periods of time, reduces crime in those areas without displacing it elsewhere (Sherman, 1996). The severities of injuries related to guns have also been reduced using the "hot spot" approach. In a controlled experiment in Kansas City, police concentrated in areas with high gun-related crime used traffic violations to increase gun seizures. Shots fired decreased 81 percent in the experimental area compared to 32 percent in the comparison area (Sherman, 1996).

Some of the literature on targeting countermeasures based on surveillance raises the question of whether the targets should be based on rates per exposure versus total numbers. For example, one report from a police service in Canada compared police-reported motor vehicle crashes and convictions of drivers by age and gender relative to a survey of kilometers driven. Based on a narrowing of differences in crashes and convictions among age and gender groupings when considering rates per kilometer driven relative to proportionate involvement, the author of that study suggested that less attention should be paid to young and/or male drivers (Mercer, 1989). Yet, from a public health standpoint, one would target the groups with the largest numbers whether or not those numbers were generated by disproportionate exposure.

Particular aspects of the motor vehicle injury problem are known to be concentrated on certain roads at certain times of day. For example, figure 12-1 presents illegal alcohol involvement in fatally injured drivers in the United States by type of road and time of day in counties where alcohol was actually measured in more than 90 percent of fatally injured drivers. While the amount of driving with illegal blood alcohol on these roads might be useful to indicate how other conditions combine with alcohol to increase or decrease individual risk, the data are clear regarding enforcement of law. If the police are to maximize the apprehension of persons with illegal blood alcohol who will be in severe crashes, they will concentrate their alcohol squads on two-lane roads at night, where 61 percent of fatal crashes with illegally intoxicated drivers occur.

Research is needed to identify other times and places that law enforcement could be concentrated. For example, sales of guns used in felonies have been found concentrated among identifiable dealers, controlling for crime rates and sociodemographic factors (Wintemute et al., 2005). Do assaults in public occur repeatedly in certain bars, in other establishments, or on certain streets during certain hours? Do domestic assaults occur repeatedly in definable households at certain times of day and days of week?

Although assault among members of households resulting in injury requiring medical attention is more frequent than assault by strangers, arrest in domestic assault cases in the 1970s was about half as likely as in cases involving strangers (Berk and Loseke, 1980–1981). A controlled experiment of the effect of arrest on specific deterrence of spouse battering was conducted in Minneapolis. In response to calls regarding domestic violence, police randomly applied one of three actions: (1) arrest of the assailant, (2) order the assailant away from the premises for eight hours, or (3) give advice or attempt mediation. Follow-up study of police records

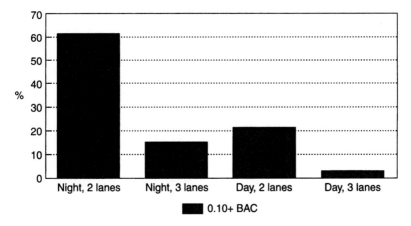

Figure 12-1. Percentage of Fatally Injured Drivers with Blood Alcohol Concentration (BAC) Greater than 0.10, by Type of Road and Time of Day

and interviews with the persons assaulted indicated that arrest was the most effective policy to reduce recidivism (Sherman and Berk, 1984).

A retrospective study of 28 months of police records in a California county, controlling for factors that affected probability of arrest, found the same result (Berk and Newton, 1985). Since time in jail has implications for job or income loss, the authors of the latter study suggested another controlled experiment with treatments, such as (1) a citation (like a traffic ticket); (2) arrest, book, and immediate release; or (3) arrest and hold for a hearing. If the first or second were found as effective in deterring battering as arrest and hold, they would be preferable.

While many cities adopted an arrest policy as a result of the research, a substantial debate ensued regarding the methods of these studies, such as reliance on police records, and unmeasured effects, such as more severe injuries from escalation of domestic disputes exacerbated by the arrest (Sherman, 1992). Replication of the Minneapolis experiment in other cities did not produce consistent results, but some evidence of efficacy was found when the various studies were compared (Buzawa and Buzawa, 1996; Christopher et al., 2001). This experience illustrates the difficulty both in policing private behavior and in learning whether or not police response has an effect because of questionable accuracy of reporting private behavior.

An example of an experimental study of detailed aspects of the effects on publicly observable behavior of a combined publicity and enforcement campaign is the research on elderly pedestrian behavior in Dade County, Florida. The experimental area was a street in Miami Beach with a high concentration of elderly residents, and the control area was a comparable street with similar-age residents in Coral Gables. Cameras mounted high above the street recorded pedestrians, and postcrossing interviews were also obtained, before, during, and after the increased enforcement of a law prohibiting jaywalking (crossing the street outside designated pedestrian crossing areas).

Prior to increased enforcement, news media coverage and speeches by police officers to 35 groups in the experimental area emphasized the law and the date of increased enforcement. During a two-week special enforcement period, extra police foot patrols were deployed, and about 300 tickets for jaywalking were issued, compared to about 40 per month ordinarily.

The results indicated that legal crossings increased during the enforcement period, more so when police were in sight, but declined to the preenforcement percentage when no police were present in the observation period after the special enforcement. Postcrossing interviews indicated that most people understood the law but preferred to rely on their own judgment regarding the movement of vehicles (Weiner, 1968). The effect on actual pedestrian collisions was not measured since too few for statistical power would be expected in a two-week period.

Cameras are also used as an enforcement tool. Cameras that identify the vehicles that run red lights or speeding result in substantial reductions in proscribed behavior compared to control areas without cameras (Retting et al., 1999; Retting and Farmer, 2003). The outcome measure did not include crashes that may or may not decline commensurate with the proscribed behavior.

WHAT TO MEASURE

Most of the studies of effects of laws and rules measure the proscribed or required behavior, or the incidence and severity of injuries that are supposedly affected by the behaviors. Preferably, both should be measured. For example, research on the effect of motorcycle helmet use included observations of helmet use by motorcyclists at selected sites in states with and without helmet use laws, as well as fatal injuries to motorcyclists in states with and without the laws before and after the laws were enforced. Since helmet use was almost universal in the states with laws requiring use, there was no question about differential use by those at differential risk after the law (Robertson, 1976a).

Just because a law results in a change in the behavior required does not mean that the law is having proportional success in injury reduction. If compliance is not universal and those who comply with the law are more or less at risk, the ultimate effect of the law on injury will not be proportional to the technical effectiveness of the required behavior. That has apparently been the case with seat belt use laws.

The expected percent change in injury rate as a result of a change in behavior is

$$P = 100 \ \frac{E(B - A)}{1 - BE}$$

where

P = expected percentage change in injury rate
B = proportion behaving in the prescribed way before the change
A = proportion behaving in the prescribed way after the change
E = the technical effectiveness of the behavioral change (Robertson, 1983b)

In Australia, where the first belt use law in a large jurisdiction (Victoria) was enacted, belt use increased from 20 to 70 percent from before to after the law. If the one-piece lap and shoulder belts used in Australia were 60 percent effective in reducing death when used, as claimed at the time, then $E = .6$, $B = .2$, and $A = .7$. Therefore, the reduction in deaths should have been about 1/3. It was actually 10 percent in rural areas and 20 percent in urban areas, based on comparison of changes in death rates in Victoria relative to provinces without the law at the time (Foldvary and Lane, 1974). Even if belts, when worn, were 45 percent effective in reducing deaths, that is, $E = .45$, the reduction should have been about 26 percent without selective use by those at less risk. Estimates of the effects of belt laws in the United States are also not compatible with 60 percent belt effectiveness when used (Cohen and Einav, 2003). See appendix 12-1 for a critique of studies claiming 60–65 percent belt effectiveness when used.

There is a hypothesis that nonusers of belts are more likely to crash at higher speeds, resulting in an overestimate of the effects of belts. Tests of the hypothesis, however, rely on data that are inadequate to support or reject the hypothesis. For example, Evans (1996) compared Δv ("delta-v") in crashes, an estimate of velocity change in the crash, from the National Automotive Sampling System (NASS) during 1982–1991, between belted and unbelted drivers. Δv was missing in 60 percent or more of cases in each of those years, and the percent missing among the injury severity codes was substantially different. Competent epidemiologists do not rely on data with such huge potential for bias in the selection of vehicles to measure Δv based on the outcome in injury severity (Farmer, in press). Evans also used a data set from North Carolina that measured injury by the police codes, combining A + K, which is biased by the overwhelming number of A injuries that are relatively trivial (see figure 6-1).

When changes occur simultaneously that could affect injury rates, then specification of changes in the behavior and specification of the injuries that should be affected by a law enacted at that time is essential for confidence in the research results. For example, multiple changing events occurred during the oil boycott that began near the end of 1972. The lack of gasoline and increased prices of fuel resulted in reduced driving, economic recession occurred, and the 55-mile-per-hour (mph) speed limit was adopted on roads that had a higher limit, primarily to reduce fuel use, all in a matter of months. In the United States, there was a very notable reduction of about 8,000 deaths related to motor vehicles per year in 1974–1975 compared to the average in the five immediately preceding years (interrupted time series), but the amount of the reduction that could be attributed to the reduced legal speed limit rather than the other factors was widely argued.

To estimate the effect of the speed limit, researchers noted that average speeds declined, particularly on rural interstates more than other roads. The percentage of drivers exceeding 65 miles per hour decreased from 59 percent in 1973 to 10 percent in 1974, and those exceeding 55 miles per hour declined from 93 percent in 1973 to 68 percent in 1974. The greatest reduction in deaths per miles traveled occurred on interstate and federal-aid primary roads—those where the speed limit was reduced. On the basis of reductions per miles traveled, about half of the total death reduction was attributed to the 55 mph limit (Kemper and Byington, 1977).

Eventually, due to an equivocal report from the Transportation Research Board (Altschuler et al., 1984) and an antiregulation Congress, the speed limits were raised. Deaths on rural interstate highways, where the limits were first raised, increased about 17 percent (Farmer et al., 1999). This is not as much as expected from the earlier research, but more crashworthy vehicles were introduced in the interim (chapter 13), perhaps moderating the effect.

Occasionally, a situation arises that allows the researcher to obtain data regarding a hypothesis that is ordinarily difficult to test. For example, a police strike in Finland provided evidence of the effect on vehicle speeds of public knowledge that police would not be on the road (Summala et al., 1980). The average speed increased only slightly, but the standard deviation increased about 20 percent. Apparently, some drivers drove faster but were almost matched by those who drove more slowly, perhaps for fear of other drivers in a period of no enforcement. Unfortunately, crash data were not included, perhaps because the strike lasted only two weeks and the numbers would have been too small for statistical power.

Generally, the effects of laws on behavior and the evaluation of the effects are enhanced if the behavior is easily observable. If the researcher can observe the behavior, so can the police. It is not surprising, therefore, that laws requiring observable behavior, such as limits on vehicle speed, child restraint use, seat belt use, and motorcycle helmet use, are usually more effective than laws directed at phenomena not observable without stopping persons—such as limits on blood alcohol of drivers or carrying concealed weapons (Robertson, 1983a).

UNINTENDED CONSEQUENCES

Generally laws that apply to publicly observable behaviors have proved more effective than nonlegal persuasive approaches (e.g., Mock et al., 1995). Few studies have paid attention to the possibility that laws requiring or proscribing a particular behavior could result in alternative behaviors that could place the individuals affected at more or less risk. For example, if children are required to be placed in child restraints while riding in cars, it is doubtful that families who could not afford child restraints would make fewer trips, resulting in the child being in a more or less safe environment, given the availability of restraint loaner programs. But if child restraints were required on commercial airplanes, it has been argued, a large enough proportion of children that now fly free in adult arms would be driven rather than flown if the airline required payment for use of a seat. Since children are so seldom killed in commercial airline crashes, the relative risk in motor vehicles compared to cars would result in more injuries to children, or so the theory goes.

Since no data are available on what people would actually do, those who argue the issue one way or another are less than well informed. One can conceive of a study in which child restraints would be required on a set of experimentally assigned air routes, and the numbers of child passengers in airplanes, motor vehicles (including busses), and trains would be counted by observers of the different modes of traffic among the experimental and randomly selected control routes before and after the restraint rule was put in effect. If there were apparent substitution of mode of travel, the net effect on risk to children could be estimated given known risk per mile by each mode of travel, and the observed use of child restraints in the two environments.

In Japan, comparison of child injuries and deaths before and after a child restraint use law revealed an increase in the child occupant death rate (Desapriya et al., 2004). The authors of the study compared that rate with the pedestrian rate, supposedly as a control for general trends in death and injury on the road. The pedestrian rate declined. They suggested misuse of child restraints as an explanation of the unexpected finding, but the more likely explanation is that the study was done when people were reducing their walking with children and increasing travel by motor vehicle. Although the study included vehicle miles traveled, it did not include number of passengers per vehicle. Without data, we do not know whether there was an increase in transportation of children in motor vehicles and, if so, whether the increase was because parents believed they were safer in child seats. Given the known effectiveness of child seats, it is not plausible that an increase in their use increased child deaths in vehicles.

Laws that proscribe participation in certain activities also raise the issue of the extent to which the alternative activities are more or less dangerous. Numerous studies were done of the effects of the minimum legal drinking age on involvement of teenagers as drivers in fatal crashes without consideration of potential effects on other injuries. Although the estimates of effects on vehicle crashes were somewhat biased toward underestimate of the effect of the laws because proxy measures for alcohol involvement (night and single-vehicle crashes) were not as indicative of alcohol in the younger drivers (Robertson, 1981), the studies usually found reduced fatal motor vehicle crashes of the drivers in the age groups affected by the laws (General Accounting Office, 1987).

These studies left open the question of what teenagers who were drinking in bars or other settings, where drinking was legal, would have been doing had they not been there. Not only did no one consider that those drinking legally were placed at risk of other injuries related to alcohol (e.g., assaults in bars), but also no one considered that if they could not drink, they might be doing something even more dangerous.

Finally, one research project, based on one state that changed its legal drinking age compared to one that did not, found no statistically significant effect of changing the drinking age on mortality from non-motor-vehicle injury (Hingson et al., 1985), but the statistical power was limited by the small sample. A larger study, based on all the states, estimated the effect of the legal minimum drinking age on all fatal injuries to persons 16 to 24 years of age and found a net beneficial effect on all injuries (Jones et al., 1992). Several potential effects were considered. Did the law affect injuries to persons younger than the drinking age, presumably because alcohol may be more easily obtained if adjacent-age peers can drink legally? Was there a spurt in injuries at the age that drinking became legal—the initiation effect? Did injuries decline as persons aged beyond the drinking age—the experience effect? The data indicated that, for most types of injuries, the higher the legal minimum drinking age, the lower the injury death rates in correlation with the number of years between the individuals' ages and the legal age. The hypothesized initiation effect was found only for homicides, and increased rather than decreased injury death rates occurred in correlation with presumed drinking experience (age at death minus legal drinking age).

Laws that prohibit alcohol sales in a limited geographic area have the potential to increase the risk of injury if the law results in driving or walking by intoxicated persons returning to the "dry" area from the "wet" area. During a brief period of legal alcohol use on an American Indian reservation, the arrests of reservation residents for intoxication in the neighboring county were reduced about one-third with no increase in such arrests on the reservation (May, 1975). Since arrests do not necessarily reflect alcohol use or the other behaviors associated with its use, the data are inadequate for a strong conclusion, but the issue is worthy of research. One study comparing retail availability of alcohol among states found no correlation between "single-vehicle" fatal crashes at night and alcohol retail outlets when other factors were taken into account (Greunewald and Ponicki, 1995).

Comprehensive study of a variety of laws among U.S. states found most alcohol laws have some effect (Villaveces et al., 2003). The imputation of alcohol in drivers in which alcohol was not measured weakens confidence in some of the results. Following the oil boycott in the mid 1970s, most U.S. states adopted a law allowing right turns at red lights at signalized intersections after stopping to assure that the turn could be made safely, unless a particular intersection was specified otherwise. The purpose of the law was to conserve fuel that was being burned during the waits for lights to change. However, observations of driver behavior indicated that the number of drivers who turned right at signalized intersections without stopping increased from 47 percent to 70 percent in one state (Baumgartner, 1981). The unintended effect was an increase in total crashes and, particularly, injuries to pedestrians and bicyclists (Zador, 1984).

A theory of unintended consequences says that drivers whose crash protection is increased will drive more riskily and endanger other road users—so-called risk compensation or risk homeostasis theory. Economists claimed to originate this theory in the 1970s (Lave and Weber, 1970; Peltzman, 1975), but it was used to oppose the requirement of safety equipment on trains in the nineteenth century (Adams, 1879). The typical study claiming to support the theory employs an ecological design: cross-sectional or time-series data on fatality rates correlated to aggregated data on seat belt use or regulation of vehicle characteristics. The latter studies are discussed in chapter 13.

Among the problems in such studies is that the drivers who were more protected were not disaggregated from those less protected, and motorcyclists were included as "pedestrians." For example, one study attempted to correlate occupant and other road user fatalities among states to belt use and factors such as vehicle miles driven, percent urban population, average speed on rural roads, alcohol sales per capita, percent youth in the population, and income per capita. States with higher belt use, according to the behavioral risk factor survey of the Centers for Disease Control and Prevention, had higher nonoccupant fatalities, controlling statistically for the other factors (Garbacz, 1990).

In the study, "nonoccupants" included all motorcyclists, many of whom were killed in single-vehicle crashes in which other drivers, belted or not, were not involved. As noted in chapter 7, the behavioral risk factor survey on belt use is not valid. Numerous differences among the states that could be confounded with belt use and fatal injuries were not considered, such as child restraint laws, motorcycle helmet use laws, and vehicle mix (large and small cars, tractor-trailer trucks, pickups, sport utility vehicles, and motorcycles).

The studies that have examined disaggregated data on the effects of belt use laws on behavior of drivers, or belt use in crashes, have not found evidence of risk compensation. Several important driving behaviors were observed on the road before and after the belt use law was enforced in Newfoundland, and in Nova Scotia during the same period without a law. Belt use increased from 16 percent to 77 percent in Newfoundland and remained virtually unchanged in Nova Scotia. Four driver behaviors—speed, stopping at intersections when the control light was amber, turning left in front of oncoming traffic, and gaps in following distance—were measured at various sites before and after the law. Changes in these behaviors in Newfoundland were similar to those in Nova Scotia, except that drivers in Newfoundland drove slower on expressways after the law, contrary to the theory (Lund and Zador, 1984). Study of interstate changes in belt use found no effect on nonoccupant fatalities (Cohen and Einav, 2003). The author has found no study of appropriately disaggregated data that showed an effect of increased driver belt use on other road users.

Detailed data from Suffolk County, New York, on all motor-vehicle-related injuries (including nonoccupants) seen in emergency departments (or that were fatal), before and during the first two quarters of the seat belt use law in New York, indicate a substantial reduction in severe injuries. Total injury cases decreased slightly in the first quarter and increased slightly in the second quarter, compared to the same periods in the year before, but larger increases were expected based on trends in Rhode Island without a law (Barancik et al., 1988; Rockett et al., 1988). In Suffolk County, the fatalities per emergency department case declined 20 percent in the first six months of the belt use law compared to the same period a year earlier, while in Rhode Island, without a law, the fatalities per case increased 24 percent. The economist who claimed that risk compensation behavior offsets the effects of belts did not mention these studies or the above-mentioned studies of the effects of belt use laws.

Changes in laws can have unintended consequences if they affect substitution of a less effective countermeasure for one having some effect. In Nassau County, New York, drivers convicted of driving while intoxicated were assigned randomly to the usual sentence or an education-rehabilitation program. The drivers who had the latter program had worse subsequent driving records than those who received the usual sentences (Preusser et al., 1976). Contrary findings occurred in an experiment in two Canadian cities. When "accidental" and violent injuries were combined, convicted drunk drivers who received rehabilitation were less likely to die in the subsequent decade (Mann et al., 1994).

The effect of law on economic incentives or disincentives may also have unintended consequences. In Quebec, Canada, the government did not subsidize driver education as was done in the United States, but required it for licensure before age 18 at a cost to the potential licensee of about $200. In 1983, the law was amended to require driver education of all newly licensed drivers. Since, thereafter, drivers could not avoid the cost of driver education whatever their age, the economic incentive to delay licensure to age 18 was removed. Licensure of 16- to 17-year-olds increased 12 percent among males and 19 percent among females in the year after the law was changed (Potvin et al., 1988).

Laws and rules regarding work practices have unintended consequences that could be changed to reduce injuries. Comparison of fatalities in the periods around the one-hour change from daylight savings and standard time indicate that some 900 fatal crashes could be avoided annually if daylight savings time were retained year round (Ferguson et al., 1995). The self-reported crash rate of hospital nurses working in rotating shifts is twice that of those working fixed shifts (Gold et al., 1992).

Unintended consequences of changes in law are not always adverse to injury control, for example, the death reductions when the 55 mph speed limit was enacted. Deposits on cans and bottles for various drinks and other uses have been required in various jurisdictions to reduce cleanup costs and for conservation. In Maryland, the adoption of such legislation was associated with a 60 percent reduction of glass-related lacerations to children (Baker et al., 1986).

Replicated quasi experiments of the effect of alcohol taxes on alcohol consumption indicate substantial effects. Increase in the cost of alcoholic beverages is associated with a reduction in motor vehicle fatalities, as well as mortality due to cirrhosis (Cook, 1981). Replication of that research is needed on the effects of alcohol taxes on other injuries, including homicide and suicide.

APPENDIX 12-1

Belt Laws and Belt Effectiveness

When belt use laws were enacted in a number of states in the United States in the mid to late 1980s, belt use increased substantially and death rates declined commensurate with a belt effectiveness of 45%, when used. That estimate controlled for changes in vehicle crashworthiness, alcohol involvement, economic conditions, vehicle size, and vehicle age (chapter 13). The regression coefficient in table 13-2 indicates a reduction of .007 in fatal crashes per 100 million vehicles miles for each percentage point increase in belt use. Belt use was approximately 53 percent in 1989 (Datta and Guzek, 1990). If the remaining 47 percent of car occupants had been restrained, the occupant fatality rate of 1.6 per 100 million miles would have been reduced by about 21 percent. This result is obtained by multiplying the coefficient in table 13-2 by the percent-unused belts ($.007 \times 47 = .329$) and dividing the result by the death rate ($.329/1.6 = 0.21$). The implied effectiveness of belts when used is 21/47, or 45 percent. While the study did not account for belt use by the occupants of the vehicles in crashes, it had the advantage that the observations of belt use by model year of vehicle in the population were independent of knowledge of the crashes.

Nineteen studies of belt effectiveness in reducing severe and fatal injuries, available by the mid 1970s, indicated estimates ranging from 7.5 percent to 82.8 percent effectiveness. That variation was examined for two potential factors that might explain it: the seriousness of the injuries included and the potential bias in claimed belt use (Robertson, 1976b).

Table 12-1 illustrates the potential biases that could occur if injuries of different severity were used, or if some people who were uninjured claimed to use belts when they actually did not. The latter was known to occur when comparing observed use in traffic and later questioning people about their belt use (Waller and Barry, 1969). As the table of hypothetical data shows, if 5 percent (500 of the 10,000 hypothetical occupants) of the persons in crashes claimed to use belts but did not, the effectiveness of belts would be overestimated. If only injured persons were considered, belt effectiveness would be underestimated. In the 19 studies examined, belt effectiveness was primarily correlated to claimed use, suggesting that the higher estimates of belt effectiveness were influenced by false claims of belt use.

Researchers who use hospitalized injuries to estimate the effects of belts and other equipment (e.g., Orsay et al., 1988) should be aware that without inclusion of the fatally injured and the uninjured, the estimates are substantially biased.

A few researchers combine fatal and "A" (supposedly disabling) injuries in state police files in their studies, for example, in the assessment of seat belt

Table 12-1. Hypothetical Data Illustrating Potential Systematic Error in Estimating Belt Effectiveness

	Belt Use		
	Belted	Unbelted	Total
All vehicle occupants in crashes	2,500	7,500	10,000
No injuries	2,040	5,700	7,740
Minor injuries	400	1,500	1,900
Severe injuries	60	300	360
Percent severe of all occupants	2.4	4.0	
Percent severe and minor of all occupants	18.4	24.0	

Estimated belt effectiveness in reducing all injuries = $\dfrac{(24 - 18.4)}{24}$ = .233 or 23 percent.

Estimated belt effectiveness in reducing severe injuries = $\dfrac{(4.0 - 2.4)}{4}$ = .40 or 40 percent.

If only injury cases are used to estimate effectiveness, estimated belt effectiveness = $\dfrac{(16.7 - 13.0)}{16.7}$

$$= .221 \text{ or } 22 \text{ percent.}$$

If 500 noninjured occupants claimed to use belts but did not:

	Claimed Belt Use	
	Belted	Unbelted
All vehicle occupants in crashes	3,000	7,000
Percent severe of all occupants	2.0	4.3

Estimated belt effectiveness = $\dfrac{(4.3 - 2.0)}{4.3}$ = .535 or 54 percent.

effectiveness (e.g., Streff, 1994; Reinfurt and Chi, 1981). Because A injuries are far more frequent than fatalities and nearly half the "A" injuries are nonserious injuries that occur to belted drivers (see figure 6-1), estimates of belt effectiveness or other factors in such studies are not valid.

In contrast to the 40–45 percent effectiveness estimate using Fatality Analysis Reporting System (FARS) data before 1986, 60–65 percent effectiveness in both older and newer model cars was found in 1986 and subsequent years using a within-vehicle comparison method. The method, called "double-pair comparison" (Evans, 1986a), attempts to control for a variety of factors. It is a variation of a case–control design applied to fatal crashes in which there is more than one occupant. The relative risk (R) of a fatality to a given set of occupants is calculated as a ratio of ratios. For example, the calculation of the relative risk of belt use for drivers and passengers is noted in table 12-2, using the cross-tabulation of who was

Table 12-2. Double-Pair Comparison of Drivers and Passengers in Fatal Crashes by Belt Use and Who Was Killed

	Passenger			
	Killed		Alive	
Driver	Belted	Unbelted	Belted	Unbelted
Killed		c		a
Belted	f	l	d	j
Unbelted				
Alive				
Belted		b		
Unbelted	e	k		
Driver $R = (a + c)/(b + c)/(j + l)/(k + l)$				
Passenger $R = (d + f)/(e + f)/(k + l)/(j + l)$				

using belts and who died, in the formula as indicated. Belt effectiveness in percent is then $100(1 - R)$. Estimates of the effectiveness of belts by this method, using FARS data for 1975–1984 car models in calendar years 1975–1983, produced a weighted average of belt effectiveness in preventing death at 41 percent, averaged among age groups (Evans, 1986b), similar to the effectiveness noted above in the study using observed belt use in the driver population.

Estimates of the effectiveness of seat belts, based on police reports or special investigator reports of use in crashes (NASS Crashworthiness Data System [CDS]; see chapter 6), have varied substantially, partly because of variations in belts or their effectiveness in crashes of different severity, and partly because of variations in research methodology. Apparently, differential misreporting of belt use of survivors of crashes, and by police and NASS investigators assuming higher belt use, became rampant after belt use laws were enacted. This misled a team of researchers to publish repeatedly the claim of 60–65 percent belt effectiveness (Cummings et al., 2002, 2003). An analyst in the National Highway Traffic Safety Administration did a thorough study of subgroups of drivers and passengers to identify potential biases and concluded that the jump in belt effectiveness estimates was biased by self-reported belt use by survivors probably because of the laws requiring use (Kahane, 2000). He indicated that the 45% estimate of belt effectiveness in passenger cars is more realistic given the potential biases in reported belt use in crashes and that changes in death rates over time in relation to observed belt use in the driving population are incompatible with 60–65 percent effectiveness. A telling commentary on police reports in that study is the finding that 65 percent of dead drivers in multiple vehicle collisions were judged culpable by police while only 32 percent of the surviving drivers in the same crashes were considered culpable (Kahane, 2000). The dead tell no tales, but apparently the survivors do.

Nevertheless, Cummings and colleagues claimed that belt effectiveness is near 60–65 percent based on analysis of data from the NASS CDS, assuming that the NASS investigator recording of use was a "gold standard" (Cummings et al.,

2003; Schiff and Cummings, 2004). Cummings (2002) compared belt effectiveness using police reports and investigations by multidisciplinary teams for the NASS, the latter supposed better investigators than police. He concluded that police reports are valid indicators of belt use because the seat belt effectiveness data using either police reports or NASS investigations are similar, particularly among the more seriously injured (Schiff and Cummings, 2004). Since these analyses produce implausible belt effectiveness coefficients based on data from each of the two groups, they merely demonstrate that NASS investigators are just as biased as the police. That does not mean that they are intentionally biased, but knowing the outcome could shade anyone's judgment. Cummings attributed the large increase in belt effectiveness estimates using within-vehicle comparisons primarily to a phenomenon called nondifferential misclassification, which means that random error in seat belt use classifications will result in an understatement of effectiveness in within-vehicle comparisons when use is low. He claims the theory is supported by trends in police-reported use in such crashes and a simulation of its effect on effectiveness estimates. What is not explained adequately by the theory is the nonrandom bias in police and NASS CDS reported belt use by the dead and survivors that was exacerbated by belt use laws in the mid-1980s.

The political push for belt use laws during the mid-1980s probably sensitized police and NASS investigators to the importance of belts. Some may have taken the illogical step of assuming that if the person died, the belts were not in use. Perhaps too much emphasis has been placed on the problem of self-reports of crash survivors and not enough emphasis on the potential bias of investigators judging the cause based on the outcome. Of course, that is why we require double-blind studies in assessing the effects and safety of drugs rather than rely on the judgments of physicians and patients who know which drug was taken and the outcome. Would that all injury prevention researchers were as careful.

An objective measure of belt use and other conditions, such as speed and crash forces in crashes, is now available. The installation of "event data recorders" in vehicles provides a measure of such conditions preserved electronically at the time of a crash. Some 40 million vehicles were equipped with them in the United States by 2004. The first data on these vehicles that appeared in the NASS CDS files indicate that in 31 percent of 213 cases where NASS investigators indicate belts as buckled in a crash, the data recorder indicated that the belt was not in use. The investigators reported 74 percent of vehicle occupants buckled up but only 54 percent of the data recorders indicated belts buckled (Gabler et al., 2004). Some of those could be buckled while the occupant sat on them. Apparently, the NASS investigators, like the police, are substantially overestimating belt use, which results in inflated estimates of effectiveness. The assumption that NASS investigators provide the "gold standard" for seat belt use (Cummings et al., 2003; Schiff and Cummings, 2004) is foolish.

Estimates of the effectiveness of air bags and other countermeasures that controlled for seat belt use using invalid police and NASS investigator reports of belt use are also likely invalid (e.g., Cummings et al., 2002). Some researchers that employ police reports of seat belt use note reporting bias in the "limitations" section of their reports but fail to acknowledge that such bias renders their estimates of belt effects on injury, and perhaps other claimed correlates of belt use, untenable (e.g., Allen et al., 2006).

As more objective data become available, particularly among the fatally injured, we will at least be able to know more precisely the effectiveness of seat belts in combination with air bags and other vehicle factors and equipment. Since there are few, if any, cars that have data recorders and no air bags, an estimate of the effectiveness of seat belt use alone based on accurate belt use data may never be available unless vehicles in countries where air bags are less prevalent are equipped with data recorders. Unless the sampling protocol for NASS is changed from one based on inaccurate police characterization of injury severity, research using that system will remain in question (see chapter 6; Farmer, in press).

References

Adams CF (1879) *Notes on Railroad Accidents.* New York, NY: G.B. Putnam's Sons.

Allen A, Zhu S, Sauter C, Layde P, and Hargarten S (2006) A comprehensive statewide analysis of seatbelt non-use with injury and hospital admissions: new data, old problem. *Acad Emerg Med.* 13:427–434.

Altschuler AA, et al. (1984). *55: A Decade of Experience.* Special Report 204. Washington, DC: Transportation Research Board.

Baker MD, Moore SE, and Wise PH (1986) The impact of "Bottle Bill" legislation on the incidence of lacerations in childhood. *Am J Public Health.* 76:1243.

Baker SP (1985) Without guns, do people kill people? *Am J Public Health.* 75:587–588.

Barancik JI, Kramer CF, Thode HC, and Harris D (1988) Efficacy of the New York state seat belt law: preliminary assessment of occurrence and severity. *Bull N Y Acad Med.* 64:742–749.

Baumgartner WE (1981) After stop, compliance with right turn on red after stop. *Inst Transport Eng J.* 51:19–27.

Becker G (1968) Crime and punishment: an economic approach. *J Polit Econ.* 76:169–217.

Berger LR, and Mohan D (1996) *Injury Control: A Global View.* Delhi, India: Oxford University Press.

Bergman AB (ed.) (1992) *Political Approaches to Injury Control at the State Level.* Seattle, WA: University of Washington Press.

Berk RA, and Newton PJ (1985) Does arrest really deter wife battery? An effort to replicate the findings of the Minneapolis spouse abuse experiment. *Am Sociol Rev.* 50:253–262.

Berk SF, and Loseke DR (1980–1981) "Handling" family violence: situational determinants of police arrests in domestic disturbances. *Law Soc Rev.* 15:317–333.

Buzawa ES, and Buzawa CG (eds.) (1996) *Do Arrests and Restraining Orders Work?* Thousand Oaks, CA: Sage.

Campbell DT (1969) Reforms as experiments. *Am Psychol.* 24:409–429.

Christopher DM, Garner JH, and Fagan JA (2001) *The Effects of Arrest on Intimate Partner Violence: New Evidence From the Spouse Assault Replication Program.* Washington, DC: U.S. Department of Justice.

Cohen A, and Einav L (2003) The effects of mandatory seat belt laws on driving behavior and traffic. *Rev Econ Stat.* 85:828–843.

Cook PJ (1981) The effect of liquor taxes on drinking, cirrhosis and auto accidents. In Moore MH, and Gerstein DR (eds.), *Alcohol and Public Policy: Beyond the Shadow of Prohibition.* Washington, DC: National Academy Press.

Cressey DR (1975) Law, order and the motorist. In Hood R (ed.), *Crime, Criminology and Public Policy.* New York, NY: The Free Press.

Cummings P (2002) Association of seat belt use with death: a comparison of estimates based on data from police and estimates based on data from trained crash investigators *Inj Prev.* 8: 338–341.

Cummings P, McKnight B, Rivara FP, and Grossman DC (2002) Association of driver air bags with driver fatality: a matched cohort study. *BMJ.* 324:1119–1122.

Cummings P, Wells JD, and Rivara FP (2003) Estimating seat belt effectiveness using matched-pair cohort methods. *Accid Anal Prev.* 35:143–149.

Datta TK and Guzek P (1990) *Restraint System Use in 19 U.S. Cities:1989 Annual Report.* Washington, DC: National Highway Traffic Safety Administration.

Desapriya EBR, Iwase N, Pike I, Brussoni M, and Papsdorf M (2004) Child motor vehicle occupant and pedestrian casualties before and after enactment of child restraint seats legislation in Japan. *Inj Contr Saf Promot.* 11:225–230.

Evans L (1986a) Double pair comparison—a new method to determine how occupant characteristics affect fatality risk in traffic crashes. *Acc Anal Prev.* 18:217–227.

Evans L (1986b) The effectiveness of safety belts in preventing fatalities. *Accid Anal Prev.* 18:229–241.

Evans L (1996) Safety belt effectiveness: the influence of crash severity and selective recruitment. *Acc Anal Prev.* 28:423–433.

Farmer CM (in press) Another look at Meyer and Finney's 'Who wants airbags' Chance.

Farmer CM, Retting RA, and Lund AK (1999) Changes in motor vehicle occupant fatalities after repeal of the national maximum speed limit. *Accid Anal Prev.* 31:537–43.

Ferguson SA, Preusser DF, Lund AK, Zador PF, and Ulmer MA (1995) Daylight savings time and motor vehicle crashes: the reduction in pedestrian and vehicle occupant fatalities. *Am J Public Health.* 85:92–95.

Fife D, and Abrams WR (1989) Firearms' decreased role in New Jersey homicides after a mandatory sentencing law. *J Trauma.* 29:1548–1551.

Foldvary LA, and Lane JC (1974) The effectiveness of compulsory wearing of seat-belts in casualty reduction. *Accid Anal Prev.* 6:59–81.

Gabler HC, Hampton CE, and Hinch J (2004) *Crash Severity: A Comparison of Event Data Recorder Measurements With Accident Reconstruction Estimates.* Paper 2004-01-1194. Warrendale, PA:Society of Automotive Engineers.

Garbacz C (1990) Estimating seat belt effectiveness with seat belt usage data from the Centers for Disease Control. *Econ Lett.* 34:83–88.

Geisel MS, Roll R, and Wettick RS Jr (1969) The effectiveness of state and local regulation of handguns: a statistical analysis. *Duke Law J.* 1969:647–676.

General Accounting Office (1987) *Drinking-Age Laws: An Evaluation Synthesis of Their Impact on Highway Safety.* Washington, DC: U.S. Congress.

Gold DR, Rogacz S, Bock N, Tosteson TD, Baum TM, Speizer FE, and Czeisler CA (1992) Rotating shift work, sleep, and accidents related to sleepiness in hospital nurses. *Am J Public Health.* 82:1011–1014.

Goldstein H (1990) *Problem Oriented Policing.* Philadelphia, PA: Temple University Press.

Goryl ME, and Bowman BL (1987) *Restraint System Usage in the Population.* Washington, DC: National Highway Traffic Safety Administration.

Greunewald PJ, and Ponicki WR (1995) The relationship of the retail availability of alcohol and alcohol sales to alcohol-related traffic crashes. *Accid Anal Prev.* 27:249–259.

Hingson R, Merrigan D, and Heeren T (1985) Effects of Massachusetts raising its legal drinking age from 18 to 20 on deaths from teenage homicide, suicide, and non traffic accidents. *Pediatr Clin North Am.* 32:221–232.

Hingson R, Howland J, Heeren T, and Levenson S (1988) Effects of legal penalty changes and laws to increase drunken driving convictions on fatal traffic crashes. *Bull N Y Acad Med.* 64:662–677.

Hingson R, McGovern T, Howland J, Heeren T, Winter M, and Zakocs R (1996) Reducing alcohol-impaired driving in Massachusetts: the Saving Lives Program. *Am J Public Health.* 86:791–797.

Hoff JC (1983) *A Practical Guide to BOX-JENKINS Forecasting.* Belmont, CA: Lifetime Learning Publications.

Houston DJ, Richardson LE Jr, and Neeley GW (2001) The effectiveness of child safety seat laws in the fifty states. *Policy Stud Rev.* 18:163–184.

Jones NE, Pieper CF, and Robertson LS (1992) The effect of the legal drinking age on fatal injuries of adolescents and young adults. *Am J Public Health.* 82:112–115.

Kahane CJ (2000) *Fatality Reduction by Safety Belts for Front-Seat Occupants of Cars and Light Trucks.* Washington, DC: National Highway Traffic Safety Administration.

Kelling GL, Pate T, Dieckman D, and Brown CE (1974) *The Kansas City Police Patrol Experiment.* Washington, DC: Police Foundation.

Kemper WJ, and Byington SR (1977) Safety aspects of the 55 mph speed limit. *Public Roads.* 41:58–67.

Lave LB, and Weber WW (1970) A cost-benefit analysis of auto safety features. *Appl Econ.* 4:265–275.

Leamer EE (1983) Let's take the con out of econometrics. *Am Econ Rev.* 73:31–43.

Li-Hui C, Baker SP, and Li G (2006) Graduated driver licensing programs and fatal crashes of 16-year-old drivers: a national evaluation. *Pediatrics.* 11118:56–62.

Lund AK, and Zador P (1984) Mandatory belt use and driver risk taking. *Risk Anal.* 4:41–53.

Magaddino JP, and Medoff MH (1984) An empirical analysis of federal and state firearm control laws. In Kates DB (ed.), *Firearms and Violence: Issues of Public Policy.* Cambridge, MA: Ballinger.

Mann RE, Anglin L, Wilkins K, Vingilis ER, MacDonald S, and Sheu WJ (1994) Rehabilitation for convicted drinking drivers (second offenders): effects on mortality. *J Stud Alcohol.* 55:372–374.

May PA (1975) Arrests, alcohol, and alcohol legalization among an American Indian tribe. *Plains Anthropol.* 20:129–134.

McLoughlin E, Marchone M, Hanger SL, German PS, and Baker SP (1985) Smoke detector legislation: its effect on owner occupied homes. *Am J Public Health.* 75:858–862.

Medoff MH, and Magaddino JP (1983) Suicides and firearm control laws. *Eval Rev.* 7:357–372.

Mercer GW (1989) Traffic accidents and convictions: group totals versus rate per kilometer driven. *Risk Anal.* 9:71–77.

Mock CN, Maier RV, Boyle E, Pilcher S, and Rivara FP (1995) Injury prevention strategies to promote helmet use decrease severe head injuries at a level I trauma center. *J Trauma.* 39:29–33.

Moore MH (1995) Public health and criminal justice approaches to prevention. In Tonry M, and Farrington DP (eds.), *Building a Safer Society: Strategic Approaches to Crime Prevention.* Chicago, IL: University of Chicago Press.

Morrisey M, Grabowski D, Dee T, and Campbell C (2006) The strength of graduated drivers license programs and fatalities among teen drivers and passengers. *Accid Anal Prev.* 38:135–141.

National Highway Traffic Safety Administration (1995) *Traffic Safety Facts 1994.* Washington, DC: U.S. Department of Transportation.

O'Connor RJ, and Gilman B (1978) The police role in deterring crime. In Cramer JA (ed.), *Preventing Crime.* Beverly Hills, CA: Sage.

Orcutt GH, Watts HW, and Edwards JB (1968) Data aggregation and information loss. *Am Econ Rev.* 58:773–787.

Orsay EM, Turnbull TL, Dunne M, Barrett JA, Langenberg P and Orsay CP (1988) Prospective study of the effect of safety belts on morbidity and health care costs in motor-vehicle accidents. *JAMA.* 260:3598–3603.

Pearn JH, Wong RK, Brown J, Ching Y, Bart R, and Hammar S (1979) Drowning and near-drowning involving children: a five-year total population study from the city and county of Honolulu. *Am J Public Health.* 69:450–454.

Peltzman S (1975) The effects of automobile safety regulations. *J Polit Econ.* 83:677–726.

Podell S, and Archer D (1994) Do legal changes matter? The case of gun control laws. In Costanzo M, and Oskamp S (eds.), *Violence and the Law.* Thousand Oaks, CA: Sage.

Potvin L, Champagne F, and Laberge-Nadeau C (1988) Mandatory driver training and road safety. *Am J Public Health.* 78:1206–1209.

Preusser DF, Ulmer RG, and Adams JR (1976) Driver record evaluation of a drinking-driver rehabilitation program. *J Safety Res.* 8:98–105.

Preusser DF, Williams AF, Zador PL, and Blomberg RD (1984) The effect of curfew laws on motor vehicle crashes. *Law Policy.* 6:115–128.

Preusser DF, Zador PL, and Williams AF (1993) The effect of city curfew ordinances on teenage motor vehicle fatalities. *Accid Anal Prev.* 25:641–645.

Reinfurt DW, and Chi GYH (1981) Automatic vs manual safety belt systems: a comparison using state accident data involving 1975–1979 model VW Rabbits. In Green RN, and Petrucelli E (eds.), *Proceedings: International Symposium on Occupant Restraints Morton.* Grove, IL: American Association for Automotive Medicine.

Retting RA, and Farmer CM (2003) Evaluation of speed camera enforcement in the District of Columbia. *Transport Res Rec.* 1830:34–37.

Retting RA, Williams AF, Farmer CM, and Feldman AF (1999) Evaluation of red-light camera enforcement in Fairfax, Va., USA. *ITE J.* 69:30–34.

Roberts WO, Brust JD, Leonard B, and Hebert BJ (1996) Fair-play rules and injury reduction in ice hockey. *Arch Pediatr Adolesc Med.* 150:140–145.

Robertson LS (1976a) An instance of effective legal regulation: motorcyclist helmet and daytime headlamp laws. *Law Soc Rev.* 10:456–477.

Robertson LS (1976b) Estimates of motor vehicle seat belt effectiveness and use: implications for occupant crash protection. *Am J Public Health.* 66:859–64.

Robertson, LS (1981) Patterns of teenaged driver involvement in fatal motor vehicle crashes: implications for policy choices. *J Health Polit, Policy Law.* 6:303–314.

Robertson LS (1983a) *Injuries: Causes, Control Strategies and Public Policy.* Lexington, MA: DC Heath.

Robertson LS (1983b) Public perception and behavior in relation to vehicle passenger restraints. In Covello VT, Flamm WG, Rodricks JV, and Tardiff RG (eds.), *The Analysis of Actual Versus Perceived Risks.* New York, NY: Plenum.

Robertson LS (1989) Blood alcohol in fatally injured drivers and the minimum legal drinking age. *J Health Polit Policy Law.* 14:817–825.

Robertson LS, Rich R, and Ross HL (1973) Jail sentences for driving while intoxicated in Chicago: a judicial policy that failed. *Law Soc Rev.* 8:55–67.

Rockett IRH, Hollingshead WH, and Lieberman ES (1988) A preliminary assessment of change in motor vehicle traffic trauma incidence and outcome in Rhode Island, 1984–1985. *Bull N Y Acad Med.* 64:750–756.

Ross HL (1960) Traffic law violations: a folk crime. *Soc Probl.* 8:231–241.

Ross HL (1982) *Deterring the Drinking Driver: Legal Policy and Social Control.* Lexington, MA: DC Heath.

Ross HL (1992) *Confronting Drunk Driving: Social Policy for Saving Lives.* New Haven, CT: Yale University Press.

Ross HL, and Blumenthal M (1975) Some problems in experimentation in a legal setting. *Am Sociol.* 10:150–155.

Ross HL, and Klette H (1995) Abandonment of mandatory jail for impaired drivers in Norway and Sweden. *Accid Anal Prev.* 27:151–157.

Sanders RS (1982) Legislative approach to auto safety: the Tennessee experience. In Bergman AB (ed.), *Preventing Childhood Injuries.* Columbus, OH: Ross Laboratories.

Schiff MA, and Cummings P (2004) Comparison of reporting of seat belt use by police and crash investigators: variation in agreement by injury severity. *Accid Anal Prev.* 36:961–965.

Sherman LW (1992) *Policing Domestic Violence.* New York, NY: Free Press.

Sherman LW (1996) The police. In Wilson JQ, and Petersilia J (eds.), *Crime.* San Francisco, CA: Institute for Contemporary Studies Press.

Sherman LW, and Berk RA (1984) The specific deterrent effect of arrest for domestic violence. *Am Soc Rev.* 49:261–272.

Smith DL, and Warren CW (1978) Use of victimization data to measure deterrence. In Cramer JA (ed.), *Preventing Crime.* Beverly Hills, CA: Sage.

Sood S (1988) Survey of factors influencing injury among riders involved in motorized two-wheeler accidents in India: a prospective study of 302 cases. *J Trauma.* 28:530–534.

Streff FM (1994) Field effectiveness of two restraint systems: the 3-point manual belt versus the 2-point-motorized-shoulder, manual lap belt. In *38th Annual Proceedings of the Association for the Advancement of Automotive Medicine.* Morton Grove, IL: Association for the Advancement of Automotive Medicine.

Summala H, Naatanen R, and Roine M (1980) Exceptional condition of police enforcement: driving speeds during the police strike. *Accid Anal Prev.* 12:179–184.

Teret S, Jones AS, Williams AF, and Wells JAK (1986) Child restraint laws: an analysis of gaps in coverage. *Am J Public Health.* 76:31.

Villaveces A, Cummings P, Koepsell TD, Rivara FP, Lumley T, and Moffat J (2003) Association of alcohol-related laws with deaths due to motor vehicle and motorcycle crashes in the United States, 1980–1997. *Am J Epidemiol.* 157:131–140.

Waller PF and Barry PZ (1969) *Seat belts: a comparison of actual and reported use.* Chapel Hill, NC: North Carolina Highway Safety Research Center.

Webster DW, and Starnes M (2000) Reexamining the association between child access prevention gun laws and unintentional shooting deaths of children. *Pediatrics.* 106:1466–1469.

Weiner EL (1968) The elderly pedestrian: response to an enforcement campaign. *Traf Saf Res Rev.* 11:100–110.

Williams AF, and Robertson LS (1975) The fatal crash reduction program: a reevaluation. *Accid Anal Prev.* 7:37–44.

Wintemute GJ, Cook P, and Wright MA (2005) Risk factors among handgun retailers for frequent and disproportionate sales of guns used in violent and firearm related crimes. *Inj Prev.* 11:357–363.

Zador PH (1984) Right-turn-on-red laws and motor vehicle crashes: a review of the literature. *Accid Anal Prev.* 16:241–245.

Zador PH, Lund AK, Fields M, and Weinberg K (1988) *Fatal Crash Involvement and Laws Against Alcohol-Impaired Driving.* Washington, DC: Insurance Institute for Highway Safety.

Zimring FE, and Hawkins G (1987) *The Citizen's Guide to Gun Control.* New York, NY: MacMillan.

13

Evaluation of Agent, Vehicle, and Environmental Modifications

Control of energy, vehicles that convey the energy, and characteristics of environments that contribute to the concentration of energy and vehicles has often been successful in reducing injury when applied. Product manufacturers and the builders of roads, housing, and other products have the opportunity to modify them to reduce the incidence and severity of injurious energy exchanges. The sources of the vast majority of serious injuries are the products of industry and builders in everyday or frequent use, among them motor vehicles, roads, guns, agricultural and industrial machines, stairs, cigarettes, matches, propane lighters, stoves and space heaters, clothing, bedding, swimming pools, and watercraft.

Many industrially developing countries are repeating the mistakes that occurred during the industrialization of Europe and the United States. Replacement of human and animal power by electrical and internal combustion engines exposes people to vastly increased energy, often with no attention to features or alternatives that would minimize harm (Berger and Mohan, 1996; Krishnan et al., 1990).

Well-designed epidemiological studies can reveal the injuries associated with the characteristics of products and environments. They can also aid in the evaluation of the effectiveness of modifications of products, protective equipment, and environments in injury control. For example, does motion detection technology used in swimming pools to detect potential drowning result in lower drowning rates (see http://www.poseidon-tech.com/us/system.html)? If so, does drowning occur in community pools significantly to justify the cost of installation, or is drowning mainly in home pools where the cost of such technology may be prohibitive for the majority of pool owners? Are there inexpensive ways to accomplish the same result?

Decisions that influence the rate of injuries associated with a given product may include design characteristics, quantity per package and type of package, quality control in manufacture or building the product, and extent and target of marketing efforts. Most of the efforts by government to influence these decisions for injury reduction have focused on standards affecting designs, or recalls of products that have design or manufacturing defects. The agreement between the U.S. Consumer Product Safety Commission and the manufacturers of all terrain vehicles that the vehicles would not be marketed for use by children, the very occasional banning of a product by the commission, and labeling requirements by various agencies are exceptions to the general lack of attention to marketing and its targets.

PRODUCT DESIGN

Research that relates product or environmental designs to injury rates and patterns can inform manufacturers, builders, and governmental regulatory agencies, although there is often resistance to the inference that injury is "caused" by the design. Such research is frequently attacked on the grounds that every conceivable behavioral factor was not controlled or was inadequately controlled. In contrast, when a behavioral factor is correlated to rates of injury, questions regarding controls for characteristics of products involved are rarely raised by scientists, much less by manufacturers or the government.

Not only is analysis of causation sometimes a diversion from adoption of effective prevention (chapter 8), but so is the argument about causation with respect to injury from product characteristics. If children are being poisoned by aspirin, what are the causes—the children's natural tendency to put things in their mouths, the parents' or others' failure to store the aspirin inaccessible to children, the attractiveness of the aspirin package, the number of pills per package, or the color of the pills?

If the number of pills per package can be reduced or the cap on the bottle can be changed to make it difficult for the child to open it, why argue about primal causation or launch expensive studies to specify the effects of various risk factors, some of which are much less controllable than a product modification? In the case of child poisonings from aspirin, the aspirin manufacturers were informed by pediatricians and consumer groups that they could make a difference in child poisonings by modification of quantity per package and type of packaging and did so. The child poisonings from aspirin declined 80 percent (Done, 1978).

The hazardous characteristics of certain products are obvious, but their consequences are often ignored. Examples are points and edges on interior and exterior surfaces of motor vehicles, sharp edges on the ends of roadside guardrails, the height of playground equipment relative to the hardness of the surface under it, the ease of use of handguns, and exposed moving parts of industrial, agricultural, and recreational machines. Product testing can reveal less obvious factors, such as the energy management capabilities of vehicles in crash tests (crashworthiness).

Clinical case studies can be a rich source of hypotheses regarding such characteristics of products, as they were historically in investigations of motor vehicles and aviation (e.g., Woodward, 1948; Gikas, 1972; Snyder, 1975; Champion et al., 1986; Clark et al., 1987). The epidemiologist can draw attention to a given problem and provide estimates of the effects of modification by correlating the incidence and severity of injuries to variations in relevant characteristics of the products or environments.

Even products that are sometimes used to injure intentionally may be changed to reduce severity. As noted in chapter 2, the physics of bullets and shotgun pellets have been described in detail (Sykes et al., 1988; Ortog et al., 1988; Karlson and Hargarten, 1997), but their relative contribution to severity of injuries in shootings has only recently been subjected to epidemiological investigation. Trends toward higher caliber weapons that remain small enough to be concealed will probably increase the fatalities per shooting (Wintemute, 1996). The companies that aggressively promoted the cheap "Saturday night specials" increased their marketing of more powerful, concealable handguns (Wintemute, 1994).

Suicide by cutting and piercing declined about 80 percent among males in England in parallel with the replacement of straight razors with safety razors (Farmer, 1992). Apparently no one studied the exact extent of razor involvement, but at least some of the reduction is likely from replacement of a potentially lethal instrument easily at hand. The removal of carbon monoxide from domestic gas was associated with a reduction of about one-third in the net suicide rate in England and Wales, but apparently not so in Scotland or the Netherlands (Kreitman, 1976; Clarke and Mayhew, 1988). In the United States, suicide by motor vehicle exhaust increased among males as that by domestic gas decreased, but there was an apparent net decrease in suicides among females (Lester, 1990).

Characteristics of products and environments that may not be obvious but are likely contributors to injury incidence or severity can be learned by review of elementary physics or chemistry (see chapter 2). Examples are energy-absorbing capability of vehicle components, as well as trees, poles, guardrail, and other roadside objects; stability of vehicles; cigarette burn rates; flammability of clothing, furniture, and bedding; and toxicity of drugs, household chemicals, and chemicals used in farming and industry. Again, the epidemiologist can learn the variations among products and, by observing the patterns of such variations in relation to relevant injury rates, estimate the effect of potential modifications (see appendix 9-1).

Biomechanical studies in the laboratory also suggest hypotheses for epidemiological investigation. Laboratory studies of simulated pedestrian collisions using bumpers of varying height indicated that bumpers 25 or more inches from the road surface produced more severe injuries (Weiss et al., 1977). Epidemiological study of the injuries to people struck on the road showed more severe injury related to higher bumper height (Ashton, 1982).

Collaboration of biomechanical and epidemiological researchers can contribute to understanding of injury tolerances of subsets of the population. For example, examinations of severity and circumstances of injuries to children in free falls and biomechanical simulations of the events were used to estimate tolerances of children to head impacts (Mohan et al., 1979).

EVALUATION OF PRODUCT CHANGES

It is also important to know whether product modifications intended to reduce risk are functioning as intended. For example, of 20 families who had antiscald devices attached to bathroom faucets, 19 had removed them within nine months because of sediment buildup in the devices (Fallat and Rengers, 1993).

Opportunities to study relatively rare phenomena sometimes arise to epidemiologists at the site for other reasons. For example, an area in Guatemala, where nutrition studies were under way, experienced an earthquake. Epidemiologists were able to correlate injury with housing characteristics and other factors (Glass et al., 1977).

Most governmental standards for products are performance standards that do not directly dictate design but set minimum limits for performance in injury reduction or, in the case of worker injuries, set standards and allow for inspections of workplaces. The U.S. Federal Motor Vehicle Safety Standards, for example, specify criteria for performance of components, such as the energy absorption of steering assemblies in frontal crashes, but do not indicate how the component is to be designed to meet the standard.

The effectiveness of a regulation depends on the technical effectiveness of the regulation relative to the performance of the regulated product, process, or environment prior to the regulation, and the degree of compliance to the regulation by manufacturers (or other relevant organizations). There is also the argument, noted in chapter 12, that persons whose risk is reduced will behave differently, offsetting the effect of laws or regulation. Another test of the hypothesis that increased protection would be offset by behavior was provided by the introduction of airbags in cars. Those drivers protected by airbags could have reduced their belt use to partly offset the reduced risk provided by the airbags, but they did not. Belt use by drivers in airbag-equipped cars was not significantly different than in cars without airbags (Williams et al., 1990).

The research on the effect of regulation includes conflicting conclusions, mainly based on differences in research methodology (appendix 13-1). These issues are instructive regarding the misleading results that are often obtained from insufficiently disaggregated data.

The evidence on the effectiveness of the initial motor vehicle safety standards does not mean that all regulation is effective or that regulation is always the most effective way to achieve injury reductions. The time necessary for unregulated products to be discarded is also a factor in accomplishing the full effects of regulation, or product changes undertaken voluntarily. In the case of passenger cars, the average life of the vehicles is more than 10 years, so it took that long for the initial regulations to have full effect as the older vehicles were scrapped. Other products, such as mattresses, may be used longer, and some, such as children's cribs, may be used for generations. Research on trends in child suffocations and strangulations suggests that standards for refrigerator or freezer entrapment and warnings on plastic bags reduced fatalities from those sources, but regulations regarding crib design have had less, if any, effect (Kraus, 1985).

EVALUATION OF PROTECTIVE EQUIPMENT AND ENVIRONMENTS

Irrespective of the means employed to obtain use of increased protection (persuasion, laws directed at individuals, regulation, or voluntary changes in products and processes), the effect of the protection in use is often worthy of epidemiological study. Engineers who design and test protective equipment can indicate precisely the energy absorbed, reduction of access to moving parts, stability, and other product characteristics, but other factors cannot always be anticipated—the range of uses and factors affecting lack of use, the amounts of energy involved in actual injuries, and the possibility of misuse. Epidemiological data on the use and effectiveness of potentially injurious energy sources can be helpful in modifications of design or attempts at changes in how the equipment is used. Unfortunately, failure to consider plausibility of results misleads some researchers to unwarranted conclusions. In that regard, the decades-long debate on the effectiveness of seat belts is recounted in appendix 12-1.

When new protective equipment is introduced, it is possible to conduct controlled experiments of effectiveness. Again, the best research design is the experimental-control design where feasible. For modifications of higher priced products, experimental-control designs are usually not feasible for sales to the general public, but if large volumes are bought for use by corporations or the government, random assignment to users in those organizations is possible. For example, the effect of the high-mounted brake light on crashes of cars while braking was studied experimentally in corporate and governmental fleets (e.g., Reilly et al., 1980).

If the government or other agencies distribute certain products, it can be done experimentally. The New York Health Department undertook an experimental-control study of potential problems with a type of child-resistant cap for medicine containers (the Palm-'N'-Turn cap) by randomly distributing them in municipal hospitals and conducting follow-up home visits in experimental and control groups (Lane et al., 1971). The substantial effect of breakaway bases on injuries to softball players was demonstrated by randomly rotating teams among fields with and without the breakaway bases (Janda, 1988).

Many studies of protective technology are case–control studies done after partial adoption of the technology. This always raises the issue of selection bias— risk-averse people may be more often early adopters. One means of estimating potential bias in selection of cases or controls is the use of more than one control group in a case–control study. An example of such a study involved estimation of the effect of bicycle helmets in reducing head injuries. Cases were persons who were seen at five hospitals for head injuries while bicycling. One comparison group was bicyclists who came to the emergency departments of the same hospitals for injuries other than to the head. Another comparison group of injured bicyclists was identified from the records of a group health plan. The claimed helmet use in the two comparison groups was nearly the same but was substantially lower in the head-injured group. Data obtained on several potential confounding factors in the three groups allowed adjustment for these factors in the estimate of helmet effectiveness given an injury while bicycling, which suggested a reduction of about 85 percent in risk of head injury of bicyclists using helmets (Thompson et al., 1989).

The researchers had no way of verifying that helmets were actually used in the groups studied. To check on claims of use versus actual use, observed users and nonusers would have to be identified unobtrusively and later questioned regarding use. To control for whether or not bicyclists who are injured are more or less likely to be using helmets, a third control group would be needed—those bicycling at the same times and places as the injured.

Modifications of environments under the jurisdiction of corporations or governments can usually be studied experimentally, but often are not. Extensive reviews of the literature on road modifications are available (Federal Highway Administration, 1982; Elvik and Vaa, 2004). Much has been learned from cross-sectional studies of road features and before–after studies of modifications. Often, the differences in crashes or severity in before–after studies of environmental modifications are so large that the reduction is unlikely due to biased study design, but the lack of control sites and the potential for regression to the mean (chapter 11), where the modifications were targeted only at high incident sites, raise doubts about the exact magnitude of some effects.

For example, installation of flashing lights at rural stop signs was associated with an 80 percent reduction in fatal crashes at those sites (Hagenauer et al., 1982). Removal of trees near roadsides or use of impact attenuators at fixed objects was estimated to reduce fatal crashes by 50–75 percent (McFarland et al., 1979).

An analysis of various studies that claimed large reductions in motor vehicle crashes at high-incidence sites (so-called black spots) claims that those with controls for regression to the mean show less or no effects (Elvik, 1997). The study did not distinguish between reduced incidence and reduced severity. For example, a guardrail may reduce severity without reducing incidence. While modifications at sites that had temporarily high incidence rates would be expected to return to the average without the modifications, studies that are based on long experience of severe injuries at particular sites show remarkable reductions over similarly long follow-up periods when the modification would be expected to have a long-term effect, such as guardrail installations (Short and Robertson, 1997).

Case–control studies have indicated criteria for selecting high-risk sites for severe crashes where vehicles left the road (chapter 8). Epidemiologists who become familiar with the literature and gain agreement with highway authorities, park administrators, and others in charge of facilities to aid in study designs could make an enormous contribution to increased precision of estimates of the effects of road and other environmental modifications.

INSPECTING HAZARDS

Regulation that provides for inspections, such as the workplace inspections of the Mine Safety and Health Administration and the Occupational Safety and Health Administration (OSHA), could have effects analogous to those discussed for legal controls of individual behavior in chapter 12—general deterrence and specific deterrence. If corporate executives in a position to make changes wish to avoid citations and fines, they could make the changes in the absence of actual inspections (general deterrence). Some may make changes only after citation by inspectors (specific deterrence), and others may not respond even under those conditions.

A substantial increase in regulation of coal mines followed the enactment of the Federal Coal Mine Health and Safety Act of 1969. Death rates of miners in the prior 10 years showed no trend, but the rates declined rapidly in the 1970s (Weeks and Fox, 1983). Apparently, no attempt has been made to study differential effects in mines inspected versus others to delineate the effects of frequency and quality of inspections. The inspections of coal mines were intense relative to other occupational settings, about 34,641 inspections of 2,131 active underground mines in 1977, for example.

The probability of inspection of workplaces regulated by the OSHA was much lower than that of mines in the 1970s and declined substantially in the 1980s. A business could expect to be inspected once per 20 years in 1977 if the inspections were random (Mendeloff, 1979). OSHA targeted industries with higher injury rates for more frequent inspections, and some plants were inspected every few years. Several econometric analyses of trends in worker injuries found no effect of OSHA (Mendeloff, 1979; Smith, 1976; Viscusi, 1979). Further analysis of disaggregated data found an effect in one instance but not significantly so in another (Smith, 1979).

One of the economists who found no effect of OSHA inspections claimed that increased protection of workers would be offset by behavior changes (risk compensation) and that fines for plants cited were too low to provide an incentive for workplace modification in any case (Viscusi, 1979). In a project originally intended to study the epidemiology of worker injuries in three metal-working plants during eight years, the author and a colleague serendipitously discovered new data on the issue of the effects on injury rates of workplace inspections (Robertson and Keeve, 1983).

Individual differences in injuries in the plants were mainly correlated to the type of work being done in specific departments, with some correlations to worker age, formal education, and number of previous employers. Using regression estimates of the effects of these factors at the individual level, the expected injury rate in a given year in a given plant was calculated and compared to the actual rate. The actual rates were separated into injuries that could be observed objectively in the plants' clinics (lacerations, burns, amputations), which we called "objective injuries," and those that were discernable as to incidence or severity primarily by patient complaint (mainly back pain), which we called "subjective injuries." Figure 13-1 shows the actual and expected rates per year in one of the plants.

Noting that the actual rates varied from the expected rather sharply in certain years, we asked ourselves what other factors might have affected the rates in a given year. Two obvious external factors were OSHA inspections and workers' compensation available to workers who missed work because of injury. When the effects of these factors were examined, "objective" injuries declined relative to those expected in the year following OSHA inspections and "subjective" injuries increased more than expected when workers' compensation increased above inflation (Robertson and Keeve, 1983).

The lack of the effect of OSHA in the previous studies of aggregated data was apparently due to failure to control for workers' compensation effects. We also examined change in lost workdays from 1975 to 1976 among industries in 20 states,

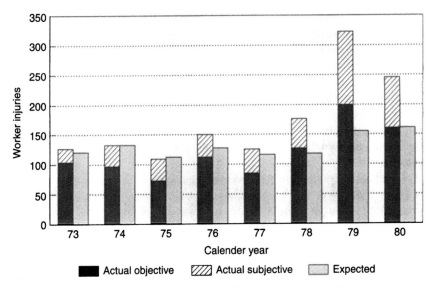

Figure 13-1. Actual Versus Expected Objective and Subjective Worker Injuries in a Metal-Working Plant

and the injuries decreased in correlation to an increase in OSHA inspections but increased in relation to increases in workers' compensation. If "risk compensation" occurred at all, it did not offset the effects of OSHA inspections, but actual compensation that allowed the workers to take time off apparently did affect their absence when they could afford to be away from work, particularly for pain and strain, when working and not working is more discretionary.

The economic theory that the fines for OSHA violations were too small for deterrence did not seem a factor in the plants studied. The researchers were given free access to correspondence regarding OSHA citations, and it was obvious that management took the citations very seriously, in some cases spending more in time and travel to persuade OSHA to reduce a fine than the amount of the fine. The deterrent effect of OSHA inspections did appear to be specific and temporary. Lagged correlations indicated no effect of an OSHA inspection beyond the first year following an inspection.

QUALITY CONTROL

Reducing hazards in products during the production phase may also be important for reducing injuries. In any manufacturing process, variances will occur in the products produced. Prudent manufacturers employ an inspection system to identify and correct safety defects from variances in manufacturing processes, as well as other aspects of quality of the product. Some manufacturers install internal checks on operability of safety and other systems even after the product is sold. For example, the airbags and some other systems in motor vehicles are checked electronically each time the vehicle is started.

An important issue in quality control of the manufacturing process, particularly for products or components that can increase injury and death, is how many to inspect and the criteria for rejection of a defective product or inspection of a total batch for defects when one or more is found in a sample. The cost of inspection is a small proportion of the cost of relatively expensive products, such as cars, but adds proportionately more to the price of inexpensive items, such as matches, propane lighters, and hand tools. Of course, many such items are inexpensive, so a proportional increase in price is affordable. In some cases, the inspection of every unit produced may not be feasible, and a sample of the products in a batch is inspected.

The probability of finding a defect or percentage of defects in a batch is highly sensitive to the size of the sample inspected. The Poisson probability distribution can be used to provide a good estimate of the probability of a proportion of defects escaping detection in inspection of a sample from each batch (Burr, 1953). Assuming that a defect found in a sample results in inspection of the entire batch and removal of all defective products found, the probability of accepting a batch with a proportion (p) of the batch being defective in samples of size n is $P = e^{-pn}$. If a sample of 100 is inspected and no defect is found in the sample, there is a 37 percent chance that one percent of the products in the batch are defective. That chance can be reduced to 14 percent if a sample of 200 is inspected, to 5 percent if 300 are inspected, to 2 percent if 400 are inspected, and to 0.7 percent if 500 are inspected. The probability of injury from the product is the risk of injury per product times P. Obviously, manufacturers can greatly reduce the injuries from their products by using larger samples in their inspection systems.

The size of samples used in quality control is proprietary to the manufacturers. The author is aware of no federal or state standards for sample size to detect defects from manufacturing variances. Motor vehicle manufacturers are required to report known design defects or defects due to manufacturing variances to the National Highway Traffic Safety Administration, but known defects have not always been reported.

A requirement that sample sizes used for detecting defects be revealed publicly, as well as the numbers found and the procedure for inspecting the batch given defects in the sample, would likely result in greater manufacturer attention to the problem. It would also give epidemiologists a tool to correlate the types of quality control and sample sizes to injury incidence and severity related to product variations.

APPENDIX 13-1

Evaluation of U.S. Motor Vehicle Safety Standards

Motor vehicles were essentially unregulated in the United States until the 1960s, except for a few consensus standards adopted by the states, such as for headlamps. Installation of lap belts in front outboard seats was required by several states in the early 1960s, and by 1964, the manufacturers installed them in passenger cars as standard equipment. The federal government required certain standards, such as energy-absorbing steering assemblies and windshields, in 1966 and later models sold to the government, and the manufacturers included these features in public sales of certain models that also were sold to the government in substantial numbers. In 1968 and subsequent model years, the federal government required numerous standards, including several to reduce energy exchanges of occupants and vehicles in crashes and several to reduce incidence, such as reduced glare in drivers' eyes, redundant brakes, and side running lights.

Since national data disaggregated by type, make, and model of vehicles in crashes were not available until FARS (now called the Fatality Analysis Reporting System) began in 1975, it was necessary to assemble state data to obtain such detailed information. The author undertook such a study using fatal crashes in Maryland to evaluate the overall impact of Federal Motor Vehicle Safety Standards. The data indicated that, during the calendar years 1972–1975, occupant deaths averaged 44 fatalities per 100,000 cars in pre-1964 model cars, 35 per 100,000 for 1964–1967 cars, and 27 per 100,000 for 1968–1975 model cars, a decline of 39 percent from unregulated pre-1964 cars to the federally regulated cars (figure 13-2). Deaths to pedestrians struck by the cars, compared by model year, were not significantly different—8 per 100,000 for pre-1964 cars, 10 per 100,000 for 1964–1967 cars, and 9 per 100,000 for 1968–1975 cars (Robertson, 1977a).

Factors such as driver age and vehicle age that later came into contention regarding the effect of regulation were not found in the author's Maryland study. Percentage of youthful drivers (in this case, younger than 26 years) was slightly less in the older, unregulated cars—opposite to subsequent conjectures that older cars had higher rates because they were driven by younger drivers. The death rate of the preregulation 1960–1963 model cars during 1972–1975 in Maryland was the same as the national death rate for passenger cars in the calendar years 1960–1963, 44 per 100,000. Therefore, age of vehicle did not explain the reductions in deaths to occupants of regulated vehicles.

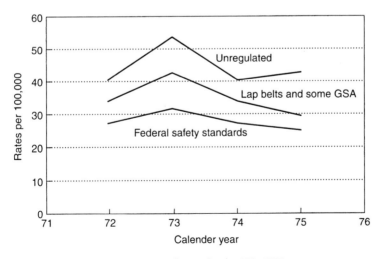

Figure 13-2. Death Rates to Car Occupants in Maryland: 1972–1975

After completion but prior to publication of the Maryland study, an economist published a study using aggregated trends in motor vehicle fatalities and other factors in an attempt to evaluate the effect of motor vehicle safety regulations on fatality rates (Peltzman, 1975). He argued that drivers with increased occupant protection would drive more "intensively"—the "risk compensation" or "risk homeostasis" hypothesis—and kill more pedestrians.

His study design involved projections of expected death rates based on correlations of death rates and trends in other aggregated data over time. He included separate regressions of total occupant and "pedestrian" death rates during 1947 to 1965, using as predictors alcohol consumption per capita, average speeds on rural roads, linear trend, ratio of younger to older persons in the population, income, and "cost of crashes" in those years. The regression equations were then used to project the expected death rates in 1966–1972 based on year-to-year indicators of the other variables during that time. The actual occupant rates were less than expected, but the "pedestrian rates" were greater than expected, the latter offsetting the former. The results, he said, supported risk compensation theory and indicated no net benefit of regulation (Peltzman, 1975).

Having found no effect of regulation on pedestrian deaths in the Maryland study, perhaps because the numbers were too small for statistical power, I obtained the data used in the econometric analysis in an attempt to account for the difference in results of the two studies. The econometric study was laced with methodological errors. Not only were regulated and nonregulated cars not separated, but also occupants of unregulated trucks and "pedestrians" struck by them were not disaggregated from regulated cars. Motorcyclists were included as "pedestrians," and single-vehicle motorcycle crashes were not disaggregated from those in collisions with other vehicles. Also, motorcycle registrations were doubling every five years, guaranteeing a substantial increase in their deaths.

There were also problems with the predictor variables. The alcohol-consumption variable excluded beer. The crash-cost index was based on the Consumer Price Index for auto repair services, which includes such things as oil changes and filters, but not the cost of auto parts damaged in crashes. The "youth" variable was ratio of 15- to 24-year-olds to older persons in the population rather than their percentage as licensed drivers or drivers in crashes, which was known for all but three of the earliest years studied. A regression equation based on 1947–1960 data did not predict the rates in 1961–1965, a simple check on the validity of the model that would have ruled out its use to evaluate regulation. Some of the predictor variables were virtually substitutes for one another, a condition called multicolinearity that distorts regression coefficients, and their correlations changed drastically in the pre- and postregulation periods, guaranteeing invalid projections (table 13-1). Although exactly what was considered "intensive" driving was not specified, the most likely candidate, speed, was used as a predictor variable rather than an outcome variable (Robertson, 1977b).

Since publication of the original Peltzman (1975) study, it has been cited frequently as gospel in the economic literature, usually without reference to the critique and other research contradicting it, including one study on similar regulations in Sweden published later in the same journal (Lindgren and Stuart, 1980).

Table 13-1. Correlation Matrix of Data Used by Peltzman (1975) to Project Fatality Rates, 1947–1965 (1966–1972 in parentheses)

	1.	2.	3.	4.	5.
1. Crash cost index	—				
2. Income/capita age 15+	−.87 (.88)				
3. Linear trend	−.92 (.80)	.97 (.95)			
4. Alcohol consumption	−.85 (.72)	.90 (.95)	.91 (.91)		
5. Average rural speed	−.89 (.68)	.98 (.88)	.98 (.85)	.89 (.96)	
6. 15- to 24-year-olds/ older population	−.34 (.78)	.29 (.95)	.37 (.99)	.57 (.91)	.32 (.99)

When the FARS data became available for a number of years (1975–1978), it was possible to examine separately data on regulated and unregulated vehicles nationally. Using a survey of mileage per vehicle age, the effects of state and federal regulations on death rates per mile of occupants and on pedestrians, motorcyclists, and pedal cyclists in collisions with specific vehicles were estimated in a regression equation, controlling for age of vehicle and type of vehicle (cars vs. trucks). The data indicated that significant reductions in car occupant death rates were associated with state regulations, and deaths both to car occupants and nonoccupants struck by cars were lower in those subject to federal safety standards. These results were consistent with the fact that state lap-belt requirements and standards for government cars in 1964–1967 models were exclusively aimed at occupant protection in crashes, while the 1968 and subsequent federal standards included crash avoidance. The occupant death reduction was similar to that found in the Maryland study, 40 percent (Robertson, 1981).

The study of the FARS data was attacked by an economist who claimed that it was inappropriate to compare cars to trucks. Because age of vehicle and model year were correlated, the critic said that the regulatory effect was greatly reduced mainly by his estimate of a vehicle-age effect (Orr, 1984). His estimate of lives preserved, however, was miscalculated by 38 percent using his own regression coefficients (Robertson, 1984).

The most misleading characterization of the alleged vehicle-age effect was presented in a conference at General Motors. Graphs of model year differences were separated by calendar year, removing rather than demonstrating the vehicle-age effect, and totally and mistakenly attributing all model-year differences to vehicle age (Adams, 1985). A simple graph shows that the primary decline in death rates occurred in relation to model year of the vehicles and not vehicle age, as indicated by calendar year in figure 13-3.

Another econometric study was published that claimed offsetting behavior (Chirinko and Harper, 1993) apparently from failure to separate passenger cars

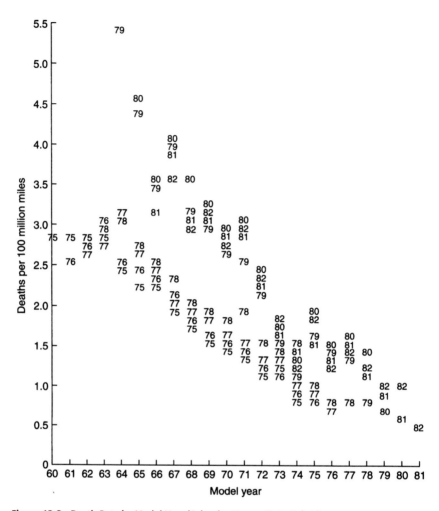

Figure 13-3. Death Rate by Model Year (Calendar Year as Data Points)

from pickup trucks and utility vehicles in a time-series analysis. This will give false results on the effects of regulation on passenger cars, not because the regulated cars are more often hitting trucks as claimed by recent proponents of the risk compensation hypothesis, but because the government failed to impose standards to reduce rollover of unstable pickup trucks and utility vehicles that have grown substantially in use (see appendix 8-1).

Since more data are accumulated each year in FARS, the opportunity to evaluate the effects of safety standards and other factors as conditions change is available. Adoption of safety standards virtually ceased from 1978 to 1987. The federal standard that required seat belts that automatically encircle front-outboard occupants, or alternatively, air bags, was rescinded by the Reagan administration. It was restored in the late 1980s only after the courts ruled that the administration had acted illegally. The National Highway Traffic Safety Administration did continue frontal crash tests of a selection of cars annually and published the results. Manufacturers were embarrassed enough by the reported forces on occupant test dummies at 35 miles per hour that on occasion they requested a retest after modifying the vehicles.

The crash tests indicated incremental improvement in crashworthiness during the 1980s, as evidenced by reduced forces on crash-test dummies. Research on fatalities to occupants in frontal crashes indicated reduced deaths in vehicles that performed well in the crash tests (Zador et al., 1984; Kahane, 1994), but the research designs of these studies did not allow for the possibility of offsetting behavior—the alleged increased risky driving. Seat belt use laws, enacted by the states from 1985 to 1990, largely accounted for more than doubling of seat belt use (National Highway Traffic Safety Administration, 1975–1991), and alcohol in fatally injured drivers declined about 20 percentage points during the 1980s (National Highway Traffic Safety Administration, 1995).

By combining FARS data with data from other sources on vehicle use and belt use, the data can be used to assess the effects of the various mentioned government policies. Death rates per 100 million miles use in which passenger cars were involved, by model year of the vehicles and whether the death was to one or more occupants of the cars, were tabulated for model years 1961–1990 in each of the calendar years 1975–1991. The miles per vehicles of a given age in a 1988 mileage survey (Energy Information Administration, 1990) were adjusted to other years by multiplying them by the ratio of average miles driven in other years to the 1988 average (Federal Highway Administration, 1975–1992). The mileage survey included periodic calls to the same households to obtain odometer readings, which is probably more valid than asking people their annual mileage. Rates were available on 254 combinations of vehicle model year and calendar year.

Two sets of rates per 100 million miles were analyzed separately: (1) occupant fatalities and (2) crashes fatal to nonoccupants (occupants of the other vehicle in multiple-vehicle crashes, pedestrians, and bicyclists). The first allows an estimate of the effects of safety standards, improved crashworthiness, and the other factors on all occupant deaths. The second examines possible effects on other road users. If there is offsetting behavior, nonoccupant death rates should increase in relation to regulation, crash test publicity, or belt use.

Since the General Services Administration imposed some safety standards in 1966 on cars sold to the government and the standards for all cars began to be imposed in 1968, the absence of standards is correlated with vehicle age. Data on the 1975–1977 models were available for a full 15 years of vehicle use. The death rates (each of the two sets separately) per mile were calculated for these model years for each year of age and averaged among the three model years. The death rates were neither linear nor monotonic as the vehicles aged (Robertson, 1996). Ten- to 15-year-old 1975–1977 models had substantially lower death rates than the 10- to 15-year-old preregulation vehicles. The 1975–1977 rate for a vehicle of a given age was used as an expected rate for a vehicle of that age to control for variation attributable to vehicle age.

Other factors considered were the "downsizing" of vehicles and economic conditions during a given calendar year, both of which have been correlated to death rates, observed seat belt use in a given calendar year, and percentage of drivers with blood alcohol greater than 0.10 percent by weight in a given calendar year. Smaller vehicles have higher occupant death rates because of less interior space to decelerate, and deaths per mile are marginally higher in years of greater economic prosperity. Wheelbase, the distance from the front to rear axle, has been shown to be the best predictor of differences in fatality rates due to vehicle size (Robertson, 1991).

To control for vehicle size, the death rates per mile in calendar year 1988 were calculated for seven categories in five-inch increments of wheelbase (from <95.1 to ≥120.1), using the 1988 mileage survey and decoded vehicle identification numbers for make and model of vehicle in the fatal file and mileage survey file. Expected fatalities were calculated by multiplying the 1988 rate for each size times the numbers of vehicles of those sizes sold in a given model year, discounted for numbers scrapped as they aged (Ward's Automotive Yearbook, 1960–1992; Flammang, 1992). The expected number was then divided by the mileage previously estimated for each model and calendar year. The Index of Industrial Production was used as an indicator of economic activity (Council of Economic Advisors, 1994). Belt use in a given model-calendar year was included from the annual survey of 19 cities and their environs, extrapolating for a few years in which the survey was not done (National Highway Traffic Safety Administration, 1975–1991). Percentage of alcohol in fatally injured drivers for each model-calendar year was obtained from FARS in states that test 80 percent or more of such drivers.

Ordinary least-squares regression was used to estimate the effects of the various factors. The variable for minimum safety standards was zero for pre-1966 models, incremented from 1 to 12 in 1966–1977 models, and assigned 12 for 1978–1991 models. As noted, the reduction in occupant death rates has been shown to be incremental in 1966–1977 models, partly because of the imposition of new standards in various years of that period and partly because of delays in meeting the standards in some models. The publication of NHTSA's 35 mph frontal crash test NCAP results began in 1979, so the NCAP variable is zero for 1961–1979 models and incremented by 1, from 1 to 11 consecutively, for 1980 to 1990 models, based on the assumption that crashworthiness was improved incrementally as the crash test results for particular makes and models became known.

The regression coefficients for the predictor variables are presented in table 13-2. Controlling for the expected effects of vehicle age and size differences, the incremental model years in which minimum standards were imposed and the model years during which NCAP tests were publicized are strong predictors of reduced occupant death rates and are somewhat related to reduced nonoccupant fatal crash rates.

In the 1966–1977 model passenger cars, the reduction was an average 0.26 deaths per 100 million vehicle miles (mvm) per model year across 12 model years for a total reduction of 3.12 deaths per 100 mvm (.26 × 12). The reduction in 1980–1990 models was .077 per model year, a total of .847 per 100 mvm in 11 model years (.077 × 11). The effect of belt use increases and alcohol reductions were much less. A 40-percentage-point increase in belt use reduced the

Table 13-2. Regression Estimates and 95% Confidence Intervals of the Effects on Passenger Car Death and Fatal Crash Rates per 100 Million Vehicle Miles, 1961–1990 Cars in 1975–1991

Variable	Occupant Deaths	Nonoccupant Fatal Crashes
Standards	−0.260 ± 0.023	−0.055 ± 0.010
NCAP publicity	−0.077 ± 0.033	−0.029 ± 0.020
% Belt use	−0.007 ± 0.006	−0.006 ± 0.004
% Alcohol > 0.10	0.007 ± 0.006	0.007 ± 0.005
Calendar year	−0.017 ± 0.036	−0.016 ± 0.022
Industrial production	0.029 ± 0.014	0.019 ± 0.009
Expected age of vehicle effect	0.444 ± 0.212	0.289 ± 0.096
Expected wheelbase effect	1.066 ± 0.454	1.252 ± 0.299
Intercept	−0.793	−1.950
R^2	0.92	0.86

rate .28 (40 × .007), and a 20-percentage-point reduction in alcohol reduced the rate .14 (20 × .007).

The rates increase marginally in more economically prosperous years as indicated by the predictive coefficient on the Index of Industrial Production. There is no significant linear trend in the rates independent of the other predictor variables as indicated by the coefficient on calendar year.

The results support the conclusion that vehicle-related fatalities were reduced substantially by increased crashworthiness and somewhat by increased seat belt use and reduced alcohol use. Contrary to offsetting behavior theory, the evidence indicates that the reduction of fatalities per mile attributable to increased crashworthiness of passenger cars and increased seat belt use was not attenuated by increased risk to others from more protected drivers. Indeed, more regulated vehicles were in fewer crashes fatal to other road users.

There are reasonable explanations for the latter. The minimum safety standards included crash avoidance standards (redundant brakes, reduced glare in driver's eyes, and side running lights) as well as crashworthiness standards. The period of NCAP tests and increased seat belt use was also the period of increased aerodynamic designs to save fuel, which may, coincidentally, reduce severity of pedestrian and cyclist impacts. The points and edges on older models were related to increased risk to pedestrians (Robertson, 1990). The "crumple zones" that absorb more energy may help reduce the velocity changes to occupants of other vehicles in crashes with the more crashworthy vehicles.

Although most of the reductions in occupant deaths are model-year specific during the period of regulation or publicized crash tests, and therefore vehicle rather than driver or environmentally based, the data do not allow the conclusion that all of the reduction is attributable to regulation or embarrassment. Some aspects of crashworthiness might have been adopted without government standards had there been no regulation, although the failure of most manufacturers to adopt available technology, until required to do so in the 1960s, and the 18-year battle against the airbag in the 1970s and 1980s suggest otherwise. And concern for sales lost to manufacturers of vehicles that had better crash indices in the NCAP tests may have motivated improvements, irrespective of embarrassment.

This discussion may seem to be only an academic quarrel over study designs, but it had more ominous results. The antiregulation administrators of federal agencies in the 1980s until today were often advised by neoclassic economists, and those who attempted some feeble extension of safety regulations were blocked by the neoclassic economists and others in the Office of Management and Budget in the White House. The long delay in the adoption of airbags was but one of many delays in regulations influenced by these intragovernmental debates.

References

Adams J (1985) Smeed's law, seat belts, and the emperor's new clothes. In Evans L, and Schwing RC (eds.), *Human Behavior and Traffic Safety.* New York, NY: Plenum.

Ashton SJ (1982) Vehicle design and pedestrian injuries. In Chapman AJ, et al. (eds.), *Pedestrian Accidents.* London: John Wiley and Sons.

Berger LR, and Mohan D (1996) *Injury Control: A Global View.* Delhi, India: Oxford University Press.

Burr IW (1953) *Engineering Statistics and Quality Control.* New York, NY: McGraw-Hill.

Champion HR, Copes WS, Craig M, Morelli S, Keast S, and Bain L (1986) *A Preliminary Study of Head and Neck Trauma of Automobile Crashes, and Their Consequences.* Washington, DC: National Highway Traffic Safety Administration.

Chirinko RS, and Harper EP (1993) Buckle up or slow down? New estimates of offsetting behavior and their implications for automobile safety regulation. *J Policy Anal Manage.* 12:270–293.

Clark CC, Jettner E, Digges K, Morris J, Cohen D, and Griffin D (1987) *Simulation of Road Crash Facial Lacerations by Broken Windshields.* Paper No. 870320. Warrendale, PA: Society of Automotive Engineers.

Clarke RV, and Mayhew P (1988) The British gas story and its criminological implications. *Crime Justice.* 10:79–116.

Council of Economic Advisors (1994) *Economic Indicators.* Washington, DC: U.S. Government Printing Office.

Done AK (1978) Aspirin overdosage: incidence, diagnosis, and management. *Pediatrics.* 59(suppl):890–897.

Elvik R (1997) Evaluations of road accident blackspot treatment: a case of the iron law of evaluation studies? *Accid Anal Prev.* 29:191–199.

Elvik R, and Vaa T (2004) *The Handbook of Road Safety Measures.* Amsterdam: Elsevier.

Energy Information Administration (1990) *Household Vehicles Energy Consumption, 1988.* Washington, DC: U.S. Department of Energy.

Fallat ME, and Rengers SJ (1993) The effect of education and safety devices on scald burn prevention. *J Trauma.* 34:560–563.

Farmer R (1992) Epidemiology of suicide. *Int Clin Psychopharmacol.* 6(suppl)6:1–11.

Federal Highway Administration (1975–1992) *Highway Statistics.* Washington, DC: U.S. Department of Transportation.

Federal Highway Administration (1982) *Synthesis of Safety Research Related to Traffic Control and Road Elements.* Washington, DC: U.S. Department of Transportation.

Flammang JM (1992) *Standard Catalog of Imported Cars, 1946–1990*. Iola, WI: Kraus Publications.

Gikas PW (1972) Mechanisms of injury in automobile crashes. *Clin Neurosurg.* 19:175–190.

Glass RI, Urrutia JJ, Sibony S, Smith H, Garcia B, and Rizzo L (1977) Earthquake injuries related to housing in a Guatemalan village. *Science.* 197:638–643.

Hagenauer GF, Upchurch D, and Rosenbaum MJ (1982) Intersections. In *Federal Highway Administration. Synthesis of Safety Research Related to Traffic Control and Roadway Elements.* Washington, DC: U.S. Department of Transportation.

Janda DH (1988) Softball sliding injuries: a prospective study comparing standard and modified bases. *JAMA.* 259:164–166.

Kahane CJ (1994) *Correlation of NCAP Performance With Fatality Risk in Actual Head-on Collisions.* Washington, DC: National Highway Traffic Safety Administration.

Karlson TA, and Hargarten SW (1997) *Reducing Firearm Injury and Death: A Public Health Sourcebook on Guns.* New Brunswick, NJ: Rutgers University Press.

Kraus JF (1985) Effectiveness of measures to prevent unintentional deaths of infants and children from suffocation and strangulation. *Public Health Rep.* 100:231–240.

Kreitman N (1976) The coal gas story. *Br J Prev Soc Med.* 30:86–93.

Krishnan R, Subramanian N, and Adnan A (eds.) (1990) *Proceedings of the First Malaysian Workshop on Accident Prevention.* Kuala Lumpur: University of Malaya.

Lane MF, Barbarite RV, Bergner L, and Harris D (1971) Child-resistant medicine containers: experience in the home. *Am J Public Health.* 61:1861–1868.

Lester D (1990) The effects of detoxification of domestic gas on suicide in the United States. *Am J Public Health.* 80:80–81.

Lindgren B, and Stuart C (1980) The effects of traffic safety regulations in Sweden. *J Polit Econ.* 88:412–417.

McFarland WF, Griffin LI, Rollins JB, Stockton WR, Phillips DT, and Dudek CL (1979) *Assessment of Techniques for Cost-effectiveness of Highway Accident Countermeasures.* Washington, DC: U.S. Department of Transportation.

Mendeloff J (1979) *Regulating Safety: An Economic and Political Analysis of Occupational Safety and Health Policy.* Cambridge, MA: MIT Press.

Mohan D, Bowman BM, Snyder RG, and Foust DR (1979) A biomechanical analysis of head impact injuries to children. *J Biomech Eng.* 101:250–260.

National Highway Traffic Safety Administration (1975–1991) *Restraint System Use in the Traffic Population.* Washington, DC: U.S. Department of Transportation.

National Highway Traffic Safety Administration (1995) *Traffic Safety Facts 1994.* Washington, DC: U.S. Department of Transportation.

Orr LD (1984) The effectiveness of automobile safety regulation: evidence from the FARS data. *Am J Public Health.* 74:1384–1389.

Ortog GJ, Wasserberger J, and Balasubramaniam S (1988) Shotgun wound ballistics. *J Trauma.* 28:624–631.

Peltzman S (1975) The effects of automobile safety regulation. *J Polit Econ.* 83:677.

Reilly RE, Kurke DS and Bukenmaier CC (1980) Validation of the Reduction of Rear-end Collisions by a High-Mounted Auxiliary Stoplamp. Washington, DC: National Highway Traffic Safety Administration.

Robertson LS (1976) Estimates of motor vehicle seat belt effectiveness and use: implications for occupant crash protection. *Am J Public Health.* 66:859–864.

Robertson LS (1977a) State and federal new-car safety regulation: effects on fatality rates. *Accid Anal Prev.* 9:151–156.

Robertson LS (1977b) A critical analysis of Peltzman's "The effect of automobile safety regulation." *J Econ Issues.* 11:587.

Robertson LS. (1981) Automobile safety regulations and death reductions in the United States. *Am J Public Health.* 71:818–822.

Robertson LS (1984) Automobile safety regulation: rebuttal and new data. *Am J Public Health.* 74:1390–1394.

Robertson LS. (1990) Car design and risk of pedestrian injuries. *Am J Public Health.* 80:609–610.

Robertson LS. (1991) How to save fuel and reduce injuries in automobiles. *J Trauma.* 31:107–109, 1991.

Robertson LS (1996) Reducing death on the road: the effects of minimum safety standards, publicized crash tests, seat belts and alcohol. *Am J Public Health.* 86:31–34.

Robertson LS (2006) Blood and oil: vehicle characteristics in relation to fatality risk and fuel economy. *Am J Public Health.* 96:1906-1909.

Robertson LS, and Keeve JP (1983) Worker injuries: the effects of workers' compensation and OSHA inspections. *J Health Polit Policy Law.* 8:581–597.

Short D and Robertson LS (1998) Motor vehicle death reductions from guardrail installation. *J Transp Eng.* 124:501–502.

Smith RS (1976) *The Occupational Health and Safety Act: Its Goals and Its Achievements.* Washington, DC: American Enterprise Institute.

Smith RS (1979) The impact of OSHA inspections on manufacturing injury rates. *J Hum Resources.* 14:145.

Snyder RG (1975) *Crashworthiness Investigation of General Aviation Accidents.* Warren, PA: Society of Automotive Engineers.

Sykes LN, Champion HR, and Fouty WJ (1988) Dum-dums, hollow-points, and devastators: techniques designed to increase wounding potential of bullets. *J Trauma.* 28:618–623.

Thompson RS, Rivara FP, and Thompson DC (1989) A case–control study of the effectiveness of bicycle safety helmets. *New Engl J Med.* 320:1361–1367.

Viscusi WK (1979) The impact of occupational safety and health regulation. *Bell J Econ.* 10:117.

Ward's Automotive Yearbook (1960–1992) Detroit, MI: Ward's Communications.

Weeks JL, and Fox M (1983) Fatality rates and regulatory policies in bituminous coal mining, United States, 1959–1981. *Am J Public Health.* 73:1278–1280.

Weiss EB, Pritz HB, and Hassler CR (1977) Experimental automobile-pedestrian injuries. *J Trauma.* 17:823–828.

Williams AF, Wells JAK, and Lund AK (1990) Seat belt use in cars with air bags. *Am J Public Health.* 80:1514–1516.

Wintemute GJ (1994) *Ring of Fire: The Handgun Makers of Southern California.* Sacramento, CA: Violence Prevention Research Program.

Wintemute GJ (1996) The relationship between firearm design and firearm violence. *JAMA.* 275:1749–1753.

Woodward FD (1948) Medical criticism of modern automotive engineering. *JAMA.* 138:627–631.

Zador PL, Jones IS, and Ginsburg M (1984) Fatal front-to-front car collisions and the results of 35 MPH frontal barrier impacts. In: *28th Annual Proceedings of the Association for the Advancement of Automotive Medicine.* Barrington, IL: Association for Automotive Medicine.

14

Evaluation of Postinjury Treatment and Rehabilitation

Research questions regarding the treatment of injuries and rehabilitation range from the profound issue of who survives trauma to the more mundane estimates of costs and payment. Only a small minority of physicians and other professionals delivering care to traumatized patients conduct research, but because of their familiarity of the treatment and rehabilitation scene, these persons are usually in a better position to ask good research questions than are academic epidemiologists (Findley, 1989).

Mortality from trauma has a trimodal distribution as a function of time after injury. Half or more of the deaths occur in the first hour, mainly from massive nervous system or heart and blood vessel damage. A second peak occurs within 1.5–2 hours, usually from internal injuries and blood loss. A third peak occurs at three to four weeks posttrauma, often due to infection or multiple organ failure. Many of the injuries to those who do not survive the first hour are not treatable, but there is substantial evidence that the timing and quality of emergency response and treatment can increase survival, particularly in the other groupings (Trunkey, 1983).

More and better research in the delivery of emergency services and on specific treatment and rehabilitation regimens can lead to increased survival and a better quality of life for those impaired by injury, when the knowledge is used. Although research on the efficacy of modes of treatment and rehabilitation has accelerated (Maier and Rhodes, 2001), many practices are based on impressions from experience rather than quantitative evidence (Basmajian and Banerjee, 1996).

Issues include placement of emergency responders to minimize response time, amount and type of treatment at the scene, safety of transportation modes (ambulances, helicopters, fixed-wing aircraft), triage to designated trauma centers, designation of trauma centers, referral to rehabilitation, and efficacy of specific treatments in acute care and rehabilitation (Committee on Trauma Research, 1985). The injury epidemiologist who becomes knowledgeable in these issues can provide assistance in study design and statistical analysis to other health and organizational researchers involved in their investigation.

EMERGENCY RESPONSE

The effect on survival of delay in treatment of injuries has been inferred from the extent of delay and survival in war (table 14-1). Bypassing field treatment and transport to MASH units in Korea and the transport directly to surgical units for definitive treatment in Vietnam are thought to be the major factors in reduced mortality (Trunkey, 1983), although controls for type and extent of wounds and improved surgical technique and technology might raise or lower the estimates somewhat. Delay in surgery for other forms of serious injury, such as hip fractures in the elderly, appears to increase risk of death, as well (Whinney, 2005).

In the United States, civilian emergency response systems have evolved from ambulance services, about half operated by morticians (who had an obvious conflict of interest), to a variety of systems based in hospitals, fire or police departments, volunteer services, and for-profit organizations (Boyd, 1983). The study of the effect of response times is complicated by the fact that response times are longer in remote rural areas where the injuries are also more severe and the quality of care upon arrival at a hospital is more often inferior. Controlling for types of motor vehicle crashes that would affect survival among rural counties in Texas, the extent of access to emergency response systems apparently reduced the ratio of mortality to disabling injuries, but the cost-effectiveness of improving systems in remote areas was questioned (Brodsky and Hakkert, 1983). A major problem is that the rural areas with the lack of adequate emergency services are often those that can least afford them (Martin et al., 1990). Leading international authorities on trauma care argue that improved initial response to injury should concentrate on response time by responders with a few basic skills to alter immediate life-threatening conditions that would reduce death substantially in parts of the world where delay and lack of skills is common (Sasser et al., 2006).

Some U.S. data on emergency response times to fatal motor vehicle crashes are available in the Fatality Analysis Reporting System, although lack of complete reporting is a problem. For fatal crashes in urban areas during 2004, the emergency service arrived an average of 6.5 minutes afterward, but the data are unreliable because 50 percent of cases had no time reported. For fatal rural crashes, arrival occurred at an average of 11.3 minutes, but 40 percent were unreported.

Table 14-1. Delay Between Injury and Surgery and Percent Mortality of the Injured in Wars

War	Delay in Hours	Percent Mortality
World War I	12–18	8.5
World War II	6–12	5.8
Korea	2–4	2.4
Vietnam	1.1	1.7

Source: Trunkey (1983).

The reporting had not improved from the previous decade despite emphasis on improved emergency response by NHTSA in the 1990s (National Highway Traffic Safety Administration, 1996, 2006).

In an area with a regionalized trauma system in which patients with severe trauma are supposed to be taken to a special treatment center, probability of survival was not directly related to time at the scene or transport time. Time at the scene averaged 16.7 minutes for survivors and 15.2 minutes for nonsurvivors. Transport time was an average 13.0 minutes for survivors and 11.9 minutes for nonsurvivors (Shackford et al., 1989). While there does not appear to be a difference in an area with the range of response times studied, that does not mean that response time would not have an effect in areas where it is longer. The possibility of real-time linking of crash severity data and location, measured on-board the vehicle, with communications directed to emergency medical responders is being considered (Champion et al., 2003).

TREATMENT AT THE SCENE

Emergency responders and the public generally should learn how to clear breathing passages, stop obvious hemorrhage, stabilize the spine, and perform cardiopulmonary resuscitation in the absence of pulse or breathing (Jacobs and Bennett, 1983). Many questions remain about the advisability of the other kinds of treatment that should be delivered at the scene of injury versus the delay involved before transport to more definitive treatment. The main controversies revolve around various practices at the scene, such as intravenous infusion of fluids, the use of the pneumatic antishock garment, endotracheal intubations, and esophageal obdurator airways (Lewis, 1983).

Many of these techniques were used by paramedics in the Viet Nam War and were adopted in civilian emergency systems, particularly early on in those manned by veteran paramedics returned to civilian life. Some have become routine, and in a few cases, at least, law mandates availability. For example, the pneumatic antishock garment was required equipment on ambulances in one-third of the states by the early 1980s despite lack of evidence of its efficacy (Lewis, 1983; for a description, see http://www.ivprehospital.com/pasg.cfm, accessed August, 2006).

A study of the use or nonuse of the pneumatic antishock garment, assigned for use in the recommended circumstance on alternating days, indicated that an average of four minutes was added to time at the scene on the days that the garment was used. Survival was 69 percent on days when the garment was used and 75 percent on days it was not used. Although the assignment was not random, as claimed, it is doubtful that day-to-day differences biased the results. The authors concluded that the use of the garment had no net positive effect on survival and possibly a negative effect (Mattox et al., 1989).

That study does not quite lay the issue to rest because survival was higher when the garment was used (38 percent vs. 29 percent when not used) among those with systolic blood pressures less than 50, although the difference was not statistically significant due to the small number of patients with those blood pressures. The remaining issue is whether more selective use of the garment on a sample and control group of sufficient size would indicate statistically significant benefit for selected patients.

Such controlled trials are unusual in the evaluation of prehospital emergency systems. The use of intravenous fluids before arrival at the hospital—studied retrospectively—indicates no advantage to trauma patients in several important subcategories of severity and clinical status. Patients taken to six hospitals in San Diego County during a 2.5-year period were studied (Kaweski et al., 1990). The use of fluids appeared to be random relative to severity of diagnosis and clinical status—some 56 percent received prehospital fluids. Time to the hospital was also similar in most severity groups, the exception being a five minute longer time among those who received fluids in the group with Injury Severity Scores (ISSs) 25–50 and systolic blood pressure greater than 90. Survival was similar in those treated with and without fluids in subgroups with various combinations of injury.

Another type of study involves retrospective review of procedures and outcomes by a committee of emergency department physicians, trauma surgeons, and neurosurgeons. For example, one such study concluded that advanced life support (the care delivered by the best trained paramedics including intravenous fluids, endotracheal intubations, and pneumatic shock garments) "appears to be beneficial in the treatment of multi-system trauma in a rural state" (Reines et al., 1988). This despite the fact that advanced life support took an average five minutes more at the scene and a 10-physician review committee judged the treatment not in compliance with recommended practice in 74 percent of cases for endotracheal intubations and 54 percent of cases for pneumatic garments. In the cases where the techniques were applied, the review committee judged advanced life support as "helpful or essential in 85 percent of cases" and harmful in less than 2 percent. A prospective multicenter study of mortality in areas with different protocols for "scoop and run" versus treatment at the scene in Canada found that treatment at the scene by emergency medical technicians could not be justified in areas with level 1 trauma centers (Liberman et al., 2003).

An ecological study found a correlation between levels of training of emergency response personnel and fatality rates per population among counties in North Carolina. Counties with advanced or paramedic training had lower fatality rates after adjusting statistically for numerous other differences among the counties. Since all of the urban counties had advanced training, however, it was not possible to totally disaggregate the possible effects of other factors (Messick et al., 1992).

Clearly, there is conflict in the results of the clinical trial and prospective studies and the results of the postinjury review study. Since the methodological power of randomized field trials and prospective studies generally is far superior to that of ecological studies and retrospective judgment, such studies must be employed to evaluate more definitively the efficacy of particular procedures. Of course, if the procedures are substantially unused even when there is a policy regarding their use, or policy guidelines are not followed, the issue is largely moot.

The efficacy of modes of transportation of injured patients is also a matter of controversy. Many hospitals have purchased helicopters ostensibly to reduce travel times, although the use in transplant programs, as well as publicity and prestige of having one, also no doubt contributed to the decision to purchase one. While the use of helicopters to transport trauma patients from remote locations is seldom questioned, research has raised doubts of its net benefit in urban areas.

For example, based on comparison of patients suffering from blunt trauma with survivable ISSs and Glascow Coma Scores, no advantage of helicopter transport in patient outcomes was indicated within a metropolitan area (Schiller et al., 1988). Other studies suggest increased survival in helicopter transfers (Schwartz et al., 1989). A complete assessment of the efficacy of the available forms of transportation would require assessment of the costs of helicopter systems as well as injury to patients and emergency personnel in crashes during transport by whatever mode. Since helicopters cannot fly in certain weather conditions or where there is insufficient landing space, they are an incremental rather than a substitutable expense. Land-based ambulance systems cannot be eliminated when a helicopter is purchased. Criteria have been suggested for choice of modes of transportation that need to be researched (Black et al., 2004).

Assessment of the effect of changing any one system component is complex because of the intercorrelation of various factors. Attempts to assess survival, length of hospital stay, and costs as a function of mode of transport and direct transport to a trauma center, versus an interim stop at another hospital, must control at least for age and injury severity. The numbers of cases in certain combinations of the factors become thin even when beginning with a large sample size. Given these limitations, the available data suggest that arrivals at a trauma center from interhospital transfers have longer length of stay and greater costs than those brought directly to the trauma center (Schwartz et al., 1989). Among spinal cord patients, the increased time in hospital is a result of increased need for acute care; time in rehabilitation is not significantly different (Oakes et al., 1990). This could be partly because only the more severe cases or cases with complications are transferred, but those who are not transferred are known to be at greater risk in many community hospitals.

TRAUMA CENTERS

Once the injured person is en route to a hospital, the hospital of choice is at issue. While time to the hospital may be a factor in outcome in some cases, if the medical care received on arrival is inadequate or misdirected, the probability of survival can be reduced. There is little doubt that the treatment received in hospitals makes a difference in chance of survival (e.g., Baker et al., 1971). Adjusted for the severity of the trauma and other factors, the survival rate of those treated in level 1 trauma centers is about 25 percent better than at other hospitals (Mackenzie et al., 2006).

Some patients are apparently dead on arrival (DOA) at the hospital, but the question of what criteria to use for attempting resuscitation remain under investigation. Based on a literature review and discussion, one trauma team defined DOA as follows:

- All blunt trauma and penetrating trauma of the abdomen, head, neck, or groin: prehospital CPR [cardiopulmonary resuscitation] > 5 minutes, age > 12 years, no pulse on arrival
- Penetrating trauma of the chest: prehospital CPR > 15 minutes, age > 12 years, no pulse on arrival

• Child with any of the above who has in-hospital CPR > 15 minutes (open or closed) without pulse (Pasquale et al., 1996)

None of 86 patients that met the DOA criteria survived despite continued resuscitative efforts on 70 at a cost of more than $4,000 each. Three of 20 patients that did not meet the criteria survived. Children were excluded from the analysis because of the small number.

The authors of the study noted that there are potential cost savings from the application of DOA criteria. They also noted that use of the criteria in their institution was "erratic." Two issues are raised by this research. First, the sample is relatively small, and a multicenter study is needed to specify factors predictive of survival probability. Second, if criteria are established, will they be followed?

The movement to designate certain hospitals as trauma centers and to transport severely injured patients to such centers evolved from the understanding that the necessary experience and training to treat severe trauma, as well as efficient use of technology, could occur only in facilities that treat large numbers of cases. While this has been accomplished in many areas, the extent of compliance with designation in a given area varies. For example, Illinois was among the first states to have regionalized trauma centers. Yet Chicago, where the fire department managed the emergency medical system, did not join the state system, and the old practice of transporting a patient to the nearest hospital continued. A study of the patients' destinations relative to their trauma scores indicated no correlation between serious injury and the probability of being taken to a trauma center (Cadigan, 1985).

One question for research in any given area is the extent to which the guidelines for transportation of patients to designated trauma centers are being followed. One surgeon has hypothesized that persons taken to community hospitals who have insurance (assessed by "wallet biopsy") are more likely to be retained there, while the rest are sent to trauma centers (Gann, 1989).

The survival rate of seriously injured patients among hospitals is inversely correlated with the volume of patients seen. In one study, for example, the survival rate was 30 percent higher in hospitals that treated more than 110 such patients per year than in those that treated 75 or fewer (Smith et al., 1990). Detailed data on severity scores were not available for more refined adjustment of the estimate, and more research incorporating such data is needed. When adjusted for injury severity within a hospital, patients treated by a trauma team were more likely to survive that those treated by others (Petrie, 1996).

Traditionally, two methods have been used in the assessment of adequacy of treatment—called the autopsy method and the clinical method (West and Cales, 1983). The autopsy method involves examination of autopsy records for certain types of cases—eliminating prehospital deaths, DOAs and central nervous system cases for which treatment is ineffective. Deaths to persons younger than 50 years, those that occurred less than six hours after arrival, those in which laparotomy or thoracotomy was not done, and deaths from hemorrhage are examined in particular detail and preventability assessed.

The "autopsy method" has identified substantial proportions of preventable deaths among the defined subsets of all deaths, a process that helped justify the designation of trauma centers and substantial reductions in deaths judged preventable in those subsets (West et al., 1983). The method is not adequate to assess the overall effect of trauma center designation, however. If the designation were to result in deaths due to longer transport times, and more deaths in emergency vehicle crashes en route due to longer travel distances, for example, those would have to be subtracted from the net lives preserved rather than eliminated from the analysis before counting.

The "clinical method" includes audit of the prehospital as well as hospital records, identification of fatalities thought to be survivable, and determination of the phase of response or treatment that failed. The use of the method is dependent on the quality of the records of paramedics, hospitals, and coroners as well as the lack of bias in those who audit the cases. Use of the method in Orange County, California, before and after the implementation of a comprehensive trauma system indicated a reduction in preventable deaths from 34 percent to 15 percent despite the fact that the average age and ISSs of the patients audited increased during the study period (West and Cales, 1983).

The use of committees to review records of deaths to judge the numbers that were preventable by treatment has been brought into serious question by reliability studies. When separate panels reviewed the same cases, the agreement was poor (MacKenzie et al., 1992; Wilson et al., 1992).

The designation of trauma centers can concentrate a cost burden on the designated hospitals that threatens their ability to continue the service. In an attempt to control rising medical care costs, insurance companies and governments use average costs in diagnosis-related groups (DRGs) to determine the amounts hospitals will receive for given diagnoses (Waller et al., 1989).

There is substantial evidence that DRGs are inadequate for determining costs of trauma treatment and certainly should not be used for quality assurance. Since only one DRG category is assigned per patient, multiple injuries are not adequately reflected as they are in more detailed classification systems (see chapter 4). Comparison of DRG classifications of trauma patients and other classifications of criteria for injury management indicate that DRGs are relatively poor predictors of cost of treatment (Young et al., 1990).

The overall impact on hospital financial status of the costs of treatment of severely injured patients compared to the amounts specified for reimbursement in DRG systems have produced conflicting results depending on case mix examined. While some studies find that the less severe injuries are reimbursed at more than cost, offsetting insufficient reimbursement of the more severe injuries (Waller et al., 1989), other hospitals have substantial net shortfalls. In the trauma center for southern New Jersey, the average cost per case in 1985 was $7,137 and the average reimbursement was $3,574, resulting in the hospital losing a total of almost $1.9 million in revenues. The research indicates that the ISS could be used to predict costs to some extent (Schwab et al., 1988).

More research from other trauma centers would perhaps lead to an adjustment of DRGs based on case-mix criteria. For example, a DRG category was added for certain burn injuries, but the categories in use apparently remain inadequate—for example, they do not distinguish substantial variations in costs of burn treatment

(Chakerian et al., 1990). Four Multiple Significant Trauma DRGs were added in 1991 to account for trauma to more than one body site. Nevertheless, a study of 49 consecutive patients that met the criteria for the new DRGs during five months found that the 38 percent of the cost of care was not covered by the DRGs, a short-fall of US$492,057 or about $10,000 per patient (Jacobs and Jacobs, 1992).

The finances of 70 trauma centers in 12 metropolitan areas with populations exceeding one million indicate that public hospitals were more likely to have "financial stress" from trauma care than are private hospitals. Any cuts in Medicaid, Medicare, or other programs that subsidize trauma centers would put many in jeopardy of survival (Bazzoli, 1996). Surveys of trauma centers that closed showed that uncompensated services, high operating costs, and inadequate reimbursement from medical assistance programs were primary factors in the closings (Dailey et al., 1992; Committee on the Consequences of Uninsurance, 2003). Attempts to control costs by "managed care" may be having an effect on prevention, as well. Suicidal patients whose care was refused or attenuated by managed care personnel who did not see the patient have allegedly resulted in suicide completions (CBS News, 1997). Research is needed on the extent of the problem.

CLINICAL STUDIES OF TRAUMA AND SPECIFIC TREATMENT

The National Research Council/Institute of Medicine's Committee on Trauma Research (1985) laid out a series of questions for research in the understanding and treatment of trauma. For example, what happens to cells in shock, and what can be done to prevent or reduce cellular dysfunction? How do metabolic systems respond to trauma, and can interventions reduce harmful reactions or optimize reactions favorable to recovery? How does the immune system react, and what can be done to control infection by augmenting the immune system or use of antimicrobials? What factors contribute to healing or failure to heal, and can healing be enhanced therapeutically? What can be done to minimize nervous system damage, and is nerve regeneration possible?

Answers to these and other questions depend on continued revision of models of anatomic systems at cellular, organ, and whole-system levels based on both animal and human studies. When a reasonable point of intervention is identified, a controlled clinical trial of a hypothesized effective intervention is warranted. Textbooks are available on experimental designs and statistical power issues in clinical trials, and all of the issues cannot be repeated here (Fleiss, 1986; Stein, 1989).

In the simplest form of a controlled clinical trial, a change in procedure, medication, or whatever is introduced in the treatment of a randomly selected experimental group while a randomly selected control group with the same medical condition receives the old accepted treatment, or a placebo if there is no extant treatment. If the effects for subsets of clinical conditions are in question, the experimental and control groups can be assigned within each group of patients with a given condition.

To avoid bias in measurement where possible, those treating the patient or obtaining measurements pre- and posttreatment should not know if the patient is in the experimental or control group. This is rather easily done in the case of drug therapy, but not in surgery or other hands-on treatment. At the least, the surgeons or others who administer obvious treatments should not be the persons to obtain measurements of outcome used in evaluation. Under certain circumstances, a cross-over design can be used in which patients in an experimental group for a period are in the control group in a succeeding period and vice versa. For example, the effects of manual and mechanized ventilator support on blood gasses were studied using such a design (Hurst et al., 1989).

Timing of treatment must also be considered in clinical trials. For example, based on animal studies, methylprednisolone was hypothesized to improve motor and sensory function of patients with acute spinal-cord injury. In a controlled clinical trial, significant improvement was found among patients given the drug within eight hours after injury, but not if delayed beyond eight hours (Bracken et al., 1990). Although the treatment is not a cure, spinal-cord patients treated within eight hours were found better able to care for themselves and otherwise lead more independent lives. Further experiments using pharmacological and other approaches to improved functioning of spinal cord patients are underway (Tator, 2002).

Nonexperimental epidemiological methods can be used to generate hypotheses regarding certain clinical issues. For example, the efficacy of surgical exploration of penetrating injuries of the spine has been questioned based on retrospective analysis of cases. The percentage whose nervous system function improved, remained the same, or deteriorated was similar with or without surgery. The proportion with complications such as infection and cerebrospinal fluid leakage, however, was significantly higher among those with surgery than without—22 percent versus 7 percent (Simpson et al., 1989).

Some clinical studies would benefit from appropriate use of multivariate analysis. For example, in a study of patients with vascular injuries in the abdomen, infection was related to low initial systolic blood pressure, number of blood transfusions, multiple injuries, and cross-clamped aorta during surgery (Wilson et al., 1989). A multivariate analysis, such as logistic regression, was not done, however, and might better isolate the potential contribution of each controlling for the others. A controlled clinical trial of the use of blood transfusions and surgical technique could be guided by the results.

Simple improvements in diagnostic tools may greatly improve clinical decisions. For example, assessment of the neurological status and possible effects of alcohol in unconscious patients is important. Epidemiologists and physicians working together showed that a device to measure concentration of alcohol in passive nasal exhalation of comatose patients is almost perfectly correlated to blood alcohol concentration (Gerberich et al., 1989).

LONG-TERM CARE AND REHABILITATION

Many people who survive traumatic injury have lost abilities because of brain and spinal damage, lost digits or limbs, lost sensory function, and distortion of tissue from burn or other scars. These patients, and their friends, family, and colleagues, are affected psychologically, socially, and economically. There is substantial anecdotal evidence of fears of being injured again, of family breakup and disruption, of dis-crimination, and of economic deprivation (Kaufman, 1989). The quantification of these effects and factors that contribute to reduced dependency and productive and personally satisfying lives is a challenge to epidemiologists and other scientists.

The Committee on Trauma Research (1985) identified numerous research issues in rehabilitation. A panel on disability expanded these (Pope and Tarlov, 1991). For example, what are the most effective methods of rehabilitation to restore activity and at the same time conserve the energies of the disabled? What are effective procedures and counseling in acute care that lead to reduction of scar contraction, muscular atrophy, and skeletal deformity, and for referral to rehabilitation and preparation of the patient for fit and use of prosthetic and cosmetic aids? What is the relative effectiveness of methods to control spasticity, optimize ventilation, improve cognitive function, and the like? What changes in the environments of persons with various handicaps would reduce their dependency or increase their productivity and satisfaction? How many persons are not receiving services that would benefit them, their families, or the community? What are the aspects of the medical care and rehabilitation systems, personal and family beliefs, or social situations of those in need of services that are barriers to use of services or benefit from them?

Studies of the posthospitalization outcomes of injury are limited by lack of representative of samples, small sample sizes, and other methodological problems. Studies are usually confined to the patients discharged from one or more hospitals serving an urban area or region. To the extent that there is selectivity of hospitals by type of injury or severity, these studies may result in over- or underestimation of the extent of a given identified problem, limitations usually recognized by the researchers.

Although not representative of the injured population, follow-up studies of discharged patients are useful in development of criteria to identify patients while in hospital that will have problems and needs thereafter. In a study of discharged patients from two trauma centers, 80 percent had problems with posthospital self-care, and an additional 12 percent who could care for themselves had problems with mobility or other physical activities. One year postdischarge, 23 percent continued to have problems with self-care, and an additional 4 percent had continued mobility or other physical problems. Only 57 percent of those who had worked before the injury had returned to full-time employment one year postdischarge. Even among those with minor to moderately severe injuries of the extremities (Abbreviated Injury Scale [AIS] codes 1–3), half to two-thirds who had been employed before their injuries had not returned to work after one year. Those with lower preinjury incomes were less likely to be working, controlling statistically for functional impairment (MacKenzie et al., 1988).

In another study, children up to age 18 in a children's hospital were followed for six months if they had one or more severe injuries (AIS codes 4–5) or two or more moderate to severe injuries (AIS codes 2–5). Of the 62 percent on whom follow-up data were obtained, about half had not returned to normal activities after six months. The authors stated that the results supported the need for more rehabilitative services, but they did not document the number and types of rehabilitation used for the children (Wesson et al., 1989). Without relating outcomes to type and degree of rehabilitation received, it is not possible to say that more such services would have made a difference.

Most of the longer term studies of patient outcomes are of small samples of patients during a few years postinjury. For example, in a follow-up study of 101 brain-injured patients 5–10.4 years postinjury, 63 were located (of which eight were deceased, including several undocumented mentions of suicide). Disability at follow-up was lower among those who had entered rehabilitation earlier, but the study did not include persons with brain injuries that were not referred to, or did not use, rehabilitation facilities.

Among patients able to respond to the survey themselves, "significant others" (spouse, other relative, or friend) rated the patients as more impaired than the patients rated themselves. Among major problems identified at follow-up were lack of social relationships (45 percent), unemployment (17 percent), physical problems, and dependency and lack of motivation (21 percent). Needs for education, support groups, and supervision were stated but not quantified (Rappaport et al., 1989).

An interesting difference in findings from retrospective and cross-sectional studies when compared to a prospective study occurred in the attempt to find risk factors for postinjury use of acute-care facilities by patients with spinal injuries. Although such factors as level of lesion, years disabled, and cigarette use were significantly correlated to hospitalization in retrospective and cross-sectional studies, a prospective study found no such correlations. Hospitalization proved unpredictable prospectively, but outpatient facility use was correlated with age, years of disability, formal education, and dissatisfaction with medical care. Those in managed care programs for independent living were less likely to use outpatient care, suggesting that the programs may reduce the cost of medical care (Meyers et al., 1989).

When psychosocial factors are assessed prior to hip fractures in the elderly, they are less predictive of institutionalization than in retrospective assessments (Marottoli et al., 1994). Apparently, postinjury assessments are influenced by the injury experience.

In a study of 756 people with traumatic brain injury, the most important predictor of involvement in rehabilitation was not physical or demographic factors but the specialization of the treating physicians (Wrigley et al., 1994). If a physical medicine and rehabilitation specialist was involved in referral decisions, the patient was more likely to receive rehabilitation, controlling for injury severity and demographic factors. Research is needed on the extent to which medical teams without this specialty are aware of the opportunities and benefits of rehabilitation.

IMPROVING OUTCOMES

Models of rehabilitation have been developed that include the effects of not only drugs and physical therapy but also social support and transitional living centers. Research on effectiveness is needed at each stage of rehabilitation (Wood and Eames, 1989). To determine the effects of treatment and rehabilitation on outcomes, there must be some consensus on expected outcomes from particular interventions. For some types of injury, for example, traumatic brain injury, a consensus on priority of outcomes has not been attained. Clients, therapists, and third-party payers have different expectations (Garner and Finlayson, 1996). The effects on families are somewhat dependent on the preinjury status of family roles (e.g., Rivara et al., 1996).

There may be substantial selection bias in choice of therapies. Results of studies of use of catheters for bladder emptying of spinal cord patients are in substantial conflict as to extent of complications (Smith et al., 1996). Clearly, individual economic situations that affect availability of skilled caretakers and living conditions would have a substantial effect on use and maintenance of catheters and infection opportunities. Such factors would also affect affordability, and likely systematic use, of prophylactic antibiotics for urinary tract infections.

One promising approach to mobility of spinal injury patients is the use of electrical stimulation. Most studies find improvements in patient physiology and mobility, but the attrition rate is high. The complexity of the current technology and the effort required from the patient relative to the noticeable improvement often is discouraging to the patients (Smith et al., 1996; Dietz and Harkema, 2004). Research is needed on the degree of improvement needed to motivate patients to continue with the effort, as well as the psychological effects of possible shattered hopes when the therapy fails to meet expectations.

The practice of physical therapy has evolved as the mix of problems presented to rehabilitation facilities has changed, and the models of the functioning of the central nervous system and musculoskeletal systems have been improved by theory and research. Increased survival of persons with central nervous system damage presents a major challenge to physical therapists (Gordon, 1987; Pinkston, 1989). Technology for potentially improving aspects of impairment must be studied relative to traditional methods of hands-on movement and exercise. The relative effectiveness of available and new methods can be discerned in controlled clinical trials.

For example, one study compared the consequences of three types of therapy among patients with incomplete cervical spinal cord injuries: physical exercise therapy supervised by a therapist (PET), electrical neuromuscular stimulation (NMS), and biofeedback with electromyography (EMG). The patients were randomly assigned to four groups, and the sequence of the different therapies was varied among three groups—EMG-PET, EMG-NMS, NMS-PET—while the fourth group received only PET. Persons unaware of the group assignment did baseline and subsequent measurement of outcomes. Although improvements in function were found among all four groups, there were no differences among the groups that suggested any advantage of one therapy over the others (Klose et al., 1990).

The evaluation of therapy and rehabilitation for impairment from trauma is substantially dependent on the reliability, validity, and prognostic predictability of measures of impairment. Epidemiologists can contribute to the development of quantified scales of such outcomes as sensation, motor ability, and balance. One such study, for example, indicated the importance of early identification of discrepancies in sensation and motor ability as diagnostic tools for patients with spinal injury (Bracken et al., 1977–1978).

The Glasgow Coma Scale is useful in acute care decisions but is not strongly correlated to long-term functioning (Zafonte et al., 1996). A battery of quantitative tests of sway among brain-injured patients has been shown to be sensitive enough to distinguish even minimal balance problems (Lehmann, 1990). Accelerometers that can be worn by the patient to monitor physical activity have been studied for reliability and validity (Kochersberger et al., 1996). Performance in an obstacle course is not adequately correlated to other balance and functional measures (maximum $R = .54$) to be used as a screening measurement (Means et al., 1996).

In addition to their use in diagnosis and rehabilitation, reliable and valid measurements could be important in prevention of repeated trauma. For example, falls are a problem among hospitalized and institutionalized patients. In a rehabilitation hospital, 12.5 percent of patients fell in a year, mainly from wheel chairs (Vlahov, 1990). The fracture rates of men in Veterans Administration (VA) nursing homes were 5–11 times those in the age-matched general population (Rudman and Rudman, 1989). The Department of Veterans Affairs has developed a "falls toolkit" for use in its own and other hospitals (Stalhandsk and Landesman, 2004). The newsletter announcing it says that there will be follow-up to see if and how it is used. It should be studied using an experimental-control design.

Potentially even more serious injuries can occur to people whose impairments are not severe enough to prevent driving but severe enough to increase probability of a crash. One study followed 22 brain-injured patients for five years after a physician, a neuropsychologist, and a driving specialist judged them fit to drive. Measurement of driving records and fitness was based on telephone interviews with the patients and "matched" control group of close friends and spouses of the patients. A neuropsychological test battery was administered to those that claimed to have driving problems. The authors concluded that the screening was adequate to identify those "fit to drive" (Katz et al., 1990).

Unfortunately, the study is wholly inadequate to reach that conclusion. The sample size is too small to obtain any statistical power in comparison of driving records. There were significantly more women than men in the control group. Self-report of crashes, violations, and other problems in driving is not an acceptable methodology without independent validation from driving records.

LENGTH OF STAY AND COSTS

The pressure from the managed care systems to reduce hospital stays may result in earlier or more frequent referral to rehabilitation facilities, which may in turn be pressured to release the patient to home or nursing home care. In a study that included patients whose impairment originated from both trauma and other conditions, length of stay was moderately correlated to an index of impairment of specific abilities (e.g., eating, toileting, bathing, and mobility), referral source, and year of admission. Type of medical insurance, gender, race, other medical conditions, and "psychological capacity" were not predictive of length of stay. Age was said to have a complex interaction with the other predictive factors and was not included in the prediction model (Stineman and Williams, 1990). The authors were appropriately cautious about generalizing the results to other facilities without similar research in those facilities. Matched for gender and injury severity, older patients require longer, more costly periods of rehabilitation to achieve the same degree of functioning (Cifu et al., 1996).

Despite the wide variation in patient needs and resultant length of stays, the DRG system has only one category for rehabilitation based on overall average cost, but exemption is allowed, which minimized the effects for hospitals that obtained exemptions. The system was used in the Department of Veterans Affairs to place its hospitals in competition for a set budget. A study from one VA hospital looked at the length of stay, readmissions, and referrals to nursing homes or home health care before and after the system was adopted. While length of stay decreased an average of three days, the discharges to nursing homes increased and those to home health care decreased significantly. The net effect may be increased costs, but costs were not assessed (Evans et al., 1990).

A study of the effect of prospective payment on treatment of hip fractures among the elderly (Palmer et al., 1989) resulted in lively debate regarding the relative efficacy and costs of rehabilitation in hospitals and skilled nursing care facilities (Lipson and Minassian, 1990). Comparison among facilities and the extent of referral to facilities may be influenced by home situations as well as medical conditions and costs (Palmer et al., 1990).

The effect of DRGs on who is treated where and who pays has been described as "squeezing the balloon": "Prospective payment systems hold the line on inpatient use and revenues, but outpatient services and spending rise dramatically" (Brown, 1988). Apparently, the relative effects of all the major potential factors on referral, outcomes in patient functioning, and costs have not been studied.

Certain programs have traditionally claimed to be cost-beneficial; that is, they return more in economic benefits to society than their costs. Vocational rehabilitation, for example, has a specific economic goal—to return the patient to gainful employment. If that employment returns more in taxes to the government than the cost of rehabilitating the person, then the investment clearly paid off, at least from the government's viewpoint, irrespective of the issues of intangible costs and benefits (more on this in chapter 15). However, vocational rehabilitation has apparently not been studied in a randomized, controlled trial. Comparisons have been done of earnings before and after rehabilitation, but with insufficient follow-up to confirm that immediate postrehabilitation earnings were sustained. Also, no comparison of types of rehabilitants was done, change in which might change the cost–benefit ratios (Berkowitz, 1988). The decline in returns on investment as increased numbers of severely disabled persons are included in the program could sway the balance of costs and benefits to the negative. Costs exceed benefits among those with certain sensory disabilities in certain age groups, for example (Gibbs, 1988). Those who live by cost–benefit could also die by cost–benefit.

References

Baker SP, Gertner HR, Rutherford RB, and Spitz WU (1971) Traffic deaths due to blunt abdominal injuries. In *Proceedings of the Fourteenth Annual Conference of the Association for the Advancement of Automotive Medicine*. Barrington, IL: Association for the Advancement of Automotive Medicine.
Basmajian JV, and Banerjee SN (eds.) (1996) *Clinical Decision Making in Rehabilitation.* New York, NY: Churchill Livingstone.

Bazzoli GJ (1996) Factors that enhance continued trauma center participation in trauma centers. *J Trauma.* 41:876–885.

Berkowitz E (1988) The cost-benefit tradition in vocational rehabilitation. In Berkowitz E (ed.), *Measuring the Efficiency of Public Programs: Costs and Benefits in Vocational Rehabitational.* Philadelphia, PA: Temple University Press.

Black J J M, Ward ME, Lockey DJ (2004) Appropriate use of helicopters to transport trauma patients from incident scene to hospital in the United Kingdom: an algorithm. *Emerg Med J.* 21:355–361.

Boyd DR (1983) Foreword. In Jacobs LM, and Bennett BR (eds.), *Emergency Patient Care: Prehospital Ground and Air Procedures.* New York, NY: Macmillan.

Bracken MB, Shepard MJ, Collins WF, Holford TR, Young W, Baskin DS, Eisenberg HM, Flamm E, Leo-Summers L, Maroon J, Marshall, LF, Perot PL Jr, Piepmeier J, Sonntag VKH, Wagner FC, Wilberger JE, and Winn HR (1990) A randomized controlled trial of methylprednisolone or naxolone in the treatment of acute spinal-cord injury. *New Engl J Med.* 322:1405–1411.

Bracken MB, Webb SB, and Wagner FC (1977–1978) Classification of the severity of acute spinal cord injury. *Paraplegia.* 15:319–326.

Brodsky H, and Hakkert S (1983) Highway fatal accidents and accessibility of emergency medical services. *Soc Sci Med.* 17:731–740.

Brown LD (1988) *Health Policy in the United States: Issues and Options.* New York, NY: Ford Foundation.

Cadigan A (1985) *An Evaluation of Trauma Center Utilization in Chicago.* Unpublished MPH thesis. New Haven, CT: Yale University.

CBS News (1997) HMO: managed or mangled. *60 Minutes*, January 5.

Chakerian MU, Demarest GB, and Paiz A (1990) Burn DRGs: effects of recent changes and implications for the future. *J Trauma.* 30:964–973.

Champion HR, Augenstein JS, Blatt AJ, Cushing B, Digges KH, Hunt RC, Lombardo LV, and Siegel JH (2003) Reducing highway deaths and disabilities with automatic wireless transmission of serious injury probability ratings from vehicles in crashes to EMS. In *Proceedings of the ESV Conference.* Washington, DC: National Highway Traffic Safety Administration.

Cifu DX, Kreutzer JS, Marwitz JH, Rosenthal M, Englander J, and High W (1996) Functional outcomes of older adults with traumatic brain injury: a prospective, multicenter analysis. *Arch Phys Med Rehabil.* 77:883–888.

Committee on the Consequences of Uninsurance (2003) *A Shared Destiny: Community Effects of Uninsurance.* Washington, DC: National Academy Press.

Committee on Trauma Research (1985) *Injury in America: A Continuing Public Health Problem.* Washington, DC: National Academy Press. Available at: http://www.nap. edu/books/0309035457/html, accessed August, 2006.

Dailey JT, Teter H, and Cowley RA (1992) Trauma center closures: a national assessment. *J Trauma.* 33:539–546.

Dietz V, and Harkema SJ (2004) Locomotor activity in spinal cord-injured persons. *J Appl Physiol.* 96:1954–1960.

Evans RL, Hendricks RD, Bishop DS, Lawrence-Umlauf KV, Kirk C, and Halar EM (1990) Prospective payment for rehabilitation: effects on hospital readmission, home care, and placement. *Arch Phys Med Rehabil.* 71:291–294.

Findley TW (1989) Research in physical medicine and rehabilitation I. How to ask the question. *Am J Phys Med Rehabil.* 68:26–30.

Fleiss JL (1986) *The Design and Analysis of Clinical Experiments.* New York, NY: John Wiley and Sons.

Gann DS (1989) Presidential address—American Association for the Surgery of Trauma, 1988 Annual Session. *J Trauma.* 29:1459–1461.

Garner SH, and Finlayson MAJ (1996) Traumatic brain injury. In Basmajian JV, and Banerjee SN (eds.), *Clinical Decision Making in Rehabilitation.* New York, NY: Churchill Livingstone.

Gerberich SG, Gerberich BK, Fife D, Cicero JJ, Lilja GP, and Van Berkom LC (1989) Analyses of the relationship between blood alcohol and nasal breath alcohol concentrations: implications for assessment of trauma cases. *J Trauma.* 29:338–343.

Gibbs E (1988) The vocational rehabilitation data base and the estimation of benefit cost ratios. In Berkowitz M (ed.), *Measuring the Efficiency of Public Programs: Costs and Benefits in Vocational Rehabilitation.* Philadelphia, PA: Temple University Press.

Gordon J (1987) Assumptions underlying physical therapy intervention: theoretical and historical perspectives. In Carr JH, et al. (eds.), *Movement Science: Foundations for Physical Therapy in Rehabilitation.* Rockville, MD: Aspen.

Hurst JM, Davis K Jr, Branson RD, and Johannigman JA (1989) Comparison of blood gasses during transport using two methods of ventilatory support. *J Trauma.* 29:1637–1639.

Jacobs BB, and Jacobs LM (1992) The effect of the new trauma DRGs on reimbursement. *J Trauma.* 33:495–502.

Jacobs LM Jr, and Bennett BR (1983) *Emergency Patient Care: Prehospital Ground and Air Procedures.* New York, NY: Macmillan.

Katz RT, Golden RS, Butter J, Tepper D, Rothke S, Holmes J, and Sahgal V (1990) Driving safety after brain damage: followup of twenty-two patients with matched controls. *Arch Phys Med Rehabil.* 71:133–136.

Kaufman S (1989) Long-term impact of injury on individuals, families and society: personal narratives and policy implications. In Rice DP, and MacKenzie EJ (eds.), *Cost of Injury in the United States: A Report to Congress, 1989.* San Francisco, CA, and Baltimore, MD: University of California Institute for Health and Aging and the Johns Hopkins University Injury Prevention Center.

Kaweski SM, Sise MJ, and Virgilio RW (1990) The effect of prehospital fluids on survival in trauma patients. *J Trauma.* 30:1215–1219.

Klose KJ, Schmidt DL, Needham BM, Brucker BS, Green BA, and Ayyar DR (1990) Rehabilitation therapy for patients with long-term spinal cord injuries. *Arch Phys Med Rehabil.* 71:659–662.

Kochersberger G, McConnell E, Kuchibhatla MN, and Pieper C (1996) The reliability, validity, and stability of a measure of physical activity in the elderly. *Arch Phys Med Rehabil.* 77:793–795.

Lehmann JF (1990) Quantitative evaluation of sway as an indicator of functional balance in post-traumatic brain injury. *Arch Phys Med Rehabil.* 71:955–961.

Lewis FR (1983) Prehospital care: the role of the EMT-paramedic. In West JG, Gazzaniga AB, and Cales RH (eds.), *Trauma Care Systems.* New York, NY: Praeger.

Liberman M, Mulder D, Lavoie A, Denis R, and Sampalis JS (2003) Multicenter Canadian study of prehospital trauma care. *Ann Surg.* 237:153–160.

Lipson MJ, and Minassian P (1990) Differences in outcome: hospital rehabilitation vs skilled nursing facility rehabilitation. *Arch Intern Med.* 150:1550–1551.

MacKenzie EJ, Rivara FP, Jurkovich GJ, Nathens AB, Frey KP, Egleston BL, Salkever DS, and Scharfstein DO (2006) A national evaluation of the effect of trauma center care on mortality. *New Engl J Med.* 354:366–378.

MacKenzie EJ, Siegel JH, Shapiro S, Moody M, and Smith RT (1988) Functional recovery and medical costs of trauma: an analysis by type and severity of injury. *J Trauma.* 28:281–297.

MacKenzie EJ, Steinwachs DM, Bone LR, Floccare DJ, Ramzy AI, and the Preventable Death Study Group (1992) Inter-rater reliability of preventable death judgments. *J Trauma.* 33:292–302.

Maier RV, and Rhodes M (2001) Trauma performance improvement. In Rivara FP, et al. (eds.), *Injury Control: A Guide to Research and Program Evaluation.* Cambridge, UK: Cambridge University Press.

Marottoli RA, Berkman LF, Leo-Summers L, and Cooney LM (1994) Predictors of mortality and institutionalization after hip fracture: the New Haven EPESE cohort. *Am J Public Health.* 84:1807–1812.

Martin GD, Cogbill TH, Landercasper J, and Strutt PJ (1990) Prospective analysis of rural interhospital transfer of injured patients to a referral trauma center. *J Trauma.* 30:1014–1020.

Mattox KL, Bickell W, Pepe PE, Burch J, and Feliciano D (1989) Prospective MAST study in 911 patients. *J Trauma.* 29:1104–1112.

Means KM, Rodell DE, and Sullivan PS (1996) Use of an obstacle course to assess balance and mobility in the elderly. *Arch Phys Med Rehabil.* 75:88–95.

Messick WJ, Rutledge R, and Meyer AA (1992) The association of advanced life support and decreased per capita trauma death rates: an analysis of 12,417 trauma deaths. *J Trauma.* 33:850–855.

Meyers AR, Branch LG, Cupples A, Lederman RI, Feltin M, and Master RJ (1989) Predictors of medical care utilization by independently living adults with spinal cord injuries. *Arch Phys Med Rehab.* 70:471–475.

National Highway Traffic Safety Administration (1996) *Traffic Safety Facts 1995.* Washington, DC: U.S. Department of Transportation.

National Highway Traffic Safety Administration (2006) *Traffic Safety Facts 2004.* Washington, DC: U.S. Department of Transportation.

Oakes DD, Wilmot CB, Hall KM, and Sherck JP (1990) Benefits of early admission to a comprehensive trauma center for patients with spinal cord injury. *Arch Phys Med Rehabil.* 71:637–643.

Palmer RM, Saywell RM Jr, Zollinger PW, et al. (1989) The impact of prospective payment systems on the treatment of hip fractures in the elderly. *Arch Intern Med.* 149:2237–2241.

Palmer RM, Saywell RM Jr, and Zollinger TW (1990) In reply. *Arch Intern Med.* 150:1551.

Pasquale MD, Rhodes M, Cipolle MD, Hanley T, and Wasser T (1996) Defining "Dead on Arrival": impact on a level I trauma center. *J Trauma.* 41:726–730.

Petrie D (1996) An evaluation of patient outcomes comparing trauma team activated versus trauma team not activated using TRISS analysis. *J Trauma.* 41:870–873.

Pinkston D (1989) Evolution of the practice of physical therapy in the United States. In Scully RM, and Barnes MR (eds.), *Physical Therapy.* Philadelphia, PA: J.B. Lippincott.

Pope AM, and Tarlov AR (1991) *Disability in America: Toward a National Agenda for Prevention.* Washington, DC: National Academy Press. Available at: http://www.nap. edu/books/0309043786/html/32.html, accessed August, 2006.

Rappaport M, Herrero-Backe C, Rappaport ML, and Winterfield KM (1989) Head injury outcome up to 10 years later. *Arch Phys Med Rehabil.* 70:885–892.

Reines HD, Bartlett RL, Chudy NE, Kiragu KR, and McKnew MA (1988) Is advanced life support appropriate for victims of motor vehicle accidents: the South Carolina highway trauma project. *J Trauma.* 28:563–570.

Rivara JB, Jaffe KM, Polissar NL, Fay GC, Liao S, and Martin KM (1996) Predictors of family functioning and changes 3 years after traumatic brain injury in children. *Arch Phys Med Rehabil.* 77:754–764.

Rudman TW, and Rudman D (1989) High rate of fractures for men in nursing homes. *Am J Phys Med Rehabil.* 68:2–5.

Sasser SM, Varghese M, Joshipura M, and Kellerman A (2006) Preventing death and disability through timely provision of prehospital trauma care. *Bull World Health Organ.* 84:507.

Schiller WR, Knox R, Zinnecker H, Jeevanandam M, Sayre M, Burke J, and Young DH (1988) Effect of helicopter transport of trauma victims on survival in an urban trauma center. *J Trauma.* 28:1127–1134.

Schwab CW, Young G, Civil I, Ross SE, Talucci R, Rosenberg L, Shaikh K, O'Malley K, and Camishion RC (1988) DRG reimbursement for trauma: the demise of the trauma center (the use of ISS grouping as an early predictor of total hospital cost). *J Trauma.* 28:939–946.

Schwartz RJ, Jacobs LM, and Yaezel D (1989) Impact of pre-trauma center care on length of stay and hospital charges. *J Trauma.* 29:1611–1615.

Shackford SR, MacKersie RC, Davis JW, Wolf PL, and Hoyt DB (1989) Epidemiology and pathology of traumatic deaths occurring at a level I trauma center in a regionalized system: the importance of secondary brain injury. *J Trauma.* 29:1392–1397.

Simpson RK, Venger BH, and Narayan RK (1989) Treatment of acute penetrating injuries of the spine: a retrospective analysis. *J Trauma.* 29:42–46.

Smith RF, Frateschi L, Sloan EP, Campbell L, Krieg R, Edwards LC, and Barrett JA (1990) The impact of volume on outcome in seriously injured trauma patients: two years' experience of the Chicago trauma system. *J Trauma.* 30:1066–1076.

Smith K, Marino RJ, and Graziani V (1996) Spinal cord injury. In: Basmajian JV and Banerjee SN (eds), *Clinical Decision Making in Rehabilitation.* New York, NY: Churchill Livingstone.

Stalhandske E, and Landesman A (2004) Introducing the new falls toolkit. *Top Patient Saf* (newsletter), no. 4 (May/June).

Stein F (1989) *Anatomy of Clinical Research.* Thorofare, NJ: Slack.

Stineman MG, and Williams SV (1990) Predicting inpatient rehabilitation length of stay. *Arch Phys Med Rehabil.* 71:881–887.

Tator CH (2002) Strategies for recovery and regeneration after brain and spinal cord injury. *Inj Prev.* 8:33–36.

Trunkey DD (1983) Trauma. *Sci Am.* 249(2):28–35.

Vlahov D (1990) Epidemiology of falls among patients in a rehabilitation hospital. *Arch Phys Med Rehabil.* 71:8–12.

Waller JA, Payne SR, and McClallen JM (1989) Trauma centers and DRGs—inherent conflict? *J Trauma.* 29:617–622.

Wesson DE, Williams JI, Spence LJ, Filler RM, Armstrong PF, and Pearl RH (1989) Functional outcome in pediatric trauma. *J Trauma.* 29:589–592.

West JG, and Cales RH (1983) Methods of evaluation of trauma care. In West JG, Gazzaniga AB, and Cales RH (eds.), *Trauma Care Systems.* New York, NY: Praeger.

West JG, Gazzaniga AB, and Cales RH (1983) Do trauma systems save lives? In West JG, Gazzaniga AB, and Cales RH (eds.), *Trauma Care Systems.* New York, NY: Praeger.

Whinney CM (2005) Do hip fractures need to be repaired within 24 hours of injury? *Cleve Clin J Med.* 72:250–252.

Wilson DS, McElligott J, and Fielding LP (1992) Identification of preventable trauma deaths: confounded inquiries? *J Trauma.* 32:45–51.

Wilson RF, Wiencek RG, and Balog M (1989) Predicting and preventing infection after abdominal vascular injuries. *J Trauma.* 29:1371–1375.

Wood RLL, and Eames P (eds.) (1989) *Models of Brain Injury Rehabilitation.* Baltimore, MD: Johns Hopkins University Press.

Wrigley JM, Yoels WC, Webb CR, and Fine PR (1994) Social and physical factors in referral of people with traumatic brain injuries to rehabilitation. *Arch Phys Med Rehabil.* 75:140–155.

Young JC, Macioce DP, and Young WW (1990) Identifying injuries and trauma severity in large databases. *J Trauma.* 30:1220–1230.

Zafonte RD, Hammond FM, Mann NR, Wood DL, Black KL, and Millis SR (1996) Relationship between Glascow Coma Scale and functional outcome. *Arch Phys Med Rehabil.* 75:364–369.

15

Injury Epidemiology and Economics

In addition to the humane reasons for injury control, there are huge cost savings to be realized. The issue in cost of injury studies is not just cost per se but also the extent of cost savings realizable by reduction of incidence and severity (Currie et al., 2000). Cost is usually measured in "human capital cost" and does not include the intangible toll in pain, grief, social disruption, and disorganization. It also does not include substitution of economic productivity with care giving to the injured by family members, which greatly reduces public costs (Rice and MacKenzie, 1989; Leigh et al., 2000; Finkelstein et al. 2006).

One of the most controversial uses of epidemiological data is the assignment of economic costs to distributions of injury and disease, and the balancing of such costs against the costs of reducing risk. The controversy arises both from repugnance on the part of some people at the notion that all aspects of injury and death can be expressed in monetary values, and from widespread disagreement over the methods when such expression is attempted.

Epidemiologists who describe sets of injuries or assess risks usually do not concern themselves with economic issues directly (other then the cost of the study and efficient study designs), but those who study the effects of programs, laws, regulations, medical care, or rehabilitation often encounter economic arguments and research. The purpose of this chapter is to alert injury epidemiologists and users of the data to some of the terminology and issues in economic analysis of injury data related to decisions regarding injury control.

THE ECONOMIC CONTEXT

Neoclassic economists promote the philosophy that people choose the risks that they take and that almost any organized attempt to reduce the risk will result in failure. As mentioned in preceding chapters, according to this theory, if people have an acceptable level of risk that they will tolerate, and their behavior offsets attempts to reduce risk (risk compensation), any attempt to reduce risk is a waste of money. As noted in chapters 12 and 13, studies in which individual behavior was actually observed in situations where risk was reduced do not support the assumption that people offset risk reduction by more risky behavior, and many attempts at injury control have had a beneficial effect.

Most economists argue that the costs of any program, including attempts at injury reduction, should not exceed the benefits. Expenditures for injury control that exceed the cost of injuries reduced is inefficient, they argue, because there is a net reduction in the goods and services available to society (e.g., Anderson and Settle, 1977). In order to balance costs against benefits, it is necessary to place a monetary value not only on the direct costs (medical care, rehabilitation, funerals) and indirect costs (lost productivity) but also on pain and suffering.

The following data are necessary to estimate costs and benefits:

$a(i)$ = number of injuries of given severity i to which an intervention applies
$b(i)$ = cost of injuries by severity i (including monetary value of pain and suffering)
$c(i)$ = proportion of each severity level i or its consequences reduced by the intervention
d = reduced costs = sum of $a(i) \times b(i) \times c(i)$, where i = each severity level
e = cost of applying or incrementing the intervention (including intangibles, e.g., inconvenience)
f = $d - e$ (i.e., benefit less cost)

Some economists use e/d, the benefit:cost ratio, but benefit less cost is more useful for comparing interventions because the amount of savings is evident.

Many health professionals and others have adopted this economic viewpoint without carefully examining its philosophical underpinnings. The welfare of a nation is the sum of its gross domestic product, according to the economic viewpoint. All of the dollars are equal, no matter what the consequences of their use. Money spent for addictive substances adverse to health such as cigarettes and alcohol is viewed just as positively as money spent for injury reduction. It does not seem to matter to many economists that some of the gross domestic product is contributing to the destruction of life-sustaining elements of the planet, nor do they consider that many of the most valued aspects of life are not reflected in the gross domestic product (Self, 1977). Perhaps the best that can be said for neoclassic economics is that it is shortsighted.

In the extreme neoclassic economic view, every good, service, intellectual or emotional satisfaction, and health risk is purchased in a market with money or some behavior the value of which can be reduced to money. The "invisible hand" of the market governs supply and demand to produce the optimal social welfare, and government is necessary only to enforce contracts and protect the public from domestic criminals and international threats.

Others recognize that society is much more complex. Organized interests at least partly control some markets, and one-sided advertising generates others. For example, in the 1930s and 1940s, General Motors conspired with Firestone

Rubber and Standard Oil of California to purchase and dismantle 46 mass transit companies that operated electric streetcars in 16 U.S. states. Although the companies were convicted of antitrust violations, their fines were minimal, and the mass transit systems were not restored (Adams and Brock, 1987).

In product advertising, benefits are often overstated, and risks are often not mentioned at all. Virtually no product advertising or user instruction gives a precise indication of risks of using a product—those that provide warnings state them in vague terms.

To do cost–benefit analysis, the monetary value of reduced risk that includes "pain and suffering" is usually assessed by research on "revealed preference," that is, implied value from behavior relative to risks, or by directly asking people what they would be willing to pay to reduce risks. To say the least, the research is problematic.

WILLINGNESS TO PAY

The introduction to a book on product labels contains the following statements: "Consumers take precautions whose benefits exceed their costs, and they forgo the other precautions. ... To estimate the benefits of precautions the consumer must assess both the effect of taking the precaution on the probability of each possible injury that it protects against and the value of the resulting reduction in the risk of injury" (Viscusi and Magat, 1987, p. 43). Two pages later, introducing the labels for two products to be studied as to consumer intent to take precautions, the report says, "Because most readers may not be familiar with the four injuries and how they arise, we briefly describe them here" (p. 45). How can one assume that the average consumer does a cost–benefit analysis on every product purchased based on the probability of injury if one assumes that readers of a book on risk, who are likely to have a better than average knowledge of risks, do not know the risks of injury from commonly used household products?

After attempting to assess the effects on intended precautions of particular labels that did not include quantitative estimates of risk, the researchers attempted to assess how much consumers would be willing to pay, per injury, to reduce them. A quantitative estimate of risk was included in information given to respondents during the willingness-to-pay phase of the study. The amounts that consumers were willing to have added to the overall costs of the products—an implied value of "$300,000 for gassings from bleach, $420,000 for child poisonings from bleach, $120,000 for hand burns from drain opener, and $360,000 for child poisonings"—were said to "appear to be excessive." They found it "implausible" that a relatively minor hand burn would be valued at $120,000, "four times the respondents' average household income" (Viscusi and Magat, 1987, p. 93).

The point missed, of course, is that the individual does not have to spend four times the family income to reduce the risk. The cost of the product modifications is spread among tens of millions of consumers, and in the aggregate, people may be willing to pay far more per product to reduce risk than economists' judgment of the worth of the risk. For the individual, the expenditure may be a few cents extra per product for household cleaners that will last weeks or months, a few dollars

extra for a child's crib that may last for generations, or a few hundred dollars extra
for a motor vehicle that will last for several years.

Also, contrary to popular belief, reduction of risk does not necessarily increase
the cost of the product. In some cases, reduction in the cost of the product can
accompany reduction of risk. For example, it takes more material and thus costs
more to make the front end of a vehicle sharp rather than smooth. Vehicles with
sharp points on their fronts have higher pedestrian death rates (Robertson, 1990).
Protruding radio knobs, air conditioning controls, and gearshift controls in
vehicles that penetrate the tissues of occupants in crashes cost more than smooth
buttons. Increased weight of a motor vehicle increases cost and risk to all road
users in the aggregate (see appendix 12-1). Designers of one of the research safety
vehicles in the mid-1970s estimated that, despite numerous features to enhance
crash avoidance and crashworthiness, the retail cost of the vehicle if mass produced would have been no more than concurrently priced compact cars (DiNapoli
et al., 1977).

Although it is claimed that the initial motor vehicle safety standards added
several hundred dollars to the cost of new cars, the increases in producer prices
of cars during the period of adoption of the standards was not as large as that for
other durable goods. During 1964–1973, the producer price index for all durable
goods rose 35 percent while the increase for cars was about half that, 17 percent
(Robertson, 1983).

If purchasers have no quantitative information on risks of a product, and some
manufacturers do not know the risks or do not attempt to reduce risks, even those
that would include reduced costs or no increased costs of the product, how can
an economist argue that the consumers' use of the product is a "revealed preference" of the balance of costs and benefits? The issue is confounded further by the
fact that the persons injured are often not the original purchasers of the product.
Certainly the pedestrian who is struck by the sharp front of a vehicle had no say
in its purchase. Based on the age of occupants injured, ownership of vehicles, and
relationship of the injured person to the owner, about 75–80 percent of persons
injured by motor vehicles were not party to the purchase (Baker, 1979).

Nevertheless, numerous economic studies attempt to assess valuation of life
and limb by calculation of premiums in wages in risky occupations, demand for
products that reduce risk relative to price, behavior implied to trade off risks and
benefits, and surveys about people's willingness to pay for reduced risk. One summary of 29 such studies, about half of which were based on wage premiums relative
to job risks, suggested a "willingness to pay" value of $2 million per life, about
the average among the studies selected, although the results of individual studies
ranged from $1 million to $3 million (Miller, 1989).

A very ambitious compendium of the effect of road injury countermeasures,
including behavior, vehicle, and environmental characteristics, applies cost–benefit
analysis to many (Elvik and Vaa, 2004). While the studies reviewed were limited
to a few journals, there are sufficient numbers of studies of countermeasures to
produce a reasonable estimate of effectiveness of some. The cost–benefit analyses were based on Norwegian economics and are more dubious for the reasons
mentioned above.

Of course, Norway is a wealthy country. A troubling aspect of cost–benefit analysis is the implications for low-income countries and low-income populations within countries. If the value of life and limb is based on the prevailing wages in a given area, there will be huge differences in the value placed on lives in those areas (Morrow and Bryant, 1995). Many countermeasures that pass a cost–benefit challenge in economically developed areas would not do so in economically poor areas. Several countermeasures used by injury control specialists in the Indian Health Service (chapter 7) have been deemed cost-beneficial using national estimates of value of life (Zaloshnja et al., 2003), but on the reservations where they occurred, unemployment is often 50 percent or more and wages of the employed are low. Fortunately, the Indian Health Service operates on the philosophy that the value of people is more than economic.

RISK–BENEFIT

A variation of cost–benefit is so-called risk–benefit analysis in which historical death rates are used to argue that risks not exceeding them are acceptable. This point is most often made by physicists and engineers who believe public opposition to certain technologies such as nuclear power generation or types of disposal of military nuclear waste is irrational. They compare the risk of these technologies to known risks, such as travel by motor vehicles and airplanes. One of the early advocates of this view said, "Automobile and airplane safety have been continuously weighed by society against economic costs and operating performance" (Starr, 1969). This anthropomorphic view of society makes no sense in the light of the history of either technology or the social processes that led to regulation or lack of regulation (Priest, 1988).

The translation of what has been tacitly accepted into what is acceptable is a prescription for disaster. Risk after risk could be added, each at or below the "acceptable" level, until a substantial number of the population are dead or disabled. Risk–benefit analysts cannot have it both ways. On the one hand, they say that risks with a history indicate what is acceptable, but on the other hand, they are fond of lists of dollars spent "per life saved," calculated for a variety of employed or proposed countermeasures to risks, to illustrate governmental irrationality in risk management. One such array showed variation from $100 per life saved for expanded immunization in Indonesia to $200,000,000 per life saved for the control of radiation in "defense high level waste." Most of the injury-related countermeasures were in a range of $20,000 to $400,000 per life saved, but coal mine safety and other mine safety was said to cost $22,000,000 and $34,000,000 per life saved (Cohen, 1980).

The accuracy of all of those estimates is unknown, but some were grossly misstated. For example, high school driver education was said to save lives, but it actually increases deaths (Robertson and Zador, 1978). The implication of a list of costs per life saved is that efficient allocation of resources should be such that the costs would be similar if rational decisions were made. Sometimes appeals are made to ethical issues such as equity; that is, if the costs per life saved are different, some people are benefiting more from resource allocations than others. Others argue that the differences represent values placed on lives that have different values. For example, much more is allocated to protect the president of the United States than for ordinary citizens (Shrader-Frechette, 1985).

Even if the estimates were accurate, the ages of the persons whose lives are preserved are very different among the technologies and programs. Cost per years of life preserved would result in a very different array for many hazards. Less value is placed on the lives of children by typical discounting to present value in cost analyses. The above-noted list of costs per life saved (Cohen, 1980) also calculated costs per 20 years of life preserved, but some of the technologies and programs affect mainly children and youth with more than 20 years expected life, while others "save" lives of people who have a life expectancy less than 20 years.

In the 1990s, a widely publicized compendium of "500 life-saving interventions" more appropriately indicated cost per year of life saved (Tengs et al., 1995). The bibliography accompanying the list may be somewhat useful to persons in a position to recommend or initiate programs, but the list is of dubious quality and should not the basis for decisions. Some of the research on which estimates are based is of doubtful validity. Many of the estimates are based on regulatory analyses by antiregulation economists or by governmental agencies. In at least one such agency, the National Highway Traffic Safety Administration (NHTSA), two regulatory analyses are often prepared on a given issue, one favorable and one unfavorable to the adoption of a given regulation. When the administrator decides which way the decision is to be made, the analysis supporting the decision is the one published. (See appendix 15-1 for the author's critique of one NHTSA cost–benefit analysis to support a do-nothing stance on vehicle stability.)

In addition, the noted list of 500 interventions is not exhaustive. For example, only a small proportion of effective highway modifications are included, and one of the most cost-effective—lighting roads at night at high-risk sites (chapter 7)—is not mentioned. The cost-effectiveness of many of the technologies and programs mentioned on the list can be increased enormously by targeting high-risk populations or environments based on surveillance (chapter 7). Depending on the extent to which certain injuries are more or less likely to cluster, the cost-effectiveness would vary enormously from that listed.

For example, based on the cluster of motor vehicle crashes identified by surveillance in Browning, Montana (chapter 7), the lighting and curb modifications that were installed in a two-mile stretch of road cost about $6,000, and the electricity to light the streets at night costs about $500 per year. The modifications undoubtedly paid for themselves in benefits to society in a few months.

Also, cost per year of life saved does not take into account the nonfatal injuries that would be prevented or reduced in severity, which varies per life saved among technologies and programs. Somehow weighting the costs as well as pain, suffering, and other consequences of nonfatal health impairment and including them with the estimates of fatality reductions is very problematic. One book on risk–benefit analysis states that the weighting is "somewhat arbitrary" (Crouch and Wilson, 1982). The authors of that book advocated a thorough risk analysis before decisions are made, but included Cohen's (1980) list of costs per life saved without the column for cost per 20 years of life.

Usually, the attempt to account for nonfatal injuries is made by monetizing both fatal and nonfatal outcomes, which turns risk–benefit back into cost–benefit. Some estimates of the cost of nonfatal injuries are based solely on the cost of medical care and lost workdays. This discriminates against children and the elderly and does not include pain and suffering. It is also difficult to evaluate lost workdays because some work is uncompensated. Also, 50 restricted activity days for a given individual is likely to have a more severe economic impact than that of five restricted workdays each for 10 people (Priest, 1988).

Another approach is to somehow adjust for quality years of life, which raises all sorts of issues (Baldwin et al., 1990). For example, do commodities consumed represent quality of life? If so, how does one deal with the quality of the commodities that is not necessarily reflected in their price? Some analysts have pointed out that characteristics of people rather than what they consume are more indicative of quality of life (Culyer, 1990), but those qualities are not indicated in any pricing system.

Questioning people can obtain estimates of the quality of life, but all of the methodological issues of reliability and validity of self-reports are involved (Petitti, 1994). Risks with equal outcomes result in different responses by respondents if presented as gains rather than as losses (Kahneman and Tversky, 1979) or in other contexts (Loomes and McKenzie, 1990). People who have not experienced given disabilities themselves cannot give informed answers about the quality of life of persons with such disabilities and their families.

UNCERTAINTY IN COSTS OF INTERVENTIONS

Costs of product modifications and other injury control programs can be estimated more easily than benefits in some cases, but such estimates are often not done. Government budgets for highway modifications, regulatory agencies, and the like are known. The total cost of regulations, however, is more difficult to estimate— particularly when the regulations are performance regulations. For example, the government standard for energy absorption by steering assemblies during frontal car crashes did not necessarily increase costs. It could have reduced costs if it resulted in attention to designs that used cheaper materials.

Cost per unit of equipment usually declines substantially as the number of units increase—called economy of scale. If cost–benefit analysis were used to make decisions, rather than its usual use to second-guess decisions after the fact of implementation, the wrong decision could be made if cost per unit were based on the originally designed equipment rather than large-scale production.

Many programs that have been suggested or implemented to some degree have not included cost studies. Researchers who evaluate the effects of interventions seldom include cost estimates of the interventions. Also, the extant costs of products or their modifications, where known, should not always be accepted as though the least costly technology is used. For example, in Sri Lanka, burnt out light bulbs are filled with kerosene and used as lamps that increase fire risk compared to more sturdy, and costly, glass lamps (Berger and Mohan, 1996). In such situations, all the alternatives for lighting, including invention of a product as cheap as or cheaper than recycled bulbs, should be considered before assuming that the situation is determined by the economics.

It is often difficult to find data on the extent of implementation of many interventions. For example, a controlled experiment in which parents in an experimental group were counseled regarding infant's falls from surfaces such as tables and beds suggests that these falls can be reduced about 41 percent by physicians' warnings and counseling (Kravitz, 1973). To estimate the benefit minus costs that could be realized from expanding such counseling, however, we need data on the extent of counseling by physicians now. Apparently, no survey of physicians to determine the extent of such counseling and its cost has been done, nor is the willingness to counsel and the compensation expected for doing so known.

OVERLAP IN EFFECTS OF INTERVENTIONS

Often, the same injuries would be prevented by more than one intervention. To the extent that there is such overlap in the effects of two or more approaches, the cost-effectiveness of each will not reflect the cost-effectiveness of applying both at the same time. For example, fatal crashes of 16- to 17-year-old drivers is increased by high school driver education (Robertson and Zador, 1978). Based on the numbers of students enrolled in 1985, a report to Congress noted that up to $2.2 billion in 1985 dollars would have been saved in that year if there were no driver education in high schools, including the $163 million cost of the program (Robertson, 1989a). Since surveys of schools to determine the numbers of students enrolled have been discontinued, it is not possible to update those estimates.

Nevertheless, if the minimum licensing age were increased to 18, virtually all of the adverse effect of driver education would be eliminated. Raising the minimum licensing age to 18 and eliminating high school driver education simultaneously would not save the sum of the injury and program costs of driver education and the cost of injuries of drivers less than 18 because an 18 age limit for licensure would reduce the same injuries and deaths as eliminating driver education. Only the cost of the driver education program could be added to the injury costs saved by raising the minimum licensing age to prevent double counting of cost savings because of the overlap in injuries reduced.

That is a very obvious example of overlap in effects of countermeasures, but there are instances in which the effects of particular interventions and the overlaps of effects are less well known, even by those in a position to find out. The NHTSA frequently issues reports on the involvement of alcohol in motor vehicle fatalities that includes seat belt use and alcohol countermeasures. In 2004, an estimated 39 percent of such fatalities were "alcohol related" and 55 percent of killed vehicle occupants were allegedly not using seat belts (National Highway Traffic Safety Administration, 2006). These claims not only are of questionable validity (chapter 12) but also are often assumed to mean that reductions in alcohol use would result in a proportionate reduction in fatalities. Indeed, the NHTSA has virtually ceased to issue standards for vehicle crashworthiness, rollover resistance, and crash avoidance, claiming that the majority of motor vehicle fatalities are related to nonuse of seat belts and use of alcohol (National Highway Traffic Safety Administration, 1994).

Since belt use is known to be lower among vehicle occupants with high blood alcohol concentrations (e.g., Foss et al., 1994), the effect of increasing belt use and reducing alcohol use cannot be additive because of the overlap. Indeed, correlation of alcohol use to Injury Severity Scores and hospital length of stay disappears when belt use is controlled (Anderson et al., 1990), indicative of confounding.

Also, if alcohol use is lower in later model cars—those that are more crashworthy (chapter 12)—and belt use is higher in such cars, some of the fatalities attributed to alcohol and nonuse of belts may be due to lack of crashworthiness of older vehicles. Alcohol involvement and belt use are correlated to vehicle age. Also, alcohol use and aggressive or impulsive behavior may be attributable to some extent to a common precursor, which suggests the possibility that at least some of the aggressive or impulsive behavior would occur in the absence of alcohol (chapter 8).

To illustrate the overlap of alcohol and belt use and the confounding of effects of other factors on assessment of the effects of belt use and alcohol, the regression model used to estimate the effects of vehicle modifications, belt use, alcohol, and other factors (see appendix 12-1) was examined in stages. First, regression coefficients of the effects of belt use and alcohol, separately and without control for other factors, were examined. They were combined without the other factors and then combined with the other factors. If the effects of belt and alcohol use are not confounded, the single estimates should not differ significantly from the effects in combination with other factors. The regression coefficients and 95 percent confidence intervals are presented in table 15-1. The estimates of belt use effects and alcohol effects, each alone, are greatly reduced when they are considered simultaneously. They are again reduced to much lower levels when the effects of safety standards, other improvements in crashworthiness (as revealed by crash tests), vehicle age, and vehicle size are all included. Note that the variance explained (R^2) is modest for seat belts and alcohol alone or in combination but that R^2 for the full model is excellent. Belt use observed in traffic was approximately 53 percent in 1991 (Datta and Guzek, 1990). If the remaining 47 percent of car occupants had been restrained, the occupant fatality rate of 1.6 per 100 million miles would have been reduced by about 21 percent. That is, multiply the coefficient in table 15-1 by the percent of unused belts ($.007 \times 47 = .329$) and divide the result by the death rate ($.329/1.6 = 0.21$).

Alcohol at 0.1% or more by weight was found in about 23.4 percent of passenger car drivers in 1991 (Klein and Burgess, 1995). Multiplying the coefficient for alcohol ($\geq 0.1\%$ by weight) by the percent involvement ($-.007 \times 23.4 = 0.164$) indicates that reducing such alcohol involvement to zero would reduce the car occupant death rate by .164, which is 10 percent of the overall rate of 1.6. Uncontrolled estimates of belt effectiveness and alcohol effects on fatal crashes are confounded by their covariation and the lower belt use and higher alcohol involvement in less crashworthy cars.

If alcohol were eliminated and belt use were 100 percent, almost two-thirds of car occupant fatalities would nevertheless occur. As a practical matter, both goals,

Table 15-1. Regression Estimates of the Effects on Passenger Car Occupant Death Rates per 100 Million Miles, in Relation to Alcohol and Seat Belt Use Without and With Controls for Other Factors

Variable	Belts Only	Alcohol Only	Belts and Alcohol	All Factors Combined
Belt use, %				
Estimated effect	−.034		−.019	−.007
95% CI	−.028, −.039		−.026, −.013	−.001, −.013
Alcohol > 0.1, %				
Estimated effect		.070	.047	.007
95% CI		.059, .080	.035, .060	001, .013
Standards				
Estimated effect				−.260
95% CI				−.237, −.283
NCAP publicity				
Estimated effect				−.077
95% CI				−.044, −.110
Calendar year				
Estimated effect				−.017
95% CI				−.052, .019
Industrial production				
Estimated effect				.029
95% CI				.015, .043
Expected from vehicle age				
Estimated effect				.444
95% CI				.656, .232
Expected from wheelbase				
Estimated effect				1.066
95% CI				.612, 1.520
Intercept	3.47	−.32	1.11	−.793
R^2	.35	.39	.46	.92

95% CI, 95 percent confidence interval.

however admirable, will not be attained. Many of the fatalities that would be prevented by increased belt use or reduction of alcohol use are the same fatalities. Any cost–benefit analysis or estimate of cost per year of life preserved, such as comparing belt use laws and alcohol crackdowns as though they were additive, would be distorted.

COST-EFFECTIVENESS AND DECISION MAKING

There are many technologies, policies, and programs to reduce injury that produce a net benefit, even by the narrow criteria of human capital costs (Robertson, 1989a). The failure to adopt them is not an issue of costs but rather one of who pays versus who benefits and who decides whether or not the intervention is used.

Many potential improvements are neglected out of sheer ignorance and inattention by policy makers. Analysis of cost/effectiveness, cost/benefit, or cost/savings (where some costs and benefits are intangible) ignores feasibility of implementation because of ideological factors and concentrated interests that may oppose certain interventions.

In the United States, the gun lobby claims that unlimited "right to bear arms" is guaranteed by the Constitution, and few citizens are informed of the falsity of the argument (Christoffel and Teret, 1993). Since those injured by guns cannot be denied treatment, the false ideology is costly to everyone. In one major trauma center, for example, 79 percent of the costs for treatment of gunshot wounds were paid from taxes. Insurers paid an additional 19 percent. Taxpayers and the insured paid for 98 percent of the treatment (Wintemute and Wright, 1992).

Policies such as government subsidization of bicycle helmet purchases, while accepted in Australia (Wood and Milne, 1988), may be difficult to implement in the United States. Although the majority of motorcyclists are in favor of helmet use laws, a vocal minority has been successful in gaining repeal in many states (Baker, 1980). Tax-supported programs, mainly Medicaid, provided 63 percent of the costs of treatment and rehabilitative care of motorcyclists in one major trauma center (Rivara et al., 1988). The data indicating huge economic losses (Hartunian, et al., 1983; Robertson, 1989a), and the evidence that the costs are paid with public monies apparently had little influence on state legislators as they repealed helmet laws when intimidated by the minority biker lobby.

The failure of the Occupational Safety and Health Administration to extend relevant regulations to reduce farm injuries is partly due to the myth that farm owners bear the risk and can take precautions they deem appropriate (Kelsey, 1994). This ignores the effects of farm injury and its costs on farmers who qualify for Medicare or Medicaid, the latter when the farm goes belly up because the farmer is no longer able to work. Also, there are many injured farm workers who are not owners, are poorly paid, and cannot afford health insurance.

Although, in the above instances, seemingly overwhelming ideological opposition or lobbying power drove the decisions, such power is not always as solid as it seems. No one familiar with Tennessee politics would have expected that state to be the first to enact a child-restraint use law, but it did, and other states followed. The gun lobby spent $6 million in an attempt to defeat gun control legislation in Maryland but was overwhelmingly defeated in a referendum in the 1988 election. The Brady Bill, providing for background checks on gun purchasers, survived the 1994–1996 U.S. Congress, many of whose members were heavily beholden to the gun lobby.

Although there is some uncertainty in each of the estimates of potential for injury reduction discussed in this book because of variation in sampling error, and the lack of good experimental design in some cases, there is no doubt that a substantial proportion of severe injuries could be reduced by a greater application of current knowledge. The potential cost savings, after accounting for the cost of injury control programs, is in the billions of U.S. dollars for many interventions for which data are available. Usually, the estimates of cost savings are far more sensitive to the difference in the estimates using the human capital and willing-ness-to-pay methods than they are to variation in estimates of effectiveness of a given intervention.

Even if all of the benefits of a given risk-reduction technology or program could be estimated accurately, it is obvious that a great deal of resource allocation will not be made based on such an analysis. If the money in the federal budget allocated to programs for dealing with "defense high-level waste" were reduced, it would not be allocated to private expenditures for safety of consumer products, much less immunization programs in Indonesia.

In those instances where a set of resources are available to a given decision maker or decision-making body, it certainly makes sense to attempt to allocate those resources to minimize human damage. One interesting issue for research is the extent to which cost–benefit or cost-effectiveness analysis actually affects decisions. In one study of future decision makers (graduate students in law and business), six experimental groups were given sets of information regarding poli-cies to reduce motor vehicle injury, and their expressed preferences were com-pared to a control group given no information. The information given to the experimental groups was varied by attributable benefit, attributable risk, and rela-tive risk. Generally, groups given data were much more likely than control groups to favor a regulatory policy (60 percent vs. 22 percent). Those given information on attributable risks and benefits in terms of injury reductions were somewhat more likely to favor regulation than those given relative risk information (64 percent vs. 52 percent). No data on costs were included, but responses varied significantly depending on attitudes regarding personal freedom and governmental regulation (Runyan and Earp, 1985).

Suppose that a set of local governments were randomly divided into experi-mental and control groups, and each government in the experimental group was presented data on the benefits less costs of adopting a set of injury control mea-sures, while each in the control group was presented the same injury control options without the cost–benefit analysis. Would the experimental communi-ties be more or less likely to take action? If both groups took action, would the experimental groups' actions be more efficient; that is, would the experimental governments achieve more reduction of injury costs per dollar spent? Similar studies of injury control for workers in private corporations would be of interest, but the likelihood of gaining access to detailed data in enough companies would be problematic.

APPENDIX 15-1

Case Study: The National Highway Traffic Safety's Cost–Benefit Analysis of a Rollover Standard

In 1972, the NHTSA successfully opposed the Army's proposed sale of surplus jeeps to the public because of evidence of instability of the vehicle. Nevertheless, the Jeep Corporation's civilian version, known as the CJ, continued to be sold—its commercials showing the vehicle going over hills with all wheels off the ground.

Ford Motor Company, also a manufacturer of military jeeps, in 1973 introduced a jeep-like Bronco for civilian use that was discontinued in 1978 (Snyder et al., 1980). In 1980, research and demonstration of the rollover propensity of the Jeep CJ-5 was featured on CBS's popular television program *60 Minutes*. The stability of other so-called utility vehicles was also of concern because of their high center of gravity relative to track width and resultant rollover rates, but attention focused on the Jeep CJ-5, which was the least stable. After hundreds of lawsuits, the CJ-5 was discontinued in 1984 and the CJ-7 in 1986.

Despite the demise of the pre-1978 Bronco and the Jeep CJs, sales of utility vehicles increased from 132,000 in 1982 to 856,000 in 1988 (Ward's Automotive Yearbook, 1983–1989). Researchers continued to document their high rollover rates (Reinfurt et al., 1981, 1984; Smith, 1982), but the government took no action other than to require a vague warning that the vehicles handle differently from other vehicles.

In 1986, a then member of the U.S. Congress, Timothy Wirth, petitioned NHTSA to adopt a stability standard for all utility vehicles based on the strong correlation of the stability ratio (track width divided by twice the height of center of gravity) and the rollover rates among vehicles (Robertson and Kelley, 1989). In 1988, the Consumers Union publicized tests of the Suzuki Samurai and petitioned the NHTSA to prohibit its further sale based on its rollover propensity. These and other petitions were rejected by the NHTSA.

In response to the Wirth petition, the NHTSA argued that choice of a specific stability ratio would be arbitrary and that the agency could not, by law, prohibit a class of vehicles (National Highway Traffic Safety Administration, 1987). Neither argument is valid. The death rate increases substantially as stability declines toward a static stability ratio of 1.2 g of lateral force, which is typical of utility vehicles but below the ratio of all but a few cars. The rollover death rate of the Jeep CJ-5 (stability, 1 g) is 19 times that of cars; the CJ-7, pre-1978 Bronco, and Bronco II (stability, 1.07–1.08 g) have rollover death rates 10–12 times that of cars, and the Samurai (stability, 1.12 g) had a rollover death rate six times that of cars (Robertson, 1989b).

Setting the stability standard at a minimum ratio of 1.2 g of lateral force would be no more arbitrary than setting the blood alcohol concentration for drivers at 0.08 percent by weight. Since the standard could be met by either lowering the center of gravity or widening the distance between the center of the tires, or both, the standard would not prohibit a class of vehicles. For example, the Jeep CJ-5 could have had a stability ratio above 1.2 by lowering its center of gravity 5.5 inches, and the other utility vehicles would have to be lowered much less than that.

The Consumers Union petition to recall the Samurai was rejected on the grounds that the Samurai was not as bad as the Bronco II (National Highway Traffic Safety Administration, 1988). Subsequently, the NHTSA announced that it would reconsider the rollover issue and specifically singled out the Bronco II because it was worse than the Samurai. In 1990, the NHTSA rejected petitions that the CJ vehicles be recalled, saying that their rollover rates were only "slightly" higher than peer vehicles. It subsequently also exonerated the Bronco II on similar grounds, stating that they were little different than peer vehicles. The leadership of the agency did not seem embarrassed by the logic of saying that a vehicle was not defective because it had an injury rate similar to vehicles with the same defect, or lying about the substantial differences among vehicles. Actually, those vehicles would have had no peers in rollover rates had the agency done something about vehicle stability when the issue was raised a decade earlier.

In June 1996, for the third time in a decade, the government refused to adopt a standard for motor vehicle stability. The NHTSA argued that the costs would exceed the benefits (National Highway Traffic Safety Administration, 1996). The NHTSA prefers to measure stability by tipping a table with the vehicle on it and observing the angle at which the upper wheels lose contact, called the tilt table angle (TTA). According to the agency, measuring center of gravity can damage a vehicle and does not account for possible effects of suspension. It said a minimum TTA standard of 46.4 degrees would result in 61 fewer deaths and 63 fewer severe injuries, an estimate that does not pass the smell test (Denmark is not the only place where something is rotten). The agency's own studies indicate that stability measured by $T/2H$ accounts for most of the variance in rollover percentages of single-vehicle crashes, controlling for behavioral and environmental factors (Harwin and Brewer, 1990; Mengert et al., 1989), and the death rate per vehicle of lower stability utility vehicles is 3–20 times that of passenger cars.

To assess the effect of lack of adoption of a vehicle-stability standard, the author conducted a study of fatal crash rates per vehicle year of use for 1989–1993 model vehicles in use during 1990–1994. The 23 vehicles with known TTA up to 47.7 degrees were included to compare the results using TTA and $T/2H$. The fatality data were extracted from the Fatality Analysis Reporting System. Vehicles in use, 1989–1993 models during 1990–1994, were obtained from published data (Insurance Institute for Highway Safety, 1995), and projected years of use were estimated from published vehicle sales (Ward's Automotive Yearbook, 1995), adjusted for known scrap rates (Oak Ridge National Laboratory, 1984).

The effect of stability on fatal rollover rates per vehicle in use was estimated by logistic regression of the rollover rates with nonrollover rates, wheelbase (distance from front to rear axle), and stability measures included as predictor variables. Nonrollover rates serve as a control for driver, vehicle, and environmental factors that affect fatality rates generally, and wheelbase has been correlated with rollover controlling for stability (Jones and Penny, 1990).

Table 15-2 presents the nonrollover and rollover death rates per 100,000 in use per year of the vehicles in the study, ranked from highest to lowest rollover rate. There is large variation in both death rates. The Amigo has a rollover death rate 16 times that of the Caravan/Voyager but a similar nonrollover rate. The logistic regression estimates are presented in table 15-3 separately for $T/2H$ (model 1) and TTA (model 2). $T/2H$ is significantly and strongly predictive of rollover when wheelbase and nonrollover rates are controlled, but TTA is not. Rollover rates are significantly higher in vehicles with shorter wheelbases and in vehicles with higher nonrollover rates.

To project the deaths attributable to vehicle instability over the expected survival of vehicles, the number of vehicles remaining after scrappage in a given year of the 20-year period after manufacture was multiplied by the difference

Table 15-2. Vehicle Parameters and Death Rates Per 100,000 Vehicles in Use 1990–1994

	Death Rate			Vehicle Parameter	
	Nonroll	Rollover	Total	T/2H	Wheelbase
1989–1993 Isuzu Amigo	7.9	35.8	43.7	1.11	92
1990–1993 Toyota 4Runner	5.0	20.3	25.3	1.08	103
1991–1993 Isuzu Rodeo	6.0	18.1	24.1	1.12	109
1989–1993 Geo Tracker	14.5	17.8	32.3	1.14	87
1989–1993 Jeep Wrangler	10.3	13.0	23.3	1.16	93
1993 Ford Ranger	14.5	12.1	26.6	1.13	125
1989–1993 GM S/T Blazer	11.1	11.4	22.5	1.10	104
1989–1993 Nissan Pickup	15.1	11.2	26.3	1.16	116
1991–1993 Ford Escort	21.5	10.5	32.0	1.38	98
1990–1993 Nissan Pathfinder	3.5	10.0	13.5	1.07	104
1989–1993 GM S/T Pickup	16.5	9.8	26.3	1.16	123
1989–1993 GM 1500 Pickup	10.2	8.9	19.1	1.14	142
1990–1993 Ford Festiva	28.6	7.9	36.5	1.34	90
1989–1993 Ford F250 Pickup	5.6	6.9	12.5	1.11	155
1989–1993 GM Astro	8.1	5.7	13.8	1.11	111
1989–1993 Ford Bronco	4.8	5.6	10.4	1.06	105
1992–1993 Ford Aerostar	5.6	5.4	11.0	1.11	119
1991–1993 Ford Explorer	4.2	5.4	9.6	1.08	107
1989–1993 Ford F150 Pickup	7.4	5.3	12.7	1.15	139
1989–1993 Mazda MPV	6.2	4.8	11.0	1.16	110
1990–1993 GM Lumina Van	6.0	3.9	9.9	1.12	110
1989–1993 Chrysler D150	10.9	3.2	14.1	1.28	115
1991–1993 Chrysler Caravan/ Voyager	6.0	2.2	8.2	1.18	119

between the rate predicted from the regression analysis for a vehicle of that stability and a vehicle with the same nonrollover rate and wheelbase but a $T/2H$ of 1.2.

Table 15-4 illustrates the calculation of preventable deaths by changing $T/2H$ using the 1991 Blazer/Jimmy ($T/2H = 1.10$) as an example. Based on the logistic coefficients in table 15-2, the expected total rollover death rate of that vehicle is

$$\text{Expected} = 1/(1 + e^{-x})$$

where $x = -3.664 + (-5.236 \times 1.10) + (-0.00435 \times 111) + (0.0740 \times 9.5)$; thus, the expected rate is .00011933. Substituting 1.2 for the $T/2H$ of 1.10 in the equation gives the expected rate at $T/2H = 1.2$, which is .00006923. The difference between the two rates (.0000501) times the number of vehicles in use in a given

Table 15-3. Logistic Regression of Rollover Rates by Stability, Wheelbase, and Nonrollover

	Coefficient	p-Value
Model 1		
Intercept	−3.66	<.01
$T/2H$	−5.24	<.01
Wheelbase	−0.00	<.01
Nonroll rate	0.08	<.01
Model 2		
Intercept	−9.43	<.01
TTA	0.01	0.61
Wheelbase	−0.01	<.01
Nonroll rate	0.03	<.01

year gives the estimate of preventable deaths in that year. Although the fractional numbers during a given year are expected values, the total is a realistic estimate. The 1991 Blazer/Jimmys would be expected to have approximately 107 fewer rollover deaths in the 20-year period after their initial sales if the $T/2H$ were 1.2.

The estimated deaths that would have been prevented in the 1990–1994 models with $T/2H < 1.2$, had the minimum standard of $T/2H = 1.2$, proposed in 1986, been adopted beginning in 1990 and subsequent models, are summarized in table 15-5. Other vehicles with $T/2H$ less than 1.2 were not included because of missing TTA. Nevertheless, approximately 5,028 preventable rollover deaths are expected in the noted vehicles for lack of a rollover standard in that five-year period. The Escort, Festiva, and Dodge D150 pickup are excluded from table 15-5 because the $T/2H$ of each is above 1.2. The rank of vehicles by numbers of preventable rollover deaths is different from the rank of fatal rollover rates mainly because of differences in sales volumes. The rate represents the risk to the occupants, while the number of preventable deaths represents the loss to society because of the combination of fatality rates and vehicle sales.

The effect on rollover fatalities of actually improved stability in a vehicle that did not change drastically in appearance is illustrated by the evolution in designs of the Jeep CJs and Wrangler. Figure 15-1 shows that fatal first-event rollover and rollover that occurred after contact with another vehicle or object declined as the $T/2H$ was gradually increased from 1.01 in the CJ-5 to 1.16 in the Wrangler. The nonrollover rate is similar among the Jeeps and is somewhat less than that of passenger cars.

Only the manufacturers know the cost of changing vehicle parameters, but it is possible to relate the relevant parameters to base price of the vehicles. Ordinary least squares regression was used to estimate the effect of center of gravity height, track width, and wheelbase on the 1993 base price of vehicles in the study (Ward's Automotive Yearbook, 1993). The base price of the 23 vehicles studied in relation to vehicle parameters is presented in table 15-6. Track width and wheelbase are not related to vehicle price when the effect of center of gravity height is

Table 15-4. Projected Deaths Preventable During 1992–2011 in the 1991 Blazer/Jimmy If *T/2H* Were 1.20

Year	Projected Vehicles in Use	Preventable Deaths
1992	152,235	7.63
1993	151,623	7.60
1994	149,787	7.51
1995	147,339	7.38
1996	144,279	7.23
1997	140,454	7.04
1998	135,864	6.81
1999	130,356	6.53
2000	123,930	6.21
2001	116,739	5.85
2002	108,936	5.46
2003	100,674	5.04
2004	92,259	4.62
2005	83,844	4.20
2006	75,735	3.79
2007	67,932	3.40
2008	60,741	3.04
2009	54,009	2.71
2010	47,889	2.39
2011	42,381	2.12
Total		107

considered. For each one-inch (2.54-cm) marginal increase in center of gravity height, there is an average $1,446 increase in base price of the vehicle.

Based on the projected 5,028 preventable deaths in five model years, each year's delay in adoption of a minimum stability standard of $T/2H = 1.2$ for light-duty vehicles in the United States resulted in the continued production of vehicles that will experience more than 1,000 preventable deaths (compared to 68 estimated by NHTSA) and huge costs from nonfatal injuries in rollovers. The government agency responsible for vehicle standards failed in its duty to analyze the problem with due diligence (Frame, 1996), and the manufacturers failed to act on what their own historic statements and experience would indicate (e.g., Stonex, 1961). Cost was not the issue.

The NHTSA's estimate of deaths prevented is based on a measure of stability (TTA), which is inferior in predicting rollover rates, as well as several false assumptions. The agency falsely assumed that increased stability only reduces single-vehicle rollovers. It claimed that most crashes would occur whether the vehicle

Table 15-5. Projected Rollover Deaths Preventable by a $T/2H$ of 1.2 in 20 Years of Use, 1990–1994 Models

Model	Preventable Deaths
Amigo	23
4Runner	135
Rodeo/Passport	66
Tracker	49
Wrangler	64
Ranger Pickup	736
Blazer/Jimmy (S/T)	696
Nissan Pickup	144
Pathfinder	131
S10/S15 Pickup	340
GM Light Pickups	592
F250 Pickup	178
Astro/Safari Van	327
Bronco	108
Aerostar Van	312
Explorer/Navajo	590
F150 Pickup	315
Mazda MPV	26
Lumina Van	78
Caravan/Voyager	118
Total	5,028

rolled or not, despite clear evidence to the contrary (e.g., figure 15-1). It used only one model year, when these vehicles are essentially unchanged in design for many years, and it failed to account for the total years of use.

Lowering the center of gravity, increasing track width, or both, can increase stability. If desired ground clearance means a high center of gravity, then appropriately increased track width can offset it. NHTSA argued that the six-inch (3.24 cm) increase in track width necessary to stabilize some of the vehicles must be accompanied by a 10-inch (25.4 cm) increase in wheelbase to retain braking stability, but that is not true with lowered center of gravity. Furthermore, most of the vehicles would require less than a six-inch (3.24 cm) extension of track to achieve $T/2H = 1.2$ given the same center of gravity. It is curious that the agency accepts a minimum ratio of wheelbase to track width to achieve braking stability but not a minimum track width to center of gravity height to achieve turning stability.

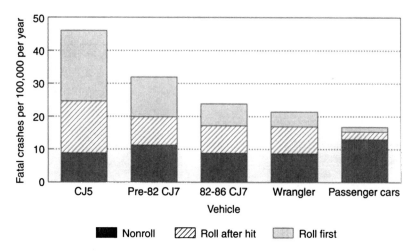

Figure 15-1. Fatal Crashes per 100,000 Vehicles per Year (Fatal Accident Reporting System, 1988–1994)

The NHTSA claims that required changes in track width and wheelbase would eliminate the "compact sport utility vehicle" class of vehicles, which they claim the agency is prohibited from doing by law. Aside from the fact that such vehicle classifications are arbitrary, the assumption is demonstrably untrue. The noted changes in the Jeep from the CJ-5 to the Wrangler did not eliminate the vehicle from the "compact sport utility" class and did not change the appearance appreciably. Extending the Wrangler's track width an additional two inches (5.08 cm) or lowering its center of gravity height by one inch (2.54 cm) to achieve a $T/2H$ of 1.2 would not eliminate the vehicle from the "compact sport utility" class.

The NHTSA official who signed the three *Federal Register* entries rejecting a rollover standard commented in a newspaper article that the total death rates in some of the less stable vehicles are less than average (Stepp, 1996). While that is obviously true because some have longer than average wheelbases and lower than average nonrollover rates, as shown in table 15-1, that is not an excuse for failure to reduce rollover rates where feasible and practicable. If a physician argued that

Table 15-6. Base Price of Vehicles in 1993 in Relation to Center of Gravity Height, Track Width, and Wheelbase (in inches)

	Coefficient	t-Value	p-Value
Intercept	−10,648	−1.32	.203
Center of gravity height	1,446	4.59	<.001
Track width	−114	−0.53	.599
Wheelbase	−53	−1.63	.119
$R^2 = 0.66$			

we should not treat cancer because heart disease is declining, the comment would not be treated seriously, even in a newspaper. The official who made the comment subsequently retired from the government and went to work for the American Motor Vehicle Manufacturer's Association, a typical "revolving door" problem between industry and government in the United States. The government official who signed the rejection of the petition to recall the Samurai retired to work for the Association of International Vehicle Manufacturers, also a Washington lobbying organization.

The NHTSA's claim that the standard would be costly also is not supported by the Jeep's history and the vehicle price data. The 1993 Wrangler's base price, U.S. $11,410, was among the lower priced vehicles for sale in the United States in that year. The correlation of price to vehicle parameters indicates that a substantial increase in price is associated with raising center of gravity when wheelbase and track width are controlled statistically. There is increased cost both in vehicle price and in death and injury to ride high. While redesign of vehicles undoubtedly bears costs, the vehicles are periodically redesigned anyway, and it is not clear that increased stability would result in net increase in costs given the apparent higher marginal price of higher center of gravity.

References

Adams W, and Brock JW (1987) Bigness and social efficiency: a case study of the U.S. auto industry. In Samuels WJ, and Miller AS (eds.), *Corporations and Society: Power and Responsibility.* New York, NY: Greenwood Press.

Anderson JA, McLellan BA, Pagliarello G, and Nelson WR (1990) The relative influence of alcohol and seatbelt usage on severity of injury from motor vehicle crashes. *J Trauma.* 30:415–421.

Anderson LG, and Settle RF (1977) *Benefit-Cost Analysis: A Practical Guide.* Lexington, MA: DC Heath.

Baker SP (1979) Who bought the cars in which people were injured? An exploratory study. *Am J Public Health.* 69:76.

Baker SP (1980) On lobbies, liberty, and the public good. *Am J Public Health.* 70:573–574.

Baldwin S, Godfrey C, and Propper C (eds.) (1990) *Quality of Life: Perspectives and Policies.* London: Routledge.

Berger LR, and Mohan D (1996) *Injury Control: A Global View.* Delhi, India: Oxford University Press.

Christoffel T, and Teret S (1993) *Protecting the Public: Legal Issues in Injury Prevention.* New York, NY: Oxford University Press.

Cohen BL (1980) Society's evaluation of life saving in radiation protection and other contexts. *Health Physics.* 38:33.

Crouch EAC, and Wilson R (1982) *Risk/Benefit Analysis.* Cambridge, MA: Ballinger.

Culyer AJ (1990) Commodities, characteristics of commodities, characteristics of people, utilities, and the quality of life. In Baldwin S, Godfrey C, and Popper C (eds.), *Quality of Life: Perspectives and Policies.* London: Routledge.

Currie G, Kerfoot KD, Donaldson C, and Macarthur C (2000) Are cost of injury studies useful? *Inj Prev.* 6:175–176.

Datta TK, and Guzek P (1990) *Restraint System Use in 19 U.S. Cities: 1989 Annual Report.* Washington, DC: National Highway Traffic Safety Administration.

DiNapoli N, Fitzpatrick M, Strother C, Struble D, and Tanner R (1977) *Research Safety Vehicle Phase II. Vol. 2, Comprehensive Technical Results.* Springfield, VA: National Technical Information Service.

Elvik R, and Vaa T (2004) *The Handbook of Road Safety Measures.* Amsterdam: Elsevier.

Finkelstein EA, Corso PS, and Miller TR (2006) *The Incidence and Economic Burden of Injuries in the United States.* New York, NY: Oxford University Press.

Foss RD, Beirness DJ, and Sprattler K (1994) Seat belt use among drinking drivers in Minnesota. *Am J Public Health.* 84:1732–1737.

Frame P (1996) Has Martinez dropped the ball at NHTSA? *Automotive News,* June 24, p. 1.

Hartunian NS, Smart CN, Willeman TR, and Zador PL (1983) The economics of safety regulation: lives and dollars lost due to repeal of motorcycle helmet laws. *J Health Polit Policy Law.* 8:76–98.

Harwin EA, and Brewer HK (1990) Analysis of the relationship between vehicle rollover stability and rollover risk using the NHTSA CARDfile accident database. *J Traffic Med.* 18:109–122.

Insurance Institute for Highway Safety (1995) Vehicle by vehicle death rate comparisons. *IIHS Status Rep.* 30:4–6.

Jones IS, and Penny MB (1990) *Engineering Parameters Related to Rollover Frequency.* SAE Technical Paper Series 900104. Warrendale, PA: Society of Automotive Engineers.

Kahneman D, and Tversky A (1979) Prospect theory: an analysis of decision under risk. *Econometrica.* 47:263–291.

Kelsey TW (1994) The agrarian myth and policy responses to farm safety. *Am J Public Health.* 84:1171–1177.

Klein TM, and Burgess M (1995) *Alcohol Involvement in Fatal Traffic Crashes, 1993.* Washington, DC, National Highway Traffic Safety Administration.

Kravitz H (1973) Prevention of falls in infancy by counseling mothers. *Ill Med J.* 144:570–573.

Leigh JP, Markowitz S, Fahs M, and Landrigan P (2000) Costs of Occupational Injuries and Illnesses. Ann Arbor, MI: The University of Michigan Press.

Loomes G, and McKenzie L (1990) The scope and limitations of QALY measures. In Baldwin S, Godfrey C, and Propper C (eds.), *Quality of Life: Perspectives and Policies.* London: Routledge.

Mengert P, Salvatore S, DiSario R, and Walter R (1989) *Statistical Estimation of Rollover Risk.* Cambridge, MA: Transportation Systems Center.

Miller TR (1989) Willingness to pay. In Rice DP, and MacKenzie EJ (eds.) *Cost of Injury in the United States: A Report to Congress, 1989.* San Francisco, CA, and Baltimore, MD: Institute for Health and Aging, University of California, and Injury Prevention Center, Johns Hopkins University.

Morrow RH, and Bryant JH (1995) Health policy approaches to measuring and valuing human life: conceptual and ethical issues. *Am J Public Health.* 85:1356–1360.

National Highway Traffic Safety Administration (1987) Federal motor vehicle safety standards; denial of petition for rulemaking; vehicle rollover resistance. *Fed Reg.* 52:49033.

National Highway Traffic Safety Administration (1988) Denial of motor vehicle safety defect petitions. *Fed Reg.* 53:34866.

National Highway Traffic Safety Administration (1994) Consumer information regulations; federal motor vehicle safety standards; rollover prevention. *Fed Reg.* 59:33254–33272.

National Highway Traffic Safety Administration (1996) Federal motor vehicle safety standards; rollover prevention. *Fed Reg.* 61:28550–28561.

National Highway Traffic Safety Administration (2006) *Traffic Safety Facts 2004.* Washington, DC: U.S. Department of Transportation.

Oak Ridge National Laboratory (1984) *Scrappage and Survival Rates of Passenger Cars and Trucks in 1970–82. Ward's Automotive Yearbook.* Detroit, MI: Ward's Communications.

Petitti DB (1994) *Meta-Analysis, Decision Analysis, and Cost-Effectiveness Analysis.* New York, NY: Oxford University Press.

Priest WC (1988) *Risks, Consensus, and Social Legislation: Forces That Led to Laws on Health, Safety and the Environment.* Boulder, CO: Westview Press.

Reinfurt DW, Li LK, et al. (1981) *A Comparison of Crash Experience of Utility Vehicles, Pickup Trucks and Passenger Cars.* Chapel Hill, NC: University of North Carolina Highway Safety Research Center.

Reinfurt DW, Stutts JC, and Hamilton EG (1984) *A Further Look at Utility Vehicle Rollovers.* Chapel Hill, NC: University of North Carolina Highway Safety Research Center.

Rice DP, and MacKenzie, EJ (eds.) (1989) *Cost of Injury in the United States: A Report to Congress, 1989.* San Francisco, CA, and Baltimore, MA: Institute for Health and Aging, University of Californiza and Injury Prevention Center, Johns Hopkins University.

Rivara FP, Dicker BG, Bergman AB, Dacey R, and Herman C (1988) The public cost of motorcycle trauma. *JAMA.* 260:221–223.

Robertson LS (1983) *Injuries: Causes, Control Strategies, and Public Policy.* Lexington, MA: DC Heath.

Robertson LS (1989a) Potential savings from injury prevention. In Rice DP, and MacKenzie EJ (eds.), *Cost of Injury in the United States.* San Francisco, CA, and Baltimore, MD: Institute for Health and Aging, University of California, and Injury Prevention Center, Johns Hopkins University.

Robertson LS (1989b) Risk of fatal rollover in utility vehicles relative to static stability. *Am J Public Health.* 79:300.

Robertson LS (1990) Car design and risk of pedestrian deaths. *Am J Public Health.* 80:609–610.

Robertson LS, and Kelley AB (1989) Static stability as a predictor of overturn in fatal motor vehicle crashes. *J Trauma.* 29:313.

Robertson LS, and Zador PL (1978) Driver education and fatal crash involvement of teenaged drivers. *Am J Public Health.* 68:959–965.

Runyan CW, and Earp JAL (1985) Epidemiologic evidence and motor vehicle policy making. *Am J Public Health.* 75:354–360.

Self P (1977) *Econocrats and the Policy Process: The Politics and Philosophy of Cost-Benefit Analysis.* Boulder, CO: Westview Press.

Shrader-Frechette KS (1985) *Risk Analysis and Scientific Method.* Boston, MA: D. Reidel.

Smith SR (1982) *Analysis of fatal rollover accidents in utility vehicles.* Washington, DC: National Highway Traffic Safety Administration.(mimeo).

Snyder RG, McDole TL, Ladd WM, and Minahan DJ (1980) *On-road Crash Experience of Utility Vehicles.* Ann Arbor, MI: University of Michigan Highway Safety Research Institute.

Starr C (1969) Social benefit versus technological risk. *Science.* 165:1232–1238.

Stepp LS (1996) Truckin' to tragedy. The Washington Post. March 1, p. D5.

Stonex KA (1961) Road design for safety. *Traffic Safety Res Rev.* 5:18–30.

Tengs TO, Adams ME, Pliskin JS, Safran DG, Siegal JE, Weinstein MC, and Graham JD (1995) Five-hundred life-Saving interventions and their cost-effectiveness. *Risk Anal.* 15:369–390.

Viscusi WK, and Magat WA (1987) *Learning About Risk: Consumer and Worker Responses to Hazard Information.* Cambridge, MA: Harvard University Press.

Ward's Automotive Yearbook (1983–1995) Detroit, MI: Ward's Communications.

Wintemute GJ, and Wright MA (1992) Initial and subsequent hospital costs of firearm injuries. *J Trauma.* 33:556–560.

Wood T, and Milne P (1988) Head injuries to pedal cyclists and the promotion of helmet use in Victoria, Australia. *Accid Anal Prev.* 20:177.

Zaloshnja E, Miller T, Galbraith M, Lawrence B, DeBruyn L, Bill N, Hicks K, Keiffer M, and Perkins R (2003) Reducing injuries among Native Americans: five cost-outcome analyses. *Accid Anal Prev.* 35:631–639.

16

Summation of Principles

Injury is a public health problem that is neglected relative to its importance in lost years of life and disability. Injury control has more immediate health and economic benefits than does chronic disease control. The infectious model—agent, carrier, host—can be applied to injuries. Interventions can reduce injuries, their severity, or consequences by modifying these factors at specific phases of the injury—before and during the acute phase and afterward.

Energy in its various forms—mechanical, thermal, chemical, electrical, and radiation—is the agent of injury. Research that focuses on modification of the agent or means of exposure to the agent will contribute most to injury control.

Research questions should focus on homogeneous subsets of severe injuries and changeable factors possibly related to incidence and severity. Certain available data sources emphasize nonchangeable factors such as age and gender and include classifications that are not useful.

Data without valid indicators of severity may be misleading because the factors relevant to reducing severe injuries are often not involved as frequently in nonsevere injuries. Improved means of quantifying severity of injury and disability are under investigation. Case identification requires knowledge of the flow of cases among treatment facilities.

Injury rates are calculated by dividing numbers of injuries by population at risk or measures of exposure, such as miles traveled for motor vehicle injuries. Rates are useful for inferring relative risk in relation to factors that can be changed to reduce risk. Rates are misleading when they are high but based on relatively rare exposures, or when they do not reflect the future exposures inherent in the lifetime exposure to a product or activity.

Surveillance of who, when, where, and how people are injured has proved to be a powerful tool for targeting injury control measures of known effectiveness. Some extant surveillance systems have quirks in the data that can mislead the user.

Missing data elements are a major problem in many. Certain data, such as police codes of injury severity and self-reported injuries and behaviors (e.g., seat belt and alcohol use), are invalid.

Specification of causal paths in complex causal sequences is often a goal of "basic" science but can be misleading in injury control. Usually, all of the potential risk factors can be ignored if a controllable necessary condition for harm is known. Since energy is the necessary and specific agent of injury, control of the energy or the way it is conveyed to the host will control the injury. A complex causal model may be useful for understanding sometimes out-of-control systems that affect injury, such as alcohol use. Generally, however, the more removed the hypothesized "cause" is from the energy that injures, the less likely that its control would reduce injury.

Commonly used epidemiological study designs—case–control, cohort—can be used to investigate factors in injury incidence or severity. Controlled experiments are the most valid methods for research but are not used in the study of injury causation for ethical reasons. They can be used to study certain interventions. Study designs that rule out false inferences and the use of statistical techniques that quantify parameters that can be changed for injury control must be learned and applied.

Injury control efforts are inordinately oriented to behavior change. Theories of behavior contain conflicting hypotheses regarding behavioral motivations and limits on individual abilities, particularly in emergency situations. Injury rates at various stages in human development are a result of changing abilities, activities contributing to differential exposures to energy, and changing susceptibility to energy.

Behavior change efforts are most successful when they decrease exposures to energy and are harmful if exposures are increased by the intervention. Response to persuasion declines in relation to frequency of behavior necessary to reduce risk. Diffusion of effort toward many behaviors dilutes the effect. Personal counseling and community-based programs, particularly if incentives are included, are more effective than impersonal approaches such as advertising.

Compliance with laws or rules aimed at reducing injury is influenced by degree of consensus regarding the justification for the law and probability of detection of a violation. If violations are not publicly observable or the behavior can be changed easily when enforcers are approaching, the effect is diluted. Severity of punishment is less important than its prominence in political debate would indicate.

Identifying clusters of violence, drunk driving, and other risky behavior in space and time, if revealed by surveillance, has been used to increase the efficiency and effects of law enforcement. Persons at increased risk of injury less often use protection required by law, which reduces the real protection to less than would be expected technically. However, evidence does not support the theory of offsetting behavior by those who do comply (risk compensation).

Changes in agents, vehicles, and environments can be made voluntarily by designers, manufacturers, and marketers of products based on the research on hazardous characteristics. Regulations to impose standards for products and processes that injure have been associated with large reductions in death rates.

Environments may affect behavior in addition to exposing people to hazards. They can be modified to reduce violence as well as exposure to inanimate energy. The best studies of reduced risk from product or environmental modifications indicate no effect on offsetting behavior, but claims for compensation are influenced by increased availability of money, above inflation, for such claims.

Well-placed and organized emergency medical systems with staff experienced in treatment of trauma increase the probability of survival of the injured that withstand the initial energy insult. Questions remain regarding the efficacy of certain treatments at the scene of injury. The existence of trauma centers, where probability of survival is increased, is threatened by evolving trends in organization and financing of medical care systems. Resolution of these issues, as well as clinical trials of acute care and rehabilitation regimes, would benefit from examination by epidemiological methods.

The results of epidemiological studies specifying factors that can be changed to reduce injuries can be used to project the effects of policies regarding those changes. Many current injury-control efforts are administered by government agencies and private organizations that seem to have no system for establishing priorities and no systematic knowledge of policies and programs that are effective. Those who learn how, when, where, and who is injured are in a position to influence the setting of priorities. Those who also learn the approaches to injury control that are effective or ineffective are in a position to increase rationality in the policy-making process.

Index

Abbreviated injury
    scale, 33, 52–53
Abilities, 120–122
Acceleration, 16
Accidents, 5
Addiction, 88
Adolescents, 123–127
Adulthood, 127
Age, 11, 23, 49, 87, 97, 101, 110, 121–122,
    127, 152, 160, 201, 209, 221
Agent, 8–9, 119, 178
Aggression, 122, 125
Air bags, 15, 89–90, 181, 185, 190
Alcohol, 8–10, 18, 21, 52–53, 60–61, 82,
    85, 88–89, 93, 97–99, 110, 123–128,
    141, 144, 153, 156, 161–162, 165,
    169, 188, 191–193, 205, 223–225, 228
    and drinking age laws, 166
Alzheimer's disease, 130
American College of Surgeons, 34
American Motor Vehicle Manufacturer's
    Association, 235
American Public Health Association, 3
Anatomic Profile, 34
    arrest, probability of, 156
Assaults, 54, 65, 77–78, 88, 99, 121,
    123–124, 153, 157, 161–162
Association of International Vehicle
    Manufacturers, 235

Aspirin package, 179
Asphyxiation, 19, 34

Back schools, 141–142
Battering, 125–126
Behavior
    group, 146–147
    pedestrian, 162
    physician, 138
    posttrauma, 130
    programs, 93, 137–148
    protective, 152–153
    theories, 120, 240
Bicyclists, 15, 144–145, 182–183
Boat propellers, 21
Brain, 15, 59, 209
Bullets, 17
Bumper height, 21, 180
Bureau of Labor Statistics, 27, 55
Burns, 18, 28, 34, 71–72

Cameras observing traffic, 162
Cancer, 19, 235
Carbon monoxide, 180
Case finding, 28–31
Causation, 6–7
    Analysis, 82–93, 240
    Henle-Koch criteria, 85
    models, 24–25, 86–89, 96, 120

Causation (*continued*)
  path analysis, 104
  types, 83–84
Cell phones, 99
Center for Auto Safety, 131
Centers for Disease Control and Prevention
    (CDC), 4, 24, 54, 57, 59, 167
  Center for Injury Control, 64
Center of gravity height, 20, 228,
    231–232, 235
Childhood, 120–123
Child pedestrians, 65, 138–139
Child restraints, 15, 20, 93, 121, 152, 154,
    165, 226
Cigarettes, 18, 178
Clinical trials, 204–205
Coast Guard, 56–57
Cohort, 96
Combat veterans, 129
Committee on Injury Scaling, 39
Committee on Trauma of the American
    College of Surgeons, 39
Community, changes, 144–145
Conflict, resolution, 146
Confounding, 24, 83, 86, 102, 112
Consumer Products Safety Commission,
    44, 56
Consumers Union, 228
Correlation, 7, 85, 105, 120
Cost-benefit, 153, 210, 217–220, 222,
    227–235
Cost-effectiveness, 24, 48, 198, 223,
    225–227
Costs, 3–4, 33, 64, 120, 188, 197, 201,
    209–210, 216–219, 222–226, 230–231
Council of State and Territorial
    Epidemiologists, 50
Counseling, 138
Crash Outcome Data Evaluation System
    (CODES), 60
Crash tests, 111, 179, 192–193
Crashworthiness Data System, 52–53, 171
Cribs, 181
Crime rates, 160
Criminal justice, 153

Data analysis, 96, 106–109
Data needs, 23–24
Daylight savings time, 168
Dead-on-arrival, criteria, 201–202

Death certificates, 49–50, 55
Deaths, 30, 34
Deceleration, 16
Defects, 185–186
Defensive driving, 140–141
Denial, 124, 127
Department of Veterans Affairs, 210
Deterrence, 153, 156
Development, stages of childhood, 88,
    120–123
Diagnosis-related groups (DRGs), 210
Diet, 139
Disability, 33, 35–38
Double-pair comparison 170–171
Drivers
  aggressive, 125, 131, 224
  education, 93, 140, 168, 220, 223
  error, 87–88
  licensing age, 159, 223
  provisional licenses, 159
Drowning 19, 43, 63, 73–74, 142, 159
Drugs, 98, 123–124

E-codes, 23–24, 49–51
Economics, 120, 188, 216–227
Economy of scale, 222
Effects, overlapping, 223
Elderly, 129
E-mail, vi
Emergency medical service, 63, 197–200,
    241
Energy, 8–11, 32, 34, 87, 178, 239–240
  absorption, 143, 180–182, 187, 193
  chemical, 18
  electrical, 19
  exchange, 25, 85–86
  mechanical, 14–17
  thermal, 18
  tolerance, 14, 85
Environment and behavior, 147–148
Epidemology, 3, 6, 87, 216
  methods, 96
  model, 8
EPPINFO, 64, 86
Equipment, protective, 153, 181–182
Ethics, 96–97
Evaluation of product changes, 180–181
Event data recorders, 172
Exercise, 143
Exposure, 41–46, 103, 140

Falls, 14, 16–17, 25, 27, 62–63, 75–76,
    83–84, 101, 129, 143, 180, 209, 223
Fatality Analysis Reporting System,
    51–52, 92, 103, 131, 144, 170, 187,
    198, 229
Federal Aviation Administration, 42
Federal Bureau of Investigation, 54
Federal Coal Mine Health and
    Safety Act, 184
Federal Highway Administration, 57, 100
Federal Motor Vehicle Safety
    Standards, 181
Feedback, 88–89, 102
Fighting, 98
Firearms, 14, 126, 159 (See also guns)
Fire/burns, 18, 28, 56, 131–132, 144
Firestone Rubber, 217–218
Fireworks, 144
Ford Motor Company, 131–132, 228
Freedom of Information Act, 60
Fuel economy, 109–115
Fuel tanks, 85–86, 131–132
Functional Capacity Index, 38

Gasoline tax, 93
Gender, 87, 97, 110, 122, 127–128, 154,
    160, 209
General Accounting Office, 46
General Estimates System, 52, 54
General Motors, 89–90, 119, 131–132,
    189, 217
General Services Administration, 191
Glasgow Coma Scale, 33, 130, 201, 208
Gold standard, 171–173
Guardrail, 65
Guns, 9, 17, 20, 98, 123, 127, 145, 154,
    157–161, 178, 180, 226 (See also
    firearms)

Haddon Matrix, 10
Harlem, 145
Hazards, 183
    inspecting, 183–186
Heart disease, 235
Health interview survey, 29
Helicopters, 197, 200–201
Helmets, 15, 145, 152–153, 163, 165,
    182–183, 226
Highway Safety Act, 93
Homicide, 54, 88, 98, 124–126, 129, 153

Hoopa Health Association Emergency
    Medical Services, 65
Horses, 147
Hospital records, 24, 42, 50, 54–56, 59–60
Hospitals, 14
Host, 25, 99
Human factors, 5, 88, 119–132, 137

Immune system, 204
Intersections, signalized, 162, 167
Impairment scale, 35–38
Indian Health Service (IHS), 51, 64–66, 220
Infants, 121, 152
Infection, 6, 197, 204–205
Injury
    children's, 121–123, 137–138
    classifications, 28–29
    clusters, 49, 51, 53, 63
    control, 83
    distributions, 197
    environmental modifications and, 178
    factors and phases, 10
    farm, 56, 226
    flow of cases, 29
    football, 30
    geographic location, 24
    intentional, 5
    lawsuits, 89
    occupational, 55
    pedestrian, 65, 144–145
    police codes, 52–53
    prevention, 3, 83
    pyramid, 41
    rates, 42–44, 101
    self-inflicted, 79–80
    severity, 5, 32–39, 169–170, 201, 217
    statistics, 41
    surveillance, 24, 32, 48–57, 59–66
    trends, 48, 51
Injury in America, 4
Injury Severity Score (ISS), 33, 53, 130,
    200–201, 224
Institute of Transportation Engineers, 148
Insurance Institute for Highway Safety,
    111, 143
Interactive Highway Safety Design Model,
    100
International Classification of Diseases,
    23, 33, 48–49
Internet, vi, 26, 90

Interrupted time series, 155–156
Interviews, 100
IQ, 130

Jeep Corporation, 227
Journal of the American Medical
    Association, 86, 90

Lap/shoulder belts, 15 (See also seat belts)
    effectiveness, 169–173
Laws, 152–167, 240
Length of stay, 209–210
Lighting, 65, 82, 148
Literature review, 26
Lobbying, 154
Logistic regression, 109

Machines, 178
Mandatory sentences, 154–155
Mass, 14–15, 87
Medical examiners, 30, 50
Medical schools, 4
Medicaid, 66, 226
Medicare, 66, 226
MEDLINE, 26
Mexican immigrants, 125, 127
Mortality rates, 152
Motorcycles, 15, 123, 147, 153, 167, 188
Motor vehicles, 14, 65, 69–70, 178
    age, 187–190
    crashworthiness, 82
    death rates, 89, 92
    electronic stability control, 115
    heads-up display, 147
    horsepower, 87
    make-model codes, 52
    rollover, 52, 87–88, 90, 100, 103–104,
        108–110, 228–235
    safety standards, 181, 186–194
    size and backed-over children, 115
    size and weight, 10, 87, 109–115
    tilt table angle, 229

N-codes, 23, 49–51
National Automotive Sampling System,
    52, 163
    investigator bias, 172–173
National Center for Health Statistics, 27,
    31, 40, 49

National Crime Surveys, 54
National Criminal Justice Reference
    Service, 54
National Fire Data Center, 56
National Fire Protection Agency, 22
National Health Interview Survey, 27, 35
National Hospital Discharge Survey, 50
National Highway Traffic Safety
    Administration (NHTSA), 51–52, 60,
    105, 119, 171, 190–191, 221, 227–235
National Institute for Occupational Safety
    and Health, 55–56
National Research Council, 121
    Committee on Trauma Research, 204
National Rifle Association, 9
National Safe Kids, 17, 22
National Safety Council, 27–28, 140–141
National Traffic and Motor Vehicle Safety
    Act, 89, 93
Native Americans, 127–128
Navajo Nation, 65
New York Health Department, 83
Nursing homes, 15

Objectives, 24
Occupational Safety and Health
    Administration (OSHA), 11, 55,
    184–185, 226
Office of Management and Budget, 194

Panel on Occupational Safety and
    Health, 31
Pediatric Trauma Score, 34–35
Physical therapy, 208
Physics, 141, 180
Pickup trucks, 90–93
Pin maps, 24
Pine Ridge Reservation, 65
Playground, 17, 65
Pluralistic ignorance, 146–147
Pneumatic antishock garment, 199–200
Poisoning, 18, 34
Police
    crackdowns, 156
    reports, 30, 50, 52, 171–172
Policy 7, 241
Potential life lost, 4
Prevalence, 35
Prevention, 83
    oriented surveillance, 62–66

Producer prices, 219
Product design, 179
Psychologists, 120
Psychopathlogy, 124
Public health, 3, 107, 153
    model, 82
Public Roads, 100
Punishment, 154, 156

Quality control, 185–186

Race, 124–125, 127, 154
Recidivism, 153
Regression coefficients, 105, 108, 112,
    188–190
Regression to the mean, 155
Regulation, 181, 188, 241
Rehabilitation, 205–207, 210
Reliability, 35, 38
Replication, 156
Research objectives, 23
Risk, 43–44, 101, 113, 123–124
Risk benefit, 220–222
Risk compensation (homeostasis) theory,
    167, 184–185, 188, 217, 240
Risk factors, 6, 24, 82, 103
    behavioral survey, 60–62, 167
    biological, 89
    changeable, 24–25
    surveillance, 60–61
Road lighting, 43, 147
Road modifications, 100, 147, 178, 183
Rules, 152–167, 240

Safe Communities, 146
Sample size, 186
Screening, 106–107, 143–144, 209
Seat belts, 20, 53, 60–61, 93, 108, 142–143,
    152–153, 163, 165, 167–173, 181,
    191–193, 223–225 (*See also* lap/
    shoulder belts)
Self reports, 60–61, 138, 146, 171, 209, 222
Selection bias, 59, 140, 146, 208
Sex, 23, 119
Sikhs, 153
Smoke detectors, 159
Snow, John, 6
Sociologists, 120
Speed, 14–15, 20, 52, 87, 147, 152,
    163–164, 188

Spinal cord injury, 15, 27, 30–31, 35, 59,
    208
Sport utility vehicles, 90–93, 110–115,
    227–235
Sports injuries, 139, 152
Stairs, 25, 178
Standard Oil of California, 218
Stapp, JP, 12, 22
Statistical power, 86
Statistics, 26, 84, 86, 106–108
Strain, 15–16
Stresses, 15
Study designs, 198, 240
    before-after, 154–155
    capture-recapture, 59
    case-control, 97–100, 170
    controlled experiments, 25, 97,
        137–143
    crossover, 205
    cross-sectional, 102–104
    ecological, 104–106, 157, 200
    interrupted time series, 155–157
    meta-analysis, 109, 141
    prospective, 101–102, 200
    retrospective, 100–101
Suicides, 5–6, 54–55, 125–126, 129, 144,
    159, 180
Swimming pools, 21, 159, 178

Technical strategies, 19–21, 48, 66
Telephone interviews, 60
Television, 139, 142
Toxicology, 18
Track width, 20, 228
Traffic control lights, 147–148
Tranquilizers, 102
Transport Canada, 93
Trauma
    brain, 207–208
    centers, 201–204
    registries, 59
    score, 33–34
Treatment 197–210
    at the scene, 199
    delay, 198
    evaluation, 197
    intravenous fluids, 199–200
    life support, 200
    long-term care, 205–207
    managed care, 209

Trucks 131
   tractor-trailer, 100
Turn distance, 111–115

Unemployment, 105
Unintended consequences,
   140, 167–168
Unit of analysis, 96–97, 105
University of the Sciences
   in Philadelphia, 13
Utah Health Department, 35

Validity, 38
Vans, 90–91, 93, 110–115
Vector, 8, 99
Vehicle, 8, 119, 178, 224
   all-terrain, 44–45
   crashworthiness, 90

defect, 229
   velocity, 16
Violation records, 110
Violence, 121, 125, 128, 139, 145, 154, 157

Washington Heights, 145
White Mountain Apache Tribal Council, 147
Willingness to pay, 218–220
Window barriers, 62–63
Wirth, Timothy, 228
Worker's
   compensation, 55, 141, 184–185
   deaths, 27
   education, 141
World Health Organization, 23, 146

Years of potential life lost, 41–42
   quality years of life, 222

LaVergne, TN USA
09 July 2010
188945LV00001B/73/P

9 780195 313840